REGIONAL CHEMOTHERAPY

CURRENT CLINICAL ONCOLOGY

Maurie Markman, MD, Series Editor

REGIONAL CHEMOTHERAPY

Clinical Research and Practice

Edited by

MAURIE MARKMAN, MD

The Cleveland Clinic Foundation, Cleveland, OH

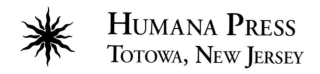

HUMANA PRESS
TOTOWA, NEW JERSEY

© 2000 Humana Press Inc.
999 Riverview Drive, Suite 208
Totowa, New Jersey 07512

For additional copies, pricing for bulk purchases, and/or information about other Humana titles, contact Humana at the above address or at any of the following numbers: Tel: 973-256-1699; Fax: 973-256-8341; E-mail: humana@humanapr.com or visit our website at http://www.humanapress.com

This publication is printed on acid-free paper. ⊚
ANSI Z39.48-1984 (American National Standards Institute)
Permanence of Paper for Printed Library Materials.

Cover design by Patricia F. Cleary.

Printed in the United States of America.   10 9 8 7 6 5 4 3 2 1

Library of Congress Cataloging-in-Publication Data

Main entry under title:

Current clinical oncology™.

Regional chemotherapy: clinical research and practice / edited by Maurie Markman.
        p.   cm.–(Current clinical oncology ; 2)
  Includes bibliographical references and index.
  ISBN 0-89603-729-0.
  1. Cancer–Chemotherapy. 2. Infusion therapy. 3. Regional perfusion (Physiology). 4. Antineoplastic agents–Administration. I. Markman, Maurie. II. Series: Current clinical oncology (Totowa, N.J.) ; 2.
  [DNLM: 1. Neoplasms–drug therapy. 2. Antineoplastic Agents–administration & dosage. 3. Perfusion, Regional.
QZ 267 R3364 2000]
RC271.C5R42   2000
616.99'4061–dc21
DNLM/DLC   99-22882
for Library of Congress   CIP

PREFACE

Regional antineoplastic drug administration is not a new concept, having been examined since the earliest days of the modern chemotherapeutic era. For example, nitrogen mustard and hemisulfur mustard were administered by the intraperitoneal route in the 1950s as a strategy to treat malignant effusions (*1,2*), while during the same time period alkylating agents were delivered by direct intraarterial instillation to treat localized tumor masses (*3*).

Over the past several decades much has been learned regarding both the potential benefits (e.g., improvement in local symptoms and quality of life, prolongation of progression-free and overall survival) and the toxicities associated with regional antineoplastic drug delivery.

Local side effects of treatment include both the direct effects of the high concentrations of drug in contact with the infused/instilled body compartment [e.g., adhesion formation following intraperitoneal therapy (*4*), blindness following intra-carotid artery delivery (*5*), biliary sclerosis following intrahepatic artery infusions (*6*)] and the complications associated with the actual drug administration (e.g., infection of catheters and bleeding following intraarterial infusion).

In a number of specific malignant disease settings, this therapeutic strategy has become the "standard of care" in patient management. Examples include the use of intravesical therapy of localized bladder cancer (*7*), and intrathecal or intraventricular antineoplastic drug delivery for treatment of meningeal leukemia (*8*). In both situations regional therapy has been established as a highly effective treatment approach.

In other areas, such as the use of intraperitoneal chemotherapy in the management of ovarian cancer, accumulating data have strongly suggested an important role for the strategy in a subset of individuals with the malignancy. Two recently reported randomized clinical trials have demonstrated that, compared to the intravenous delivery of cisplatin, the intraperitoneal administration of the agent as initial chemotherapy of small volume residual disease results in an improvement in both progression-free and overall survival (*9,10*).

Finally, promising and highly innovative approaches to the management of malignant disease that employ regional drug delivery have been reported during the past several years from a number of major research centers throughout the world. These include the direct delivery of antineoplastic agents into body cavities (peritoneal cavity, pleura, pericardium, bladder, meninges) and arterial blood vessels, utilizing both cytotoxic and biological agents.

In *Regional Chemotherapy: Clinical Research and Practice* we have been extremely fortunate to assemble many leading clinicians and clinical investigators in the rapidly expanding arena of regional antineoplastic drug delivery from around the world, to contribute to a discussion of the current state-of-the-art, as well as new developments in this important area of oncologic care and research.

Although some of the approaches to be discussed remain highly experimental, it can reasonably be hoped and anticipated that many of these imaginative and innovative strategies will ultimately be recognized as "standard treatment" for patients with malignant disease confined to specific regions of the human body.

Maurie Markman, MD

References

1. Weisberger AS, Levine B, Storaasli JP. Use of nitrogen mustard in treatment of serous effusions of neoplastic origin. *JAMA* 1955; **159**:1704–1707.
2. Green TH. Hemisulfur mustard in the palliation of patients with metastatic ovarian cancer. *Obstet Gynecol* 1959; **13**:383–393.

AUG 23 2000

3. Sullivan RD, Jones R, Jr., Schnabel TG, et al. The treatment of human cancer with intra-arterial nitrogen mustard (methylbis(2-chloroethyl)amine hydrochloride) utilizing a simplified catheter technique. *Cancer* 1953; **6**:121–134.

4. Markman M, George M, Hakes T, et al. Phase 2 trial of intraperitoneal mitoxantrone in the management of refractory ovarian carcinoma. *J Clin Oncol* 1990; **8**:146–150.

5. DeWys WD, Fowler EH. Report of vasculitis and blindness after intracarotid injection of 1,3 bis(2-chloroethyl)-1-nitrosurea (BCNU), NSC-409962 in dogs. *Cancer Chemother Rep* 1973; **57**:33–40.

6. Hohn DS, Rayner AA, Economou JS, et al. Toxicities and complications of implanted pump hepatic arterial and intravenous floxuridine infusion. *Cancer* 1986; **57**:465–470.

7. Zincke H, Utz DC, Taylor WF, et al. Influence of thiotepa and doxorubicin instillation at time of transurethral surgical treatment of bladder cancer on tumor recurrence: a prospective, randomized, double-blind, controlled trial. *J Urol* 1983; **129**:505–509.

8. Bleyer WA. Intrathecal methotrexate versus central nervous system leukemia. *Cancer Drug Deliv* 1984; **1**:157–167.

9. Alberts DS, Liu PY, Hannigan EV, et al. Intraperitoneal cisplatin plus intravenous cyclophosphamide versus intravenous cisplatin plus intravenous cyclophosphamide for stage III ovarian cancer. *N Engl J Med* 1996; **335**:1950–1955.

10. Markman M, Bundy B, Benda J, et al. Randomized phase 3 study of intravenous (IV) cisplatin/paclitaxel versus moderately high dose IV carboplatin followed by IV paclitaxel and intraperitoneal cisplatin in optimal residual ovarian cancer: An Intergroup Trial (GOG, SWOG, ECOG). *Proc Am Soc Clin Oncol* 1998; **17**:361a.

CONTENTS

CONTRIBUTORS

SUBHI ABU-ABEID, MD, *Department of Surgery, Tel Aviv Sourasky Medical Centre, Tel Aviv, Israel*

DAVID S. ALBERTS, MD, *Section of Hematology and Oncology, Department of Medicine and Pharmacology, Arizona Cancer Center, University of Arizona, Tucson, AZ*

H. RICHARD ALEXANDER, MD, *Head, Surgical Metabolism Section, Surgery Branch, National Cancer Institute/NIH, Bethesda, MD*

JYOTI ARYA, MD, *Department of Surgery, Tulane University School of Medicine, New Orleans, LA*

OMAR T. ATIQ, MD, *Associate Clinical Professor of Medicine, University of Arkansas for Medical Sciences, and Medical Director, Cancer treatment Program, Jefferson Medical Center, Pine Bluffs, AR*

RICHARD R. BARAKAT, MD, *Gynecology Service, Department of Surgery, Memorial Sloan-Kettering Cancer Center, New York, NY*

DAVID L. BARTLETT, MD, *Surgical Metabolism Section, Surgery Branch, National Cancer Institute/NIH, Bethesda, MD*

JONATHAN S. BEREK, MD, *Vice Chairman, Department of Obstetrics and Gynecology, UCLA School of Medicine, Los Angeles, CA*

MARY S. BRADY, MD, *Gastric and Mixed Tumor Service, Department of Surgery, Memorial Sloan-Kettering Cancer Center, New York, NY*

MICHAEL BURT, MD, PhD, *Thoracic Service, Department of Surgery, Memorial Sloan-Kettering Cancer Center, New York, NY*

DANIEL G. COIT, MD, *Department of Surgery, Memorial Sloan-Kettering Cancer Center, New York, NY*

OLIVER DORIGO, MD, *UCLA Women's Gynecologic Oncology Center, Department of Obstetrics and Gynecology, Jonsson Comprehensive Cancer Center, UCLA School of Medicine, Los Angeles, CA*

JOHN C. ELKAS, MD, *UCLA Women's Gynecologic Oncology Center, Department of Obstetrics and Gynecology, Jonsson Comprehensive Cancer Center, UCLA School of Medicine, Los Angeles, CA*

EMILY FISHER, MS, *Southwest Oncology Group Statistical Center, Seattle, WA*

SHIGERU FUJIMOTO. MD, *Director, Social Insurance, Funabashi Central Hospital, Funabashi, Japan*

AGUSTIN GARCIA, MD, *Kaplan Comprehensive Cancer Center, New York University Medical Center, New York, NY*

DAVA J. GARCIA, BA, *Arizona Cancer Center, Tucson, AZ*

ROBERT J. GINSBERG, MD, *Chief of Thoracic Surgery, William G. Caban Chair of Surgery, Memorial Sloan-Kettering Cancer Center, New York, NY*

SUSAN GROSHEN, PhD, *Kaplan Comprehensive Cancer Center, New York University Medical Center, New York, NY*

MORDECHAI GUTMAN, MD, *Department of Surgery, Tel Aviv Sourasky Medical Centre, Tel Aviv, Israel*

SUSAN JEFFERS, RN, *Kaplan Comprehensive Cancer Center, New York University Medical Center, New York, NY*

MATT E. KALAYCIO, MD, *Department of Hematology and Medical Oncology, The Cleveland Clinic Foundation, Cleveland, OH*

DAVID P. KELSEN, *Chief, Gastrointestinal Oncology Service, Department of Medicine, Memorial Sloan-Kettering Cancer Center, New York, NY*

NANCY E. KEMENY, MD, *Professor of Medicine, Cornell University Medical College, and Attending Physician and Member, Memorial Sloan-Kettering Cancer Center, New York, NY*

ALEXANDER W. KENNEDY, MD, *Department of Gynecology, The Cleveland Clinic Foundation, Cleveland, OH*

KERRY L. KILBRIDGE, MD, *Division of Hematology–Oncology, University of Virginia, Charlottesville, VA*

JOSEPH M. KLAUSNER, MD, *Professor and Head of Surgery, Tel Aviv Sourasky Medical Centre, Tel Aviv, Israel*

ERIC A. KLEIN, MD, *Head, Section of Urologic Oncology, Department of Urology, The Cleveland Clinic Foundation, Cleveland, OH*

DINA LEV-CHELOUCHE, MD, *Department of Surgery, Tel Aviv Sourasky Medical Centre, Tel Aviv, Israel*

STEVEN K. LIBUTTI, MD, *Surgical Metabolism Section, Surgery Branch, National Cancer Institute/NIH, Bethesda, MD*

DAVID LIU, MD, *Thoracic Service, Department of Surgery, Memorial Sloan-Kettering Cancer Center, New York, NY*

P. Y. LIU, PhD, *Southwest Oncology Group Statistical Center, Seattle, WA*

MAURIE MARKMAN, MD, *Director, The Cleveland Clinic Taussig Cancer Center, and Chairman, Department of Hematology/Medical Oncology, The Cleveland Clinic Foundation, Cleveland, OH*

JAMES H. MUCHMORE, MD, *Associate Professor of Surgery, Department of Surgery, Tulane University School of Medicine, New Orleans, LA*

FRANCO M. MUGGIA, MD, *Division of Oncology, Kaplan Comprehensive Cancer Center, New York University Medical Center, New York, NY*

EILEEN M. O'REILLY, MD, *Clinical Assistant Attending Physician, MSKCC Instructor in Medicine, Cornell University Medical Center, New York, NY*

BETH A. OVERMOYER, MD, *Ireland Cancer Center, University Hospitals of Cleveland, Cleveland, OH*

ROBERT J. PELLEY, MD, *Department of Hematology and Medical Oncology, The Cleveland Clinic Foundation, Cleveland, OH*

DAVID M. PEEREBOOM, MD, *Department of Hematology and Medical Oncology, The Cleveland Clinic Foundation, Cleveland, OH*

BRAD A. POHLMAN, MD, *Department of Hematology and Medical Oncology, The Cleveland Clinic Foundation, Cleveland, OH*

TAMAR SAFRA, MD, *Kaplan Comprehensive Cancer Center, New York University Medical Center, New York, NY*

DAVID R. SPRIGGS, MD, *Developmental Chemotherapy Service, Department of Medicine, Memorial Sloan-Kettering Cancer Center, New York, NY*

GLEN STEVENS, PhD, DO, *The Cleveland Clinic Foundation, Cleveland, OH*

PAUL H. SUGARBAKER, MD, *Washington Cancer Institute, Washington Hospital Center, Washington, DC*

MAKOTO TAKAHASHI, MD, *Social Insurance, Funabashi Central Hospital, Funabashi, Japan*

DONALD W. WIPER, MD, *Department of Gynecology, The Cleveland Clinic Foundation, Cleveland, OH*

1
Principles of Regional Antineoplastic Drug Delivery

Maurie Markman

The principal aim of all attempts to administer antineoplastic agents regionally is to increase the exposure of cancer cells to the drugs beyond what can be achieved safely through systemic drug delivery *(1–5)*. There are several ways in which this overall goal of therapy can be accomplished through regional drug delivery, as briefly outlined in Table 1. Depending on specific biological characteristics of the anticancer agent(s), as defined through evaluation of the drugs in preclinical experimental systems, one or more of these techniques of increasing exposure may have the potential to optimize the antineoplastic effects of the drug(s) considered for therapy of a particular tumor type.

It is important to remember that the ability to expose cancer to higher concentrations of an anticancer agent is, by itself, insufficient reason to do so. If a tumor exhibits a high degree of inherent resistance to a chemotherapeutic or biological agent, the significantly increased drug concentrations achievable through regional delivery may be unable to make a clinically relevant improvement in the extent of tumor cell kill. Preclinical experimental systems can be helpful in suggesting whether or not a particular drug(s) exhibits sufficient evidence of a dose–response effect to justify the initiation of clinical trials of regional delivery in a particular disease setting.

One of the most important principles of regional anticancer drug therapy is that any pharmacokinetic advantage associated with the approach is limited to the first pass of the agent through the perfused/infused area. If the drug subsequently enters the systemic circulation, there will be exposure of the tumor to the agent through capillary flow, but there will be no advantage associated with this added exposure, compared to simply administering the drug intravenously at standard dose levels.

The pharmacokinetic advantage for regional antineoplastic drug instillation is determined by comparing the amount of the drug reaching the target tissue through this route of administration, to that achieved with systemic drug delivery. Similarly, the extent of systemic exposure associated with regional drug instillation will need to be compared to that attained following intravenous administration, to evaluate the relative advantage of the local approach in decreasing the amount of the agent entering the systemic compartment. It is possible to express these two concepts, which define the overall pharmacokinetic advantage associated with regional antineoplastic therapy, by the mathematical equations shown in Table 2. The overall pharmacokinetic advantage

From: *Current Clinical Oncology: Regional Chemotherapy: Clinical Research and Practice*
Edited by: M. Markman © Humana Press Inc., Totowa, NJ

Table 1
Opportunities to Optimize Efficacy
Through Regional Administration of Antineoplastic Agents

1. Increase exposure time of tumor to minimally or moderately active cytotoxic agents (both peak drug levels and area-under-the-concentration-vs-time curve (AUC).
2. Prolong exposure of tumor to cycle-specific cytotoxic agents.
3. Decrease systemic toxicity associated with iv drug delivery.
4. Enhance opportunity for concentration-dependent synergy between two or more antineoplastic drugs.

Table 2
Pharmacokinetic Advantage of Regional Antineoplastic Drug Administration

Equation 1:
$$R_{local} = C_{local} \text{ (regional)}/C_{local} \text{ (iv)}$$

Equation 2:
$$R_{systemic} = C_{systemic} \text{ (regional)}/C_{systemic} \text{ (iv)}$$

Equation 3:
$$R = \frac{R_{local}}{R_{systemic}} = \frac{C_{local} \text{ (regional)}/C_{local} \text{ (iv)}}{C_{systemic} \text{ (regional)}/C_{systemic} \text{ (iv)}}$$

R_{local} = relative increased exposure to infused/perfused region; $R_{systemic}$ = relative decreased exposure to systemic compartment; C_{local} (regional) = local concentration following regional drug delivery; C_{local} (iv) = local concentration following systemic drug delivery; $C_{systemic}$ (regional) = systemic concentration following local drug delivery; $C_{systemic}$ (iv) = systemic concentration following systemic delivery; R = overall pharmacokinetic advantage associated with regional drug delivery.

of regional drug delivery is defined as the ratio of the concentration of drug reaching the perfused/infused body region to the concentration reaching the systemic compartment (Table 2, Eq. 3).

Careful examination of this formula leads to one of the most important principles of regional drug delivery: The relative advantage of this form of therapy, compared with systemic delivery, will be significantly enhanced as regional drug clearance is reduced, or as systemic drug removal is increased.

A variety of methods can be proposed to increase the pharmacokinetic advantage associated with regional therapy, as outlined in Table 3. Several of these approaches have become standard clinical practice, most notably the use of leucovorin rescue following intrathecal methotrexate, to prevent systemic toxicity of the cytotoxic drug. This strategy is of particular value in a patient heavily pretreated with systemic chemotherapy (e.g., induction chemotherapy for acute lymphocytic leukemia), when bone marrow reserve may be quite limited.

In the selection of agents for regional administration, particular characteristics of the drugs, in addition to their activity in the cancer being treated, may be important in the success of this therapeutic strategy. For example, in the case of hepatic arterial or portal vein infusion, agents that are rapidly metabolized during their first passage through the liver will exhibit the most favorable pharmacokinetic advantage for regional perfusion of this organ.

The property of rapid and extensive hepatic metabolism is one of the major reasons fluorodeoxyuridine has been the agent most commonly utilized in trials of hepatic arterial infusion of colon cancer metastatic to the liver *(6)*. Approximately 90–95% of the

Table 3
Methods to Increase Pharmacokinetic Advantage
Associated with Regional Antineoplastic Drug Delivery

1. Removal of drug within the perfused organ (e.g., intrahepatic arterial infusion).
2. Removal of drug following regional perfusion, but prior to entry into the systemic compartment (e.g., isolation–perfusion of extremity tumors).
3. Systemic delivery of an antagonist for the regionally administered cytotoxic drug, aimed at neutralizing the agent as it enters the systemic compartment to prevent systemic toxicity (e.g., systemic leucovorin following intrathecal methotrexate).
4. Use of a material to slow blood flow through the perfused organ (e.g., starch microspheres during intrahepatic arterial perfusion).

floxuridine is removed during its first passage through the liver, providing a significant pharmacokinetic advantage associated with use of this agent during this method of regional chemotherapy.

In contrast, if a drug is not metabolized or removed prior to its entry into the systemic compartment, there will be a far more limited pharmacokinetic advantage associated with regional delivery. A potentially important exception to this statement might occur if blood flow through the region of tumor is quite sluggish (increasing the relative time of exposure), and clearance of the agent from the systemic compartment is rapid. These factors may increase the relative exposure of the tumor, compared to the rest of the body, so that the utilization of such a strategy can be justified.

The absolute magnitude of the difference between regional and systemic exposures required to improve clinical outcome is an important and difficult question. For many tumor types, a 20-fold, or even 50-fold, increase in exposure will have little clinical relevance. In contrast, for other malignancies, preclinical data have suggested a rather steep dose–response curve for the moderately active chemotherapeutic agents available to oncologists *(7)*. A 10-fold, or even five-fold, increase in tumor exposure to these drugs, which would not be achievable following systemic delivery, may be possible with regional treatment *(8)*. Further, this increased exposure has the realistic potential to result in enhanced cytotoxicity and improved therapeutic outcome.

In addition, there is an important theoretical advantage to maintaining systemic concentrations of the antineoplastic agent at the same levels that would be achieved with standard intravenous delivery. With minimal removal of the drug before its entry into the systemic circulation, there will be less chance of a decrease in the therapeutic efficacy of the treatment program because of a lower concentration of active drug reaching macroscopic or microscopic tumor outside the perfused region *(9)*.

The toxicities associated with regional drug delivery can be both local and systemic. If the local toxic effects of a particular regional treatment program are not dose-limiting, it is possible to escalate the amount of drug delivered to the point at which as much of it reaches the systemic compartment as when the agent is administered intravenously. Thus, the extent of systemic exposure following regional drug delivery will depend to a significant extent on the drug(s) used, the specific route(s) of drug administration employed, and the local toxicity potential of each agent.

Any advantage of this method of drug administration will be relative, rather than absolute. In fact, the limited experimental data available support the concept that there will be only a modest increase in tissue and intratumor drug concentrations at the local site following regional drug delivery, despite rather dramatic increases in the level of drug measurable within the vascular or body compartment into which the drugs are infused/perfused. This is because of the limited penetration of drugs directly into tumor or normal tissue *(10–17)*. Thus, although regional drug delivery may significantly enhance the clinical activity of antineoplastic agents with known effectiveness against a particular tumor type, this strategy will probably be unable to convert a totally inactive drug against a specific cancer into a highly useful cytotoxic agent.

REFERENCES

1. Collins JM. Pharmacokinetic rationale for regional drug delivery, *J. Clin. Oncol.,* **2** (1984) 498–504.
2. Chen H-S and Gross JF. Intra-arterial infusion of anticancer drugs: theoretic aspects of drug delivery and review of responses, *Cancer Treat. Rep.,* **64** (1980) 31–40.
3. Dedrick RL, Myers CE, Bungay PM, et al. Pharmacokinetic rationale for peritoneal drug administration in the treatment of ovarian cancer, *Cancer Treat. Rep.,* **62** (1978) 1–9.
4. Sculier JP. Treatment of meningeal carcinomatosis, *Cancer Treat. Rev.,* **12** (1985) 95–104.
5. Wolf BE and Sugarbaker PH. Intraperitoneal chemotherapy and immunotherapy, *Recent Results Cancer Res.,* **110** (1988) 254–273.
6. Kemeny N, Daly J, Reichman B, et al. Intrahepatic or systemic infusion of fluorodeoxyuridine in patients with liver metastases from colorectal carcinoma: a randomized trial, *Ann. Intern. Med.,* **107** (1987) 459–465.
7. Frei E and Canellos GP. Dose: a critical factor in cancer chemotherapy, *Am. J. Med.,* **69** (1980) 585–594.
8. Alberts DS, Young L, Mason N, et al. In vitro evaluation of anticancer drugs against ovarian cancer at concentrations achievable by intraperitoneal administration, *Semin. Oncol.,* **12 (Suppl 4)** (1985) 38–42.
9. Markman M: Intraperitoneal therapy of ovarian cancer, *Semin. Oncol.,* **25** (1998) 356–360.
10. Ozols RF, Locker GY, Doroshow JH, et al. Pharmacokinetics of adriamycin and tissue penetration in murine ovarian cancer, *Cancer Res.,* **39** (1979) 3209–3214.
11. Los G, Mutsaers PHA, van der Vijgh WJF, et al. Direct diffusion of cis-diamminedichloroplatinum(II) in intraperitoneal rat tumors after intraperitoneal chemotherapy: a comparison with systemic chemotherapy, *Cancer Res.,* **49** (1989) 3380–3384.
12. Stewart DJ, Benjamin RS, Luna M, et al. Human tissue distribution of platinum after cis-diamminedichloroplatinum, *Cancer Chemother. Pharmacol.,* **10** (1982) 51–54.
13. Stewart DJ, Mikhael NZ, Nair RC, et al. Platinum concentrations in human autopsy tumor samples, *Am. J. Clin. Oncol.,* **11** (1988) 152–158.
14. Stewart DJ, Leavens M, Maor M, et al. Human central nervous system distribution of cis-diamminedichloroplatinum and use as a radiosensitizer in malignant brain tumors, *Cancer Res.,* **42** (1982) 2474–2479.
15. Carlson JA Jr, Litterst CL, Grenberg RA, et al. Platinum tissue concentrations following intra-arterial and intravenous cis-diamminedichloroplatinum II in New Zealand white rabbits, *Am. J. Obstet. Gynecol.,* **148** (1984) 313–317.
16. Vennin P, Hecquet B, Poissonnier B, et al. Comparative study of intravenous and intraarterial cisplatinum on intratumoral platinum concentrations in carcinoma of the cervix, *Gynecol. Oncol.,* **32** (1989) 180–183.
17. West GW, Weichselbau R, and Little JB. Limited penetration of methotrexate into human osteosarcoma spheroids as a proposed model for solid tumor resistance to adjuvant chemotherapy, *Cancer Res.,* **40** (1980) 3665–3668.

2 Intrahepatic Chemotherapy for Metastatic Colorectal Cancer

Nancy E. Kemeny and Omar T. Atiq

1. INTRODUCTION

Colorectal cancer (CRC) is the fourth most common malignancy in the United States *(1)*. Approximately 130,000 new patients will be diagnosed with this cancer in 1999. It is the second leading cause of cancer death, with 55,000 patients expected to die of it. Most patients die of metastatic disease. The vast majority of them have liver as the dominant site of metastases *(2)*. Approximately 30% of patients with metastatic CRC have disease confined to the liver; 10–25% of patients undergoing resection of primary CRC have synchronous hepatic metastases.

Potentially curative resection is possible in a minority of patients with hepatic disease. Systemic chemotherapy produces response rates of 15–30%, with median survival of 10–12 mo. It is estimated that 30,000 patients are candidates for regional hepatic therapy each year. Thus, the impact of this malady is substantial.

The anatomic and pharmacokinetic advantage of intraarterial chemotherapy in patients with hepatic disease makes it an attractive therapeutic option. Regional hepatic arterial infusion (HAI) chemotherapy can be administered via a hepatic arterial port

From: *Current Clinical Oncology: Regional Chemotherapy: Clinical Research and Practice*
Edited by: M. Markman © Humana Press Inc., Totowa, NJ

or a percutaneously placed intraarterial catheter connected to an external or totally implantable pump. Operative complications and hepatobiliary toxicity have been a hindrance to the widespread use of regional intrahepatic therapy. However, improvements in surgical technique and newer chemotherapy combinations have decreased the complication rate of this treatment modality.

2. RATIONALE FOR HAI

The rationale for HAI chemotherapy is based on both anatomic and pharmacologic factors. Even though colorectal metastases appear to migrate to the liver via the portal vein, they derive their blood supply almost exclusively from the hepatic artery, once they are greater than 1 cm in diameter (3). On the other hand, the normal liver hepatocytes derive their blood supply primarily from the portal circulation. Thus, the administration of chemotherapy into the hepatic artery allows for selective drug delivery to the tumor, with relative sparing of normal hepatocytes.

The pharmacologic basis of intrahepatic therapy is well-defined. Certain drugs are extracted mostly by the liver during the first pass through the arterial circulation, which results in high local concentrations of the drug, with minimal systemic toxicity (4). Because hepatic arterial blood flow has a high regional exchange rate (100–1500 mL/min), drugs with a high total body clearance and short plasma half-life are more useful for hepatic infusion. If a drug is not rapidly cleared, recirculation through the systemic circulation diminishes the advantage of hepatic arterial delivery. The area under the concentration vs time curve (AUC) is a function not only of drug clearance, but also of hepatic arterial flow.

Another rationale for HAI chemotherapy, especially for patients with metastatic CRC, is the concept of a stepwise pattern of metastatic progression (5). According to this theory, hematogenous spread occurs first via the portal vein to the liver, then from the liver to the lungs, and then to other organs of the body. Therefore, aggressive treatment of metastases confined to the liver may prolong survival for some patients.

3. CHEMOTHERAPEUTIC AGENTS

Drugs with a steep dose–response curve are more useful when given by the intrahepatic route because small increases in the concentration of the drug result in a large improvement in response. Ensminger et al. (6) demonstrated that 94–99% 5-fluorodeoxyuridase (FUDR) is extracted during the first pass, compared to 19–55% of 5-fluorouracil (5-FU), which makes FUDR an ideal drug for HAI chemotherapy. Although, after injection of FUDR into either the hepatic artery or portal vein, mean liver concentrations of drug do not differ because of the route of injection, the mean tumor FUDR levels are 15-fold higher when the drug is injected via the hepatic artery. The pharmacological advantage of various chemotherapeutic agents used for HAI is summarized in Table 1.

4. ACCESS FOR HAI

4.1. Approach

Regional HAI can be done by using either hepatic arterial port or a percutaneously placed catheter connected to an external pump, or to a totally implantable pump. Early studies with percutaneously placed hepatic artery catheters produced high response rates, but clotting of the catheters and the hepatic artery, as well as bleeding, led physicians to abandon this method (7). The development of a totally implantable pump

Table 1
Drugs for HAI

Drug	Half-life (min)	Estimated increased exposure by HAI (-fold)
Fluorouracil	10	5–10
5-Fluoro-2-deoxyuridine	<10	100–400
Bischlorethylnitrosourea	<5	6–7
Mitomycin C	<10	6–8
Cisplatin	20–30	4–7
Adriamycin (doxorubicin hydrochloride)	60	2

allowed long-term HAI with good patency of the catheter and the hepatic artery, and a low incidence of infection. One study compared three groups: surgical placement of hepatic artery catheter, percutaneous placement of hepatic artery catheter, and an operative implantable reservoir connected to the hepatic artery catheter. The reported ability of each technique to administer chemotherapy for the three groups was 31, 25, and 115 d, respectively *(5).*

The goals of pump placement are to enable bilobar hepatic perfusion with chemotherapy, and to prevent administration of chemotherapy to the stomach or duodenum. Although this appears straightforward, the complication rate with pump placement may be unacceptably high in inexperienced hands *(8).* Even with experienced surgeons, extrahepatic disease must be ruled out radiographically, with meticulous care. Celiac and superior mesenteric artery arteriograms should be done to identify arterial anatomy of the liver and vessels to the stomach, duodenum, and pancreas, preoperatively. Portal vein must be patent and portal lymph nodes should be biopsied intraoperatively, to rule out extrahepatic disease. The catheter is placed into the gastroduodenal artery, and not directly into the hepatic artery, which can lead to thrombosis. The catheter is secured with nonabsorbable ties. The arterial collaterals to stomach, duodenum, and pancreas are identified and ligated, and the liver perfusion, as well as absence of perfusion to other vital organs, is confirmed intraoperatively with fluorescein injection and Wood's lamp. A cholecystectomy is performed at the same time, to avoid drug-induced cholecystitis. Postoperative (PO) macroaggregated albumin scan should be performed through the side port of pump, to check for perfusion of the liver, and to ensure absence of extrahepatic perfusion *(9).* Careful attention to these details is important to avoid unnecessary surgery and to minimize the risks of complications, including gastrointestinal (GI) ulceration and hemorrhage.

4.2. Complications

Early PO complications include arterial injury leading to hepatic artery thrombosis; incomplete perfusion of the entire liver caused by the lack of recognition of an accessory hepatic artery; misperfusion to the stomach, duodenum, or pancreas; and pump pocket hematoma *(10).* Late complications tend to be more common, and include pump pocket infections, catheter thrombosis, and peptic ulceration. Review of data from Memorial Sloan-Kettering Cancer Center (MSKCC) over an 8-yr period showed relative lack of serious complications, in experienced hands. During this period, 303 infusion pumps were inserted for intrahepatic therapy. There were only two deaths. Arterial catheter

Table 2
Hepatic Arterial FUDR With Internal Pump: Responses

Investigator	Ref.	No. Patients	Prior Chemotherapy (%)	Partial Response (%)	Decrease in CEA (%)	Median Survival (mo)
Niederhuber	(11)	70	45	83	91	25
Balch	(12)	50	40	–	83	26
Kemeny, N.	(13)	41	43	42	51	12
Shepard	(14)	53	42	32	–	17
Cohen	(15)	50	36	51	–	–
Weiss	(16)	17	85	29	57	13
Schwartz	(17)	23	–	15	75	18
Johnson	(18)	40	–	47	–	12
Kemeny, M.	(19)	31	50	52	–	22
Lorenz	(20)	26	–	52	–	16

–, not stated.
CEA = carcinoembryonic antigen.

thrombosis occurred in 14 (4.7%) patients. Extrahepatic perfusion was seen in six (3%) patients. Incomplete perfusion occurred in five (1.7%), with the remaining complications occurring rarely, including gastric ulcers, hemorrhage, pneumonia, pocket infection, and faulty pump. Overall morbidity was seen in 34 of 303 patients (11.8%). Of the two patients who died, one died of myocardial infarction and the other died of progressive disease. The second patient underwent a laparotomy for resection of the colon primary and synchronous insertion of a pump. Although the operation was technically successful, without any significant complications, the extent of liver disease precluded a successful outcome. Patients who have more than 70% liver involvement may not benefit from surgical placement of hepatic artery pump for chemotherapy.

5. NONRANDOMIZED STUDIES OF HAI

5.1. Single-Agent Therapy

The development of a totally implantable infusional pump allowed for the safe administration of HAI chemotherapy in the outpatient setting. Early trials using an implantable pump and continuous FUDR therapy produced a median response rate of 45%, and a median survival of 17 mo (Table 2).

5.2. Combination Chemotherapy

Several phase II trials evaluating combination chemotherapy via HAI were conducted in the early 1990s. In a study at the University of California at San Francisco (21) (UCSF), 34 patients were treated with FUDR alternating with 5 FU, to take advantage of the different pharmacokinetics and toxicities of infusional FUDR and bolus 5 FU. FUDR was infused at a dose of 0.1 mg/kg/d for 7 d. Bolus 5 FU was given through the pump side port on d 15, 22, and 29 of each 5-wk cycle. There was a 50% response rate, with median survival exceeding 2 yr for previously untreated patients. Hepatobiliary toxicity was minimal with this regimen. However, progressive hepatic disease was the initial site of failure and cause of death in the majority of patients.

In a series of successive studies at MSKCC, Kemeny et al. (22) attempted modulation of FUDR by various agents, to improve response rate and decrease toxicity. In one trial, six different regimens were explored. The FUDR dose ranged from 0.25 to 0.3 mg/kg/d for 14 d, along with 15–30 mg/m^2/d leucovorin (iv). Despite a 12% incidence of biliary cirrhosis, the median survival of 42 patients treated in the second phase was 24.2 mo. In a subsequent trial, Kemeny et al. *(23)* administered 0.3 mg/kg/d FUDR and 15 mg/m^2/d LV for 14 d with 20 mg dexamethasone (DEX) through the side port of the pump on day 1: 33 patients were treated on this regimen. Response rate was 78% and median survival was 24.8 mo. Strict dose-reduction protocol reduced the incidence of biliary cirrhosis to 3%. Liver was the initial site of failure in two-thirds of the patients.

6. RANDOMIZED STUDIES
OF HAI VERSUS SYSTEMIC CHEMOTHERAPY

One of the first randomized trials was conducted at MSKCC by Kemeny et al. *(24)*. Prior to randomization, patients were stratified for extent of liver involvement by tumor and baseline lactic dehydrogenase (LDH), based on data showing them to be important prognostic indicators of survival. This prospective randomized trial compared HAI to systemic infusion of FUDR on a 14-d schedule. The dose of FUDR was 0.3 mg/kg/d in the HAI group and 0.125 mg/kg/d in the systemic group. The high dose given in the intrahepatic group was not tolerable by the systemic route. All patients underwent exploratory laparotomy, not only for pump placement, but to ensure the comparability of the two study groups, by accurately defining the extent of liver involvement, and assuring the absence of extrahepatic disease. The patients randomized to HAI had the hepatic artery catheter connected to the Infusaid pump (Shiley Infusaid, Norwood, MA). In patients randomized to systemic therapy, the hepatic artery catheter was connected to a subcutaneously implanted access port, and the pump was connected to an additional catheter placed in the cephalic vein. The study design allowed a crossover from systemic therapy to HAI by a minor surgical procedure, i.e., ligation of the systemic catheter, followed by connection of the pump with the hepatic artery catheter, in the event of tumor progression on systemic therapy. Of 178 patients referred, 12 refused randomization and four had an inadequate arterial blood supply; therefore, 162 were randomized. At laparotomy, 63 patients were excluded; 33 had extrahepatic disease, 25 had their tumor resected, four had no tumor, and one had an abdominal infection. Of the 99 evaluable patients, there were two complete responses (CRs) and 23 partial responses (PRs) (53%) in the group receiving HAI, and 10 partial responses (21%) in the systemic group ($P = 0.001$) (Table 3). Of the patients randomized to systemic therapy, 31 (60%) crossed over to HAI after tumor progression. Of these patients, 25% went on to a PR after the crossover, and 60% had a decrease in carcinoembryonic antigen levels. Toxicity differed between the two groups. In the HAI group, toxicity was predominantly hepatic and GI. An increase in hepatic enzymes and serum bilirubin (Bili) levels occurred in the intrahepatic group. In the systemic group, diarrhea occurred in 70% of the patients, with 9% requiring admission for iv hydration; mucositis occurred in 10% of patients.

The median survival for the HAI and systemic groups was 17 and 12 mo, respectively ($P = 0.424$). The interpretation of survival is difficult in this study, because 60% of the patients in the systemic group crossed over and received intrahepatic therapy after tumor progression on systemic therapy. Those who did not crossover usually had clotting of the hepatic arterial catheter, and had a median survival of only 8 mo, compared to 18 mo for those who crossed over to HAI ($p = 0.04$). An analysis

Table 3
MSKCC Study: Randomized HAI vs Systemic FUDR Infusion

	HAI (n = 48)	Systemic (n = 51)	P
Complete response	2	0	
Partial response	23 (52%)	10 (20%)	0.001
>50% decrease in CEA	29	13	
Extrahepatic metastases	27	19	0.09
Toxicity			
Ulcer	8	3	
Elevated enzymes	20 (42%)	12	
Bilirubin >3 mg/dL	9	2	
Diarrhea	1	36 (70%)	
Survival			
Total	17 mo	12 mo	0.424
Crossover		18 mo	
No crossover		8 mo	0.04

of baseline characteristics and the crossover and noncrossover groups revealed no significant differences.

A similar randomized study conducted by the North Carolina Oncology Group also used FUDR infusion in both HAI and systemic groups (25). Prior to randomization, the patients were stratified by extent of liver involvement, based on computed tomography (CT) scans, baseline bilirubin values, and performance status. The doses of FUDR were 0.2 and 0.075 mg/kg/d for 14 d in the HAI and systemic groups, respectively. These were the actual doses administered, because recalculation was done that took into account the residual volume in the pump. A total of 143 patients were entered, but only 117 were eligible. A 42% CR and PR rate was reported in the HAI group, and 10% in the systemic group ($P < 0.0001$). The median time to progression was 401 d in the HAI group and 201 d in the systemic group ($P = 0.0009$). The median survival was 503 and 484 d for the hepatic and systemic groups, respectively. Although a crossover design was not built into the study, 43% of the systemic group patients received intrahepatic therapy, possibly obscuring any difference in survival. Another factor that makes interpretation of survival difficult is that patients with metastases to hepatic lymph nodes were included in both study groups.

A National Cancer Institute study compared HAI to systemic infusion of FUDR in 64 patients (26). There was a significantly improved response rate for HAI, compared to the systemic therapy (62 vs 17%, respectively; $P < 0.003$). Interpretation of survival data is difficult because 11 (34%) patients of the HAI group never received chemotherapy, and 8% of the HAI group had positive portal lymph nodes. Despite these limitations, in the subset of patients without extrahepatic disease, the 2-yr survival was 47% in the HAI group vs 13% in the systemic group ($P = 0.03$).

Another small study conducted by the Mayo Clinic compared HAI FUDR (0.3 mg/kg/d for 14 d) to systemic bolus 5 FU (500 mg/m^2 iv for 5 d) (27). The trial only permitted entry of symptomatic patients, and did not allow a crossover to an alternative treatment; 69 patients were entered. Objective tumor response was observed in 48% of the patients receiving HAI FUDR, and in 21% of patients receiving iv 5 FU ($P = 0.02$). The time to hepatic progression was significantly longer in the HAI group (15.7 vs 6 mo; $P = 0.0001$). Despite the increased response rate and time to hepatic progression,

Table 4
Randomized Studies
of Intrahepatic vs Systemic Chemotherapy for Hepatic Metastases from CRC

Group (ref.)	No. patients	Response (%)			Survival (mo)		
		HAI	Sys	P	HAI	Sys	P
MSKCC *(24)*	162	52	20	0.001	18[a]	12	
NCOG *(25)*	143	42	10	0.0001	16.6	16	
NCI *(26)*	64	62	17	0.003	20	11	
Consortium *(31)*	43	58	38	–	–	–	
City of Hope *(30)*	41	56	0	–	–	–	
Mayo Clinic *(27)*	69	48	21	0.02	12.6	10.5	
French *(28)*	163	49	14	–	15	11	0.02
English *(29)*	100	50	0	0.001	13	6.3	0.03

–, not stated.
*Updated.

survival was similar in the two groups (12.6 mo for the HAI vs 10.5 mo for systemic therapy). Again, several factors must be considered regarding survival data. First, this was a small trial, and the power to detect survival advantage was very low. Second, of the 36 patients in the HAI group, five (14%) never received treatment, seven (19%) had extrahepatic disease, three (9%) had hepatic artery thrombosis, and two (6%) had pump malfunction. All of these patients were included in the survival analysis, even though 48% were not adequately treated or had extrahepatic disease. The investigators report that the survival of patients with extrahepatic disease is significantly shorter than those without extrahepatic disease ($P = 0.04$); therefore, inclusion of these patients in the HAI group will have a negative impact on survival. There is no comment in the report on the survival in the adequately treated patients.

In a large multicenter trial in France *(28),* 163 patients were randomized either to hepatic arterial FUDR for 14 d or to systemic bolus 5 FU for 5 d every 4 wk. The groups had comparable clinical and laboratory characteristics, including percentage of liver involvement and baseline LDH levels. In patients with measurable disease, the response rate was 49% in the HAI group and 14% in the systemic group. The median time to hepatic progression was 15 mo for the former group and 6 mo for the latter group. Median survival was 14 vs 10 mo, favoring the HAI group. The 2-yr survival was 22% for the hepatic group and 10% for the systemic group ($P < 0.002$).

In a similar study done in England *(29),* 100 patients were randomized to HAI FUDR vs systemic 5-FU. Patients were only treated if they were symptomatic. Quality of life and survival were significantly improved for the HAI group. Median survival was 405 d vs 198 d for the HAI and systemic groups, respectively ($P = 0.03$).

6.1. Summary of Randomized Studies

There are now eight randomized trials demonstrating a significantly high response rate for HAI chemotherapy compared to systemic therapy in patients with hepatic metastases from CRC (Table 4). In every study, the CR and PR rates were higher for HAI group. Whether this increase in response rate translates into increased survival remains controversial. Several factors complicate this issue. First, most of the trials contain relatively few patients, so that the power to observe differences in survival is low. Second, because of the early successes with intrahepatic infusion, some of these

Table 5
Randomized Study of HAI vs Systemic Chemotherapy

					Survival (%)			
	1 yr		2 yr		<1 yr		<2 yr	
Group (ref.)	HAI	Sys	HAI	Sys	Crossover	No crossover	Crossover	No crossover
MSKCC (24)	60	50	25	20	60	28	25	14
NCOG (25)	60	42	30	20	78	42	40	17
NCI[a] (26)	85	60	44	13				
France (28)	61	44	22	10				
Mean	66	49	30	18	69	35	37	15

[a]Excluding patients with hepatic lymph nodes.

studies allowed patients in the systemic arm to crossover to intrahepatic therapy after tumor progression on systemic therapy. This crossover may have negated any difference in survival between the two groups. The studies do demonstrate a survival advantage for the groups who receive subsequent HAI treatment, with a mean 1-yr survival of 69% for the patients who crossed over from systemic therapy to HAI vs 35% for the group who did not (Table 5).

7. ROLE OF ADJUVANT HAI

At the City of Hope, a randomized trial was conducted for patients who underwent resection of hepatic metastases from CRC (30). A total of 91 patients were entered in three different groups. In group A, after resection of solitary metastases, patients were randomized either to no further treatment (AI) or to HAI (AII). In Group B, after a resection of multiple metastases, the patients were randomized to no further treatment (BII) or HAI (BI). In Group C, there was no resection, and patients were randomized to HAI (CI) or systemic 5-FU followed by HAI (CII). In the group with solitary liver metastasis, the time to failure was 9 mo in the resection-alone group (Group AI) and 31 mo in the resection + HAI (AII) (P < 0.003). In Group B, 30% of patients who had resection + HAI were alive at 5 yr vs 7% of those receiving resection alone. Thus, this study suggests a benefit for HAI in patients who have undergone resection of liver metastases.

An ongoing Eastern Cooperative Oncology Group study (45) randomized fully resected patients to observation vs a combination of HAI FUDR and infusional 5-FU. At 5 yr, actuarial survival is 63% for those treated with HAI vs 32% in the control group. At MSKCC, 15 resected patients were randomized to HAI + systemic vs systemic alone. At 2 yr, 85% are alive in the HAI group vs 69% in the systemic group (P < 0.02). The actuarial 5 yr survival is 60% and 45%, respectively (46). Other pilot studies are exploring the role of HAI FUDR-based chemotherapy in conjunction with partial debulking of liver metastases, either via surgical resection or cryosurgery. Neoadjuvant HAI chemotherapy is also a consideration, but, like PO adjuvant HAI therapy, it must be considered investigational.

8. TOXICITY OF INTRAHEPATIC THERAPY

The most common problems with HAI are peptic ulceration and hepatic toxicity (13,32). Severe ulcer disease results from the inadvertent perfusion of the stomach and duodenum via small collateral branches from the hepatic artery, and can be prevented via careful dissection of these collaterals at the time of pump placement. However, even without radiologically visible perfusion of the stomach and duodenum, mild gastritis and duodenitis can occur. This toxicity can be reduced by careful dose reductions when any GI symptoms occur. Hepatobiliary toxicity is the most problematic toxicity seen with HAI chemotherapy. Although there is some evidence of hepatocellular necrosis and cholestasis on liver biopsies, most studies point to a combined ischemic and inflammatory effect on the bile ducts as the most important etiology of this toxicity. The bile ducts are particularly sensitive to HAI chemotherapy, because, like hepatic tumors, the bile ducts derive their blood supply almost exclusively from the hepatic artery. Pettavel et al. *(33)* prospectively studied 21 liver biopsies and four autopsy specimens of 13 patients, in whom biliary toxicity developed after HAI treatment with FUDR. The liver biopsies were characterized by portal or diffuse inflammatory changes that were predominantly mononuclear. Other changes included focal atrophy of hepatocytes and increased collagen formation. The autopsy specimens showed gross bile duct damage and intimal fibrous thickening of the small arteries, with narrowing or obstruction of the lumina.

Clinically, biliary toxicity is manifested as elevations of aspartate aminotransferase (AST), alkaline phosphatase, and Bili levels. Elevation of AST level is an early manifestation of toxicity; elevation of the alkaline phosphatase or bilirubin is evidence of more severe damage. In the early stages of toxicity, hepatic enzyme elevations will return to normal when the drug is withdrawn and the patient is given a rest. In more advanced cases, jaundice does not resolve.

In patients with severe toxicity, endoscopic retrograde cholangiopancreatography (ERCP) demonstrates lesions resembling primary sclerosing cholangitis. Because the ducts are sclerotic and nondilated, sonograms are usually unhelpful. In some patients, the strictures are more focal, usually worse at the bifurcation, and drainage procedures, either by ERCP or transhepatic cholangiography, may be helpful. Duct obstruction from metastases should first be excluded by CT scan of the liver.

Close monitoring of liver function tests is necessary to avoid biliary sclerosis. If the serum Bili level becomes elevated, no further treatment should be given until it returns to normal, and then only with a small test dose (0.05 mg/kg/d). In patients who cannot tolerate even a low dose for 2 wk, it may be possible to continue treatment by giving the FUDR infusion for 1 wk, rather than the usual 2 wk. At MSKCC, the serum AST level was found to be a useful laboratory test to monitor hepatic toxicity *(13)*. A review of the liver function tests obtained every 2 wk revealed that, in 23 of the original 45 patients, the AST level increased at the end of FUDR infusion (2 wk after treatment began), and then returned to normal, or almost normal, levels prior to the next dose (4 wk after treatment began). This pattern occurred in all patients who later developed severe hepatic toxicity (Bili >3 mg/dL). In some studies with excessive biliary sclerosis, liver function tests were only checked monthly. These investigators may have missed the 2-wk elevation, and therefore may not have reduced doses appropriately at the time of next treatment. At MSKCC, the dose of HAI chemotherapy is modified as outlined in Table 6. In older trials, cholecystitis occurred in up to 33% of patients receiving HAI chemotherapy. In more recent series, the gallbladder was removed at the time of catheter placement, to prevent this complication, and to avoid the confusion of these symptoms with other hepatic side effects of chemotherapy.

The side effects of systemic chemotherapy are almost never observed with HAI. Myelosuppression does not occur with intrahepatic FUDR. Although intrahepatic mitomycin C or carmustine (BCNU) may depress platelet counts, the absolute depression

Table 6
FUDR Dose Modification Schema

SGOT Reference Value:[a]	≤50 u/L	>50 u/L	
	SGOT at pump emptying or day of planned treatment (whichever is higher)		
			FUDR Dose
	0 to <3 × reference	0 to <2 × reference	100%
	3 to <4 × reference	2 to <3 × reference	80%
	4 to <5 × reference	3 to <4 × reference	50%
	≥5 × reference	≥4 × reference	Hold[b]
AP Reference Value:[a]	≤90 u/L	>90 u/L	
	AP at pump emptying or day of planned retreatment (whichever is higher)		
			FUDR Dose
	0 to <1.5 × reference	0 to <1.2 × reference	100%
	1.5 to <2 × reference	1.2 to <1.5 × reference	50%
	≥2.0 × reference	≥1.5 × reference	Hold[c]
Total Bili Reference Value:[a]	≤1.2 mg/dL	>1.2 mg/dL	
	Total Bili at pump emptying or day of planned retreatment (whichever is higher)		
			FUDR Dose
	0 to <1.5 × reference	0 to <1.2 × reference	100%
	1.5 to <2 × reference	1.2 to <1.5 × reference	50%
	≥2.0 × reference	≥1.5 × reference	Hold[d]

[a]Reference value is defined as the value obtained on the day the patient received the last FUDR dose. To determine if an FUDR dose modification is necessary, compare the reference value either to the value obtained on the day that the pump was emptied or to the value on the day of planned pump filling, whichever is higher.

Recommencing Treatment After Hold

[b]After treatment has been held because of elevated SGOT, chemotherapy cannot be restarted until the value has returned to within 4 × reference value (if reference ≤50 u/L) or within 3 × reference value (if reference >50 u/L). Then chemotherapy may be restarted using 50% of the last FUDR dose given.

[c]After treatment has been held because of elevated AP, chemotherapy cannot be restarted until the value has returned to within 1.5 × reference value (if reference ≤ 90 u/L) or within 1.2 × reference value (if reference >90 u/L). Then chemotherapy may be restarted, using 25% of the last FUDR dose given.

[d]After treatment has been held for elevated total Bili, chemotherapy cannot be restarted until value has returned to within 1.5 × reference value (if reference ≤1.2 mg/dL) or within 1.2 × reference value (if reference >1.2 mg/dL). Then chemotherapy may be restarted, using 25% of the last FUDR dose given.

Important: If the patient has experienced a marked elevation in Bili between the reference value and pump emptying (i.e., 2 × reference value, if reference value <1.2 mg/dL; 1.5 × reference value, if reference value >1.2 mg/dL), the patient must not receive chemotherapy on the date of the next planned pump filling, even if Bili has returned to normal. The pump should be filled with heparinized saline, and the patient's laboratory work should be reevaluated in 14 d. If, at that time, Bili is still not evaluated, and enzymes are within the range for treatment, the pump then may be filled with 25% FUDR of the last dose FUDR dose.

AP = Alkaline phosphatase; FUDR = floxuridine; SGOT = serum glutamic oxaloacetic transaminase; Total Bili = Total bilirubin.

and frequency of depression is less than with systemic administration. Nausea, vomiting, and diarrhea do not occur with HAI FUDR. If diarrhea does occur, shunting to the bowel should be suspected.

NEW APPROACHES TO DECREASE HEPATIC TOXICITY

New approaches to decrease hepatic toxicity induced by HAI FUDR are being studied. Because portal triad inflammation may lead to ischemia of the bile ducts, the HAI administration of Dex may decrease biliary toxicity. In patients with established hepatobiliary toxicity from HAI, Dex promotes resolution of liver function abnormalities. A prospective, double-blind randomized study of intrahepatic FUDR with DEX vs FUDR alone was conducted at MSKCC *(34)*, in order to determine whether the simultaneous administration of DEX with FUDR would prevent biliary toxicity, and thereby allow for administration of higher doses of chemotherapy. Although a significant increase in administered FUDR dose was documented, the response rate in 49 evaluable patients was 71% for the FUDR + DEX group vs 40% for FUDR alone. Survival also favored the FUDR + DEX group: 23 vs 15 mo. In addition, there was a trend toward decreased Bili elevation in patients receiving FUDR + DEX, compared to the group receiving FUDR alone (9 vs 30%; $P = 0.007$).

Use of circadian modification of hepatic intra-arterial FUDR infusion is another method to decrease hepatic toxicity. In a retrospective, nonrandomized study at the University of Minnesota *(35)*, a comparison of constant infusion vs circadian-modified HAI FUDR was conducted in 50 patients with CRC. The initial dose was 0.25–0.30 mg/kg/d for a 14-d infusion. The group at circadian modification received 68% of each daily dose between 3 and 9 PM, 2% between 3 and 9 AM, and 15% between each of the adjacent 6-hr periods. Over nine courses of treatment, the patients with circadian-modified infusion tolerated almost twice the daily dose of FUDR (0.79 vs 0.46 mg/kg/d). Circadian-modified infusion resulted in 46% of patients having no hepatic toxicity vs 16% of patients after constant FUDR infusion. Unfortunately, the authors do not present information on response rates achieved in both groups.

Another approach to decrease toxicity from HAI is to alternate drugs such as intra-arterial FUDR and intra-arterial 5-FU. Weekly intra-arterial bolus 5-FU has a similar activity to intra-arterial FUDR, and does not cause hepatobiliary toxicity; however, it frequently produces treatment-limiting systemic toxicity or arteritis. In a trial conducted by Stagg et al. *(21)*, FUDR by HAI was alternated with bolus intra-arterial 5-FU. No patient had treatment terminated because of drug toxicity. Metzger et al. *(36)*, using an infusion of 5-FU and mitomycin C, found that sclerosing cholangitis did not occur, but that mucositis and leukopenia did. Median survival was 18 mo, with a PR rate of 57%. Catheter complications occurred, which led to premature termination of treatment in one-third of patients.

10. METHODS TO INCREASE RESPONSE RATE

Because systemic combination chemotherapy regimens are more effective than single agents, the potential benefit of multidrug arterial therapy is being evaluated. In an early study using mitomycin C, BCNU, and FUDR, Cohen et al. *(37)* reported a 69% PR rate. In a randomized trial at MSKCC, comparing this three-drug regimen with FUDR alone, there was a slight increase in response rate and survival with the three-drug regimen *(38)*. In the 67 patients who entered this trial, all of whom had received prior systemic chemotherapy, the response rate was 45% for the three-drug regimen and

32% for FUDR alone. The median survival from the initiation of HAI therapy was 18.9 and 14.9 mo, respectively. It should be noted that the response rates in both arms are much higher than would be expected with the second systemic regimen. Thus, in addition to its role as a frontline treatment, HAI should also be considered in patients who have failed systemic therapy.

In another attempt to improve survival and response rate, a combination of HAI FUDR and LV was evaluated by Kemeny et al. *(39)*. This study was based on the success of systemic 5-FU/LV regimens, as well as on laboratory studies that suggested that LV may actually be a better modifier of FUDR than 5-FU. Sixty-four patients were treated at five dose levels. The overall response rate was 62%, but 15% of patients developed biliary sclerosis. Nevertheless, 75% of the patients were alive after 1 yr, 66% after 2 yr and 33% after 3 yr. FUDR + LV appears to have a high response rate in the treatment of hepatic metastases from CRC, but hepatic toxicity appears greater than previously reported with FUDR alone.

11. COMBINED HAI AND SYSTEMIC CHEMOTHERAPY

Extrahepatic disease develops in 40–70% of patients undergoing HAI. Such metastases can occur even when the patient is still responding in the liver, and, in many patients, it can result in death. Safi et al. *(40)* studied the ability of concomitant systemic chemotherapy to reduce the development of extrahepatic metastases in patients receiving HAI therapy. Ninety-five patients were randomized to either intra-arterial FUDR (0.02 mg/kg/d) or a combination of intra-arterial FUDR (0.21 mg/kg/d) and iv FUDR (0.09 mg/kg/d) given concurrently, for 14 of 28 d. The response rates were 60% for both arms of the study. However, the incidence of extrahepatic disease was significantly less in patients receiving the intra-arterial/iv treatment, compared with intra-arterial treatment alone (56 vs 79%; $P < 0.001$). No significant difference in survival was found between the two groups ($P = 0.08$). In the study conducted by Lorenz et al. *(41)*, combined HAI + iv therapy did not increase survival or decrease the development of extrahepatic disease (60% for HAI–systemic therapy vs 62% HAI alone).

A pilot study of HAI FUDR alternating with systemic 5-FU and LV was conducted at MSKCC *(42)*. Eight patients had liver metastases that were resected completely. FUDR was given at a dose of 0.25 mg/kg/d for 14 d. Systemic chemotherapy consisted of 200 mg/m² LV and 280 mg/m² 5-FU, using a bolus dose of 5-FU for 5 d, with escalation of the 5-FU dose in separate patient cohorts. The maximally tolerated 5-FU dose was 325 mg/m². The median survival was 16 mo, with a PR rate of 56%. The level of hepatic toxicity was similar to that in previous studies done at MSKCC. One patient had documented biliary sclerosis. All eight patients treated with adjuvant therapy were alive without disease after a median follow-up of 23 mo.

12. FUTURE DIRECTIONS

During the past 20 yr, there has been no change in the survival for metastatic CRC. More than 2000 patients have been randomized to 5-FU + LV vs 5-FU alone. A meta-analysis of these studies demonstrated a median survival of 11 mo, and a 2-yr survival of less than 20% for both treatment groups *(43)*. Recently, new drugs have been developed for the treatment of CRC: irinotecan *(47)*, a Camptothecian derivative; Tomudex, a new thymidylate synthase inhibitor; and Oxaliplatin *(48)*, a new platinum compound. All of these drugs produced response rates similar to those obtained with 5-FU and LV. In many studies of these new agents, survival is similar, with 20% of patients alive at 2 yr. Whether combinations of these agents will increase survival is yet to be tested.

In three recent studies of HAI using FUDR + LV, FUDR + DEX, and FUDR + LV and DEX, the median survivals were 23, 23, and 27 mo, respectively. The 2-yr survival rates in these studies were 61, 44, and 47%, respectively *(22,23,34)*.

Because of this apparent survival advantage of HAI chemotherapy, compared to systemic chemotherapy, a new randomized study was initiated by the Cancer and Leukemia Group B (CALGB) to ascertain whether these results can be reproduced. In that study, patients are first staged radiographically, to verify the absence of extrahepatic tumor. This staging includes a chest X-ray, CT scan of the abdomen and pelvis, and colonoscopy. Only patients with less than 70% of the liver involved by tumor are eligible. Patients are stratified according to the extent of liver involvement, prior chemotherapy, and presence or absence of synchronous disease. Patients are randomized either to HAI FUDR at a dose of 0.18 mg/kg/d and 10 mg/m^2/d LV for 14 d, with 20 mg DEX and 50,000 U heparin or to systemic chemotherapy consisting of 425 mg/m^2/d 5-FU following 20 mg/m^2/d LV, for five consecutive days. This cycle is repeated every 28 d. Crossover to the alternative treatment at the time of progression is strongly discouraged. The goal is 340 patients.

This CALGB study will address the following questions: Does HAI therapy improve survival in comparison to systemic chemotherapy? Is there a difference in the quality of life between the two treatments? Is there a difference in financial cost over the entire course of therapy? The lack of a crossover may provide a conclusive answer to these questions.

It has been shown that 24-h HAI infusion of 5-FU confers significant pharmacological advantage compared to iv infusions or intra-arterial bolus administration. Further evidence suggests that modulation of regional 5-FU administered with LV confers significant therapeutic advantage. Combining both approaches, a study was undertaken in which a fixed dose of 200 mg/m^2 LV iv over 2 hr was followed by a loading dose of 400 mg/m^2 5-FU over 15 min, followed by a 22-h infusion of 1.6 gm/m^2 5-FU, repeated on d 2 *(44)*. This cycle was repeated every 2 wk. Fifty-nine patients, with histologically proven metastases confined to the liver, received the therapy. The response rate of evaluable patients was 48%, with predicted median survival of 19 mo. The site of first progression was relatively balanced between hepatic and extrahepatic sites (42 vs 58%), respectively. The systemic toxicity was low, and so was the treatment complication rate. The therapeutic potential for this 5-FU-based HAI regimen vs systemic 5-FU–LV is being tested in a United Kingdom Medical Research Council (UK MRC)-sponsored phase III clinical trial in patients with disease confined to the liver. The conclusions from this trial will also help define the role of HAI chemotherapy in the management of unresectable hepatic metastatic disease.

13. CONCLUSION

There are several advantages to HAI. From a pharmacological standpoint, HAI is more effective than systemic therapy, because high drug levels are achieved at the sites of metastatic disease. Utilizing agents with high hepatic extraction results in minimal systemic toxicity. The high response rates obtained in trials of HAI FUDR in the treatment of CRC have not been matched by systemic trials. In eight randomized trials, the response rate was high with HAI, compared to systemic therapy. The time to hepatic progression was significantly longer in the HAI groups vs the systemic groups. None of these studies was adequately designed to evaluate the issue of survival. The results of the randomized, phase III CALGB and UK MRC trials are expected to place the worth of HAI therapy in its proper perspective.

REFERENCES

1. Landis SH, Murray T, Bolden S, and Wingo PA. Cancer Statistics, 1999, *CA Cancer J. Clin.,* **49** 8–31.
2. Kemeny N and Fong Y. Treatment of Liver Metastases, In Holland J, Frei E, Bast R, et al. (eds), *Cancer Medicine.* Williams and Wilkins, Baltimore, MD, 1996, pp. 1–15.
3. Breedis C and Young C. Blood supply of neoplasms in the liver, *Am. J. Pathol.,* **30** (1954) 969.
4. Ensminger WD and Gyves JW. Clinical pharmacology of hepatic arterial chemotherapy, *Semin. Oncol.,* **10** (1983) 176–182.
5. Weiss L. Metastatic inefficiency and regional therapy for liver metastases from colorectal carcinoma, *Reg. Cancer Treat.,* **2** (1989) 77–81.
6. Ensminger WD, Rosowsky A, and Raso V. Clinical pharmacological evaluation of hepatic arterial infusions of 5-fluoro-2-deoxyuridine and 5-fluorouracil, *Cancer Res.,* **38** (1978) 3784–3792.
7. Tandon RN, Bunnell IL, and Copper RG. Treatment of metastatic carcinoma of liver by percutaneous selective hepatic artery infusion of 5-fluorouracil, *Surgery,* **73** (1973) 118.
8. Campbell CA, Burns RC, Stizmann JV, et al. Regional chemotherapy devices: effect of experience and anatomy on complications, *J. Clin. Oncol.,* **11** (1993) 822–826.
9. Ziessman HA, Thrall JH, Yang PJ, et al. Hepatic arterial perfusion scintigraphy with Tc-99m-MAA, *Radiology,* **152** (1984) 167–172.
10. Kemeny NE and Sigurdson ER. Intra-arterial chemotherapy for liver tumors, In Blumgart LH (ed), *Surgery of the Liver and Biliary Tract.* Churchill Livingstone, New York, 1994, pp. 1473–1491.
11. Niederhuber JE, Ensminger W, Gyves J, et al. Regional chemotherapy of colorectal cancer metastatic to the liver, *Cancer,* **53** (1984) 1336.
12. Balch CM and Urist MM. Intra-arterial chemotherapy for colorectal liver metastases and hepatomas using a totally implantable drug infusion pump, *Recent Results Cancer Res.,* **100** (1986) 123–147.
13. Kemeny N, Daly J, Oderman P, et al. Hepatic artery pump infusion toxicity and results in patients with metastatic colorectal carcinoma. *J. Clin. Oncol.,* **2** (1984) 595–600.
14. Shepard KV, Levin B, Karl RC, et al. Therapy for metastatic colorectal cancer with hepatic artery infusion chemotherapy using a subcutaneous implanted pump, *J. Clin. Oncol.,* **3** (1985) 161.
15. Cohen AM, Kaufman SD, Wood WC, et al. Regional hepatic chemotherapy using an implantable drug infusion pump, *Am. J. Surg.,* **145** (1983) 529–533.
16. Weiss GR, Garnick MB, Osteen RT, et al. Long-term arterial infusion pump of 5-fluorodeoxyuridine for liver metastases using an implantable infusion pump, *J. Clin. Oncol.,* **1** (1983) 337–344.
17. Schwartz SI, Jones LS, and McCune CS. Assessment of treatment of intrahepatic malignancies using chemotherapy via an implantable pump. *Ann. Surg.,* **201** (1985) 560–567.
18. Johnson LP, Wasserman PB, and Rivkin SE. FUDR hepatic arterial infusion via an implantable pump for treatment of hepatic tumors, *Proc. Am. Soc. Clin. Oncol.,* **2** (1983) 119.
19. Kemeny MM, Goldberg D, Beatty JD, et al. Results of a prospective randomized trials of continuous regional chemotherapy and hepatic resection as treatment of hepatic metastases from colorectal primaries, *Cancer,* **57** (1986) 492.
20. Lorenz M, Hottenrott C, Maier P, Reimann M, Inglis R, and Encke A. Continuous regional treatment with fluoropyrimidines for metastases from colorectal carcinomas: influence of modulation with leucovorin, *Semin. Oncol.,* **19** (1992) 163–170.
21. Stagg RJ, Venook AP, Chase JL, et al. Alternating hepatic intra-arterial floxuridine and fluorouracil: a less toxic regimen for treatment of liver metastases from colorectal cancer. *J. Natl. Cancer Inst.,* **83** (1991) 423–428.
22. Kemeny N, Seiter K, Conti JA, et al. Hepatic arterial floxuridine and leucovorin for unresectable liver metastases from colorectal carcinoma, *Cancer,* **73** (1994) 1134–1142.
23. Kemeny N, Conti JA, Cohen A, et al. Phase II study of hepatic arterial floxuridine, leucovorin, and dexamethasone for unresectable liver metastases from colorectal carcinoma, *J. Clin. Oncol.,* **12** (1994) 228–229.

24. Kemeny N, Daly J, Reichman B, Geller N, Botet J, and Oderman P. Intrahepatic or systemic infusion of fluorodeoxyuridine in patients with liver metastases from colorectal carcinoma: a randomized trial. *Ann. Intern. Med.,* **107** (1987) 459–465.

25. Hohn D, Stagg R, Friedman M, et al. A randomized trial of continuous intravenous versus hepatic intra-arterial floxuridine in patients with colorectal cancer metastatic to the liver: the Northern California Oncology Group trial, *J. Clin. Oncol.,* **7** (1989) 1646–1654.

26. Chang AE, Schneider PD, Sugarbaker PH, Simpson C, Culnane M, and Steinberg SM. Prospective randomized trial of regional versus systemic continuous 5-fluorodeoxyuridine chemotherapy in the treatment of colorectal liver metastases, *Ann. Surg.,* **206** (1987) 685–693.

27. Martin JK Jr., O'Connell MJ, Wieand HS, et al. Intra-arterial floxuridine versus systemic fluorouracil for hepatic metastases from colorectal cancer. A randomized trial, *Arch. Surg.,* **125** (1990) 1022.

28. Rougier P, Laplanche A, Huguier M, et al. Hepatic arterial infusion of floxuridine in patients with liver metastases from colorectal carcinoma: long-term results of a prospective randomized trial. *J. Clin. Oncol.,* **10** (1992) 1112–1118.

29. Allen-Mersh TG, Earlam S, Fordy C, Abrams K, and Houghton J. Quality of life and survival with continuous hepatic-artery floxuridine infusion for colorectal liver metastases, Lancet, **344** (1994) 1255–1260.

30. Wagman LD, Kemeny MM, Leong L, et al. Prospective randomized evaluation of the treatment of colorectal cancer metastatic to the liver, *J. Clin. Oncol.,* **8** (1990) 1885–1893.

31. Niederhuber JE. Arterial chemotherapy for metastatic colorectal cancer in the liver. Conference Advances in Regional Cancer Therapy. Giessen, West Germany, 1985.

32. Hohn DC, Stagg RJ, Price DC, et al. Avoidance of gastroduodenal toxicity in patients receiving hepatic arterial 5-fluoro-2′deoxyuridine, *J. Clin. Oncol.,* **3** (1985) 1257–1260.

33. Pettavel J, Gardiol D, Bergier N, et al. Necrosis of main bile ducts caused by hepatic artery infusion of 5-fluoro-2-deoxyuridine. *Reg. Cancer Treat.,* **1** (1988) 83–92.

34. Kemeny N, Seiter K, Niedzwiecki D, et al. Randomized trial of intrahepatic infusion of fluorodeoxyuridine with dexamethasone versus fluorodeoxyuridine alone in the treatment of metastatic colorectal cancer, *Cancer,* **69** (1992) 327–334.

35. Hrushesky W, von Roemelling R, Lanning R, and Rabatini J. Circadian-shaped infusions of floxuridine for progressive metastatic renal cell carcinoma, *J. Clin. Oncol.,* **8** (1990) 1504–1513.

36. Metzger U, Weder W, Rothlin M, and Largiader F. Phase II study of intra-arterial fluorouracil and mitomycin-C for liver metastases of colorectal cancer, *Recent Results Cancer Res.,* **121** (1991) 198–204.

37. Cohen A, Kaufman SD, and Wood W. Treatment of colorectal cancer hepatic metastases by hepatic artery chemotherapy. *Dis. Colon Rectum,* **28** (1985) 389–393.

38. Kemeny N, Cohen A, Seiter K, et al. Randomized trial of hepatic arterial FUDR, mitomycin and BCNU versus FUDR alone: effective salvage therapy for liver metastases of colorectal cancer, *J. Clin. Oncol.,* **11** (1993) 330–335.

39. Kemeny N, Cohen A, Bertino JR, Sigurdson ER, Botet J, and Oderman P. Continuous intrahepatic infusion of floxuridine and leucovorin through an implantable pump for the treatment of hepatic metastases from colorectal carcinoma, *Cancer,* **65** (1990) 2446–2450.

40. Safi F, Bittner R, Roscher R, et al. Regional chemotherapy for hepatic metastases of colorectal carcinoma (continuous intraarterial versus continuous intraarterial/intravenous therapy), *Cancer,* **64** (1989) 379–387.

41. Lorenz M, Hottenrott C, Inglis R, and Kirkowa-Reiman M. Prevention of extrahepatic disease during intra-arterial floxuridine of colorectal liver metastases by simultaneous systemic 5-fluorouracil treatment? A prospective multicenter study, *Gam-To-Kaga-ku Ryoho,* **12** (1989) 3662–3671.

42. Kemeny N, Conti JA, Sigurdson E, et al. Pilot study of hepatic artery floxuridine combined with systemic 5-fluorouracil and leucovorin, *Cancer,* **71** (1993) 1964–1971.

43. Advanced Colorectal Cancer Meta-Analysis Project. Modulation of fluorouracil by leucovorin in patients with advanced colorectal cancer: evidence in terms of response rate, *J. Clin. Oncol.,* **10** (1992) 896–903.

44. Warren HW, Anderson JH, O'Gorman PO, et al. Phase II study of regional 5-FU infusion with intravenous infusion of folinic acid, *Br. J. Cancer,* **70** (1994) 677–680.

45. Kemeny M, Sadak A, Lipsitz S, Gray J, MacDonald J, Benson AB. Results of the Intergroup [Eastern Cooperative Oncology Group (ECOG) and Southwest Oncology Group (SWOG)] Prospective Randomized Study of Surgery Alone Versus Continuous Hepatic Artery Infusion of FUDR and Continuous

Systemic Infusion of 5FU After Hepatic Resection for Colorectal Liver Metastases, *ASCO,* **18** (1999) 264a.

46. Kemeny N. Randomized study of hepatic arterial infusion (HAI) and systemic chemotherapy (SYS) versus SYS alone as adjuvant therapy after resection of hepatic metastases from colorectal cancer, *ASCO* **18** (1999) 2.

47. Conti JA, Kemeny N, Saltz L, Huang Y, Tong WP, Chou TC, Pulliam S, Gonzalez C. Irinotecan (CPT11) is an active agent in untreated patients with metastatic colorectal cancer. *J Clin Oncol,* **14**(3) (1996) 709–75.

48. Cvitkovic FB, Jami A, Ithzaki M, Depres Brummer P, Brienza S, Adam R, Kunstlinger F, Bismuth H, Misset JL, Levi F. Biweekly Intensified Ambulatory Chronomodulated Chemotherapy with Oxaliplatin, Fluorouracil, and Leucovorin in Patients with Metastatic Colorectal Cancer, *J Clin Oncol,* **14**(11) (1996) 2950–2958.

3 Regional Hepatic Arterial Infusion Chemotherapy for Hepatic Colorectal Metastases

Robert J. Pelley

CONTENTS

1. INTRODUCTION

Colorectal carcinoma (CRC) is one of the most common cancers in industrialized countries. In 1999, there were over 130,000 new cases of CRC diagnosed in the United States, making it the most prevalent of the gastrointestinal (GI) cancers, and accounting for 15% of cancer deaths in American adults *(1)*. At diagnosis, 20% of patients will already have distant metastases, and another 40% will present with regional spread, which is associated with a significant recurrence rate. The liver is the dominant site for recurrence, with over 60% of relapsing patients eventually having hepatic metastases *(2)*. Nearly 40% of patients will have isolated liver metastases, but few will have disease amenable to resection and potential cure. Although survival varies tremendously for patients with unresectable liver disease, median survival is measured in months rather than years.

A logical approach to treating metastatic CRC localized to the liver has been hepatic arterial infusion (HAI) of chemotherapy. High-dose regional chemotherapy offers the hope of increased drug delivery with decreased systemic toxicity, thereby increasing the chances for tumor response and improved survival. The concept is not new, and was first reported by Bierman et al. in 1951 *(3)*. The technique suffered initially from a multitude of technical complications. However, the advent of totally implanted infusion

From: *Current Clinical Oncology: Regional Chemotherapy: Clinical Research and Practice*
Edited by: M. Markman © Humana Press Inc., Totowa, NJ

Table 1
Need Table Title

Drug	Single-pass extraction	Hepatic systemic ratio	Ref.
Floxuridine	0.7–0.92	100–400	(7)
5-Fluorouracil	0.22–0.45	5–10	(7)
Mitomycin-C	0.23	2.5–3.6	(8)
Cisplatin	–	4–7	(9)
BCNU	–	6–7	(78)

devices led to a large number of studies in the 1970s and 1980s with multiple large randomized trials. This chapter summarizes some of this experience, with emphasis on studies over the past two decades, which have utilized totally implanted ambulatory infusion pumps in the treatment of colorectal metastases.

2. HAI RATIONALE

The attractiveness of any regional therapy is the possibility of achieving higher concentrations of chemotherapy at the tumor site, while minimizing systemic toxicity. The pharmacokinetic advantages of intra-arterial chemotherapy have been extensively studied (4). The advantage for such regional therapy is dependent on the blood flow rate to the target organ, and on the total clearance of drug from the body. Mathematical models for the advantage (R_d) of such therapy have been formulated (5,6), and can be expressed by the equation:

$$R_d = \frac{1 + Cl_{TB}}{Q \, (1 - E)}$$

where Cl_{TB} is the total body clearance of drug, Q is the blood flow to the target organ, and E is the extraction ratio of the drug by the target organ. This equation would predict that drugs with the largest advantage would have high total body clearance and high rates of extraction on first pass through the target organ. A slower blood flow through the target organ will improve the theoretical advantage for regional delivery, by maximizing drug extraction, since high flow rates and high drug delivery might saturate mechanisms of drug removal.

The pharmacokinetics of most chemotherapy agents active in GI cancers have been tested in HAI systems. Table 1 summarizes data for the principal agents utilized for HAI for CRC. The most favorable drug is floxuridine (FUDR), which has both a high first-pass extraction rate and a short systemic half-life. Ensminger et al. (7) have demonstrated high hepatic-to-systemic ratios of 100–400 for FUDR. These ratios allow for high regional doses of FUDR, while maintaining systemic drug concentrations below levels that produce systemic toxicity. Additional drugs that hold theoretical advantages include 5-fluorouracil (5-FU), mitomycin-C (8), and cisplatin (9), all of which have been tested in clinical trials. A final factor, which acts as a practical advantage for HAI, involves the dual blood supply of the liver. Macroscopic hepatic metastases (3 mm and larger) derive more than 75% of their blood flow from the hepatic arteries. In contrast, normal hepatic parenchyma derives 80% of its blood flow from the portal venous system (10). Therefore, arterial infusions in the liver tend to spare normal hepatic tissue, while maximizing delivery of drug to metastases.

3. EARLY STUDIES

Initial efforts at performing HAI in the 1950s and 1960s utilized percutaneously placed hepatic artery catheters that required hospitalization and cumbersome pump devices (for review, *see ref. 11*). Complications from repeated arterial punctures, infections, and misperfusion of organs, secondary to catheter migrations, all resulted in poor patient compliance and results *(12)*. In several series, more than one-third of patients failed to complete sufficient treatment courses for evaluation *(13,14)*. Ultimately, hospitalization and bed confinement make percutaneous catheters cost-ineffective *(15)*.

Arterial ports placed at surgery, with direct arterial cannulation, presented a significant advance in patient convenience and practicality. Linked to a portable infusion pump, they could deliver chemotherapy for 4–14 d *(16)*. However, catheter and hepatic artery thrombosis occurred in up to 40% of patients, limiting the duration of infusion and use.

HAI did not become practical until the development of totally implanted infusion pumps in the 1970s. Two pump models were extensively tested: a programmable model (Syncromed, Medtronic, Minneapolis, MN) and a nonprogrammable pump (Infusaid 400, Strato/Infusaid, Norwood, MA *[17,18]*). Because of reliability and simplicity, the nonprogrammable pumps have been used more frequently. A side port injection site allows for bolus infections of both chemotherapy and imaging agents, making for easy assessment of catheter placement and hepatic perfusion.

The earliest efforts at performing HAI in the ambulatory setting utilized a mixture of devices and techniques that evolved over a 10-yr period *(19–23)*. Brachial artery approaches were frequently used with angiography catheters, which frequently cracked (up to 25%) or led to hepatic artery thrombosis (30%) *(19,20)*. One large series had a 4% mortality from complications alone *(19)*. The technical results of these efforts led to the near-universal acceptance of laparotomy for catheter placement, with careful preoperative angiographic assessment of the hepatic vasculature. Also, most investigators adopted the use of Silastic and Teflon catheters, as well as the silent implantable Infusaid pump.

4. EFFICACY OF HAI WITH FUDR

Refinements in HAI led to a series of phase II trials, which evaluated the effectiveness and toxicity of FUDR in patients with metastatic CRC. Table 2 summarizes results from these studies *(24–29)*. All series used the Infusaid 400 pump model with FUDR infusions. Almost all studies used a starting dose of FUDR at 0.3 mg/kg/d for 14 d, alternated with saline for 14 d. All series had greater than 40 patients, but each used varying methods for evaluating tumor response, including physical exam and serum carcinoembryonic antigens.

Because these trials accrued patients who were highly selected, response and survival data varied tremendously. Response rates ranged from 15 to 88%, with higher rates reported in series using less-stringent response criteria. The majority of series recorded response rates of greater than 50% in previously untreated patients. There were also responses in patients who had filed systemic 5-FU therapy. Likewise, median survival varied significantly, and ranged from 15 to 26 mo. This was substantially greater than median survivals of unselected, untreated patients with metastatic disease.

The improved morbidity and limited mortality from HAI chemotherapy in these series reflected a learning curve. In large series, mortality was minimal, with no deaths in 180 pump or port placements *(30)*, and only two deaths in 303 pump placements

Table 2
Effectiveness of Hepatic Arterial Chemotherapy with Implantable Pump

Ref.	Year	No. patients evaluable	Response Rate (%)	Median survivor (mo)
Balch et al. *(24)*	1983	81	88 (CEA)	26
Cohen et al. *(27)*	1983	41	51	–
Kemeny et al. *(25)*	1984	41	35	–
Neiderhuber et al. *(26)*	1984	93	78	18
Schwartz et al. *(28)*	1985	25	75 (CEA)	n = 50
		20	15 (CT)	15
Shepard et al. *(29)*	1985	53	32	17

CEA = carcinoembryonic antigen; CT = computed tomography.

Table 3
Severe Toxicity of Hepatic Arterial Chemotherapy with Implantable Pump

Ref.	No. Patients	Gastric Ulcers (%)	Schlerosing Cholangitis (%)	Pump failure Catheter Breast Thrombosis Infection (%)
Balch et al. *(79)*	50	6	0	0
Cohen et al. *(27)*	50	16	–	4
Kemeny et al. *(25)*	41	29	5	–
Neiderhuber et al. *(26)*	93	3	–	6
Schwartz et al. *(28)*	30	–	–	10
Shepard et al. *(29)*	62	18	0	0

(31). Table 3 summarizes severe toxicity and morbidity from these phase II trials. Pump failure, catheter breakage, thrombosis, and serious infections occurred in less than 10% of patients, reflecting refinements in the hardware technology. Generally, routine systemic side effects of chemotherapy, such as myelosuppression, mucositis, and diarrhea, did not occur unless hepatic shunting was present. On the other hand, duodenal and gastric ulcers occurred frequently, despite increasing awareness of the need to ligate gastroduodenal arterial branches, in order to prevent back perfusion of chemotherapy. Careful hepatic artery dissection, with ligation of the right gastric artery and the small branches in the hepatoduodenal and hepatogastric ligaments, can prevent back perfusion of the bowel *(32)*. Nevertheless, nearly 30% of patients still suffered GI complaints, including nausea, vomiting, and gastritis.

Hepatobiliary toxicity is the most common and serious side effect of HAI. Most of the studies above reported reversible jaundice in 20–25% of patients, with chemical hepatitis in up to 50% of patients. It was rapidly recognized that frequent treatment interruptions and dose adjustments were needed to prevent hepatic toxicity. Although not reported in these initial series, sclerosing cholangitis, fibrosis, and necrosis of the biliary tree were found in subsequent follow-up studies, and proved to be the dose-limiting toxicity for HAI with FUDR *(33,34)*.

Despite these toxicities, the results of these early studies demonstrated that HAI with implantable pumps could be performed in a majority of selected patients, with minimal mortality or severe toxicity. The average response rates of 50% were at least

Table 4
Randomized Studies of Hepatic Arterial Chemotherapy for Colorectal Liver Metastases

Ref.	Trial	Year	No. patients	Response rate		Median survival (mo)	
				Sys (%)	HAI (%)	Sys	HAI
Chang et al. (36)	NCI	1987	64	17	62	15	22
Kemeny et al. (37)	MSKCC	1987	93	20	50	12	17
Hohn et al. (38)	NCOG	1989	143	10	42	16	17
Martin et al. (39)	NCCTG	1990	69	21	48	11	13
Rongier et al. (40)	France	1992	163	9[a]	43	11[a]	15
Allen-Marsh et al. (41)	UK	1994	100	–	–	8[a]	15

[a]Systemic chemotherapy given ad lib to 50% of control patients.

3× the response rates achievable with the best available systemic therapy at the time, namely, iv 5-FU. These studies led directly to the design of multiple randomized trials in both Europe and North America.

5. RANDOMIZED TRIALS OF HIA

A number of randomized trials have studied HAI treatment in patients with metastatic CRC. One early study is worthy of mention: In the 1970s, the Central Oncology Group conducted a prospective randomized trial comparing systemic 5-FU to HAI of 5-FU, using arterial ports and external pumps (35). Although HAI generated a better response rate (34 vs 23%), the difference was not statistically significant, and there was no survival difference. Toxicity and complications were substantially greater in the HAI arm, and underscored the difficulty of giving HAI with nonimplantable pumps.

Six major trials have compared HAI using FUDR and Infusaid pumps to systemic FUDR or 5-FU (36–41). Patients were highly selected for these trials, having liver-only disease, good performance status, and no previous treatment. Again, all HAI patients were treated with FUDR and implantable pumps. Table 4 summarizes response rates and survival from these trials. All trials demonstrated superior response rates for HAI therapy, with at least a doubling in tumor response rates. All trials also showed longer median survivals for patients receiving HAI. However, survival in the American trials was, statistically, not significantly different for HAI treatment vs systemic fluoro-pyrimidines. Two trials did allow crossover of systemically treated patients to HAI treatment, which confounded survival analysis. Theoretically, this crossover may have favored systemically treated patients who benefited from both treatment modalities. However, not every trial analyzed survival on the basis of intention to treat, and thus some poor-prognosis patients with extrahepatic disease were censored from the HAI arms. Both European trials showed survival advantages for patients treated with HAI. Both trials were unique, in that the patients in the control groups received systemic chemotherapy in an ad libitum manner at the discretion of their physicians. Fewer than 50% of patients in the control groups received any chemotherapy, and those who did, frequently received it as terminal palliative care. The English study (41) contained a quality-of-life analysis, and demonstrated a dramatic improvement for patients receiving HAI therapy vs palliative controls (42).

The data from these randomized trials have been analyzed in aggregate as part of two meta-analyses (43,44). The first analysis, by the Met-Analysis Group in Cancer, confirmed a statistically significant increase in response rate for HAI compared to systemic therapy (41 vs 14%). Overall, there was a 3-mo survival advantage for patients receiving HAI. However, this result did not persist when the European studies, which inconstantly used chemotherapy in the control arms, were excluded from analysis. A second analysis, by Harmantas et al. (44), found similar results, with a 6% survival advantage at 2 yr for patients treated with HAI. Again, when the European studies were excluded, the results were not statistically significant for survival. The Meta-Analysis Group in Cancer also performed an economic analysis (45). This study calculated that HAI prolonged survival at a cost of approx $70,000/life yr, compared to the cost of systemic chemotherapy (in 1995 dollars). This ranks HAI in the range of such technical treatments as renal dialysis in terms of cost.

An analysis of these randomized phase III studies confirms a number of specific points about regional therapy and general points about solid tumors. The major advantages of regional chemotherapy were realized, in that chemotherapy could be dose-intensified without systemic toxicity. FUDR proved to be a superior drug, and performed as its pharmacologic profile would predict. Unfortunately, despite a marked improvement in tumor response rate, survival was only minimally prolonged. This too might be predictable, because patient survival prolongation with many tumor types is associated with complete responses and durable remissions, and not necessarily with partial responses or stable disease. In these studies, although partial response rates were increased, they served as better surrogates of palliation, rather than survival. Nevertheless, a number of lessons were learned from these randomized trials:

1. Surgical expertise is essential in placing pumps, and directly impacts on morbidity. This has been emphasized by a number of investigators (46).
2. Extrahepatic disease is not controlled by regional therapy, and accounted for 55% of initial sites of progressive disease. Although most patients eventually succumbed to hepatic failure, new strategies, designed to control extrahepatic disease, were needed.
3. Hepatobiliary toxicity remains the dose-limiting toxicity for HAI of FUDR. When doses are attenuated, response rates decrease (41). Obviously less toxic schedules for FUDR administration were needed.

Regional toxicity from HAI still remains one of the most difficult problems to address. Long-term follow-up of patients receiving HAI during the 1980s made it apparent that FUDR frequently resulted in irreversible biliary toxicity. Elevations in alkaline phosphatase and transaminases, first thought to be secondary to chemical hepatitis, proved to be early signs of sclerosing cholangitis, which could be detected in up to 50% of patients treated with four cycles of FUDR at 0.3 mg/kg/d (46,47). The etiology of this process is probably a combination of direct perfusion of biliary ducts, which derive their blood supply from the hepatic arteries, and concentration of metabolized chemotherapy removed during first-pass extraction (46,48).

Toxicity could be avoided by early interruption and dose reduction in FUDR. However, biliary toxicity occurred on the steep portion of the dose–response curve, as evidenced by lower tumor response rates when 0.2 mg/kg/d of FUDR was utilized (41). Thus, the same pharmacodynamics that produced regional advantage and tumor response were also responsible for a dose-limiting toxicity. Therefore, a series of phase II studies was initiated to find less-toxic alternative schedules of HAI chemotherapy. Many of these issues have been addressed in clinical trials over the past 5 yr.

6. SECOND-GENERATION TRIALS TO DECREASE TOXICITY

Kemeny et al., at Memorial Sloan-Kettering Cancer Center, initiated a series of trials to find less-toxic HAI chemotherapy. The mechanism of biomodulation of 5-FU by reduced folates, such as leucovorin (LV) was well understood in the 1980s (49,50). An initial trial using LV as a biomodulator of FUDR was initiated, but met with substantial toxicity and early closure (51). In an effort to decrease hepatobiliary toxicity by decreasing the inflammatory response, which accompanies sclerosing cholangitis, dexamethasone (DEX) was added to FUDR infusions. This second trial randomized 50 patients to either FUDR alone or FUDR with 20 mg DEX (52). Although there was a threefold decrease in elevated bilirubin levels, there was no effect on transaminases or alkaline phosphatase levels. Despite comparable amounts of FUDR being delivered in both groups (61 FUDR + DEX vs 52% FUDR alone planned dose), tumor response rates for the combination treatment were almost doubled that of the control group (71 vs 40%).

These results remained unexplained, but led to a reopening and completion of the FUDR and LV trial, with more tolerable dosing schedules (53). The best schedule (0.3 mg/kg/d FUDR and 30 mg/m^2/d LV for 14 d every 28 d) resulted in a 75% tumor response rate, and acceptable hepatobiliary toxicity. There was a significant survival of patients at 3 and 5 yr. As a result, both treatments were combined, and a third trial was undertaken, in which patients were treated with all three agents (54). Tumor response rate was 78%, with a median survival of 25 mo. Careful monitoring of hepatic toxicity, with treatment interruptions and adjustments, resulted in only 2 of 62 treated patients developing biliary sclerosis. Because DEX has no intrinsic cytotoxic activity against CRC cells in vitro (55), it has been postulated that its angiostatic properties may have played an important role in generating increased response rates.

7. TRIALS TO CONTROL SYSTEMIC DISEASE

The second major limitation of HAI is its failure to control extrahepatic disease progression. Because this is an intuitive limitation of any regional therapy, concern over systemic disease progression does emphasize the success of HAI in achieving regional control. A number of clinical trials addressed this issue by combining HAI of FUDR with systemic chemotherapy. Evidence that systemic administration of chemotherapy can contribute to systemic control of disease was supplied by Safi et al. (56). In a randomized study of 44 patients, pumps with dual arterial and venous catheters administered HAI of FUDR, with or without intravenous (iv) FUDR. The addition of iv FUDR lowered the occurrence of extrahepatic first relapse from 61 to 33%. However, overall survival was not improved, perhaps because FUDR was a less effective systemic chemotherapy regimen. In a study by Stagg et al. (57), low-dose FUDR (0.1 mg/kg/d for 7 d) was alternated with weekly hepatic arterial 5-FU administered as a bolus via the catheter side port. Results were promising, with a 50% response rate and more than 24-mo median survival. Hepatobiliary toxicity was low, but disease progression within the liver occurred in the majority of patients, and was the cause of death in most. The same treatment regimen was used in 57 additional patients at M.D. Anderson Cancer Center (58). Results were nearly identical, with 54% tumor response rate, and 30% extrahepatic disease as site of first progression.

A pilot phase I trial from MSKCC combined HAI with iv 5-FU/LV (59). A 5-d iv bolus schedule of 5-FU/LV was used. The maximum tolerated dose (MTD) of 5-FU defined (280 mg/m²) was significantly lower than other regimens using 5-FU/LV without HAI (425–450 mg/m² *[60]*). Again, tumor responses were average (56%), but the rate of extrahepatic disease as the site of first recurrence was no different than other MSKCC trials (40%). Although systemic 5-FU/FA added to systemic toxicity, it was unclear from this trial that systemic chemotherapy added any benefit.

An alternative strategy to the use of iv systemic chemotherapy is to exploit pharmacokinetic properties of hepatic metabolism. The hepatic elimination of 5-FU is nonlinear because higher doses of drug can saturate the liver's ability to metabolize drug. Systemic spillover of 5-FU can be induced by administering doses near the MTD. This strategy is feasible only because regional administration of high-dose 5-FU has far less hepatic toxicity than FUDR *(61)*.

A number of studies have used HAI of 5-FU in this way. Warren et al. *(62)* reported on the treatment of 31 patients with a 24-h infusion of 5-FU (HAI 1.5 gms/m²/wk) with LV (iv 400 mg/m²/wk) *(62)*. Response rates were typical (48%), but extrahepatic sites accounted for first site of recurrence in 58% of patients. Dose escalation of 5-FU to 2.0 gm/m² was met with dose-limiting diarrhea and vomiting *(63)*. A second study by Derr et al. *(64)* established a similar MTD for 5-FU (1.6 gm/m²). Again, the response rate was almost identical. Alternative schedules of infused 5-FU, with or without LV, met with a similar or lower response rate and systemic toxicity limitations *(65–67)*. The addition of either cisplatin or carboplatin to fluoropyrimidines also failed to either increase tumor responses or improve systemic control *(68,69)*.

The results of these and other trials have advanced understanding of regional therapy of colorectal liver metastases, since the completion of the HAI randomized trials. By incorporating steroids, HAI regimens can utilize near-maximal doses of FUDR, while avoiding the devastating complication of sclerosing cholangitis. DEX has been used in a number of reported trials, and is currently being tested in a new randomized trial sponsored by the Cancer and Leukemia Group B. This trial compares HAI to systemic 5-FU/LV, and discourages any crossover treatment of patients. Although accrual of patients has been slow, it is ongoing. In contrast, control of systemic disease has been disappointing. Combinations of HAI and systemic chemotherapy strategies have not resulted in improvements in patient survival. This fact has led to a continuation of investigations searching for more effective agents that might be used for HAI, or in conjunction with it.

8. NOVEL AGENTS USED IN HAI

Although fluoropyrimidines have the best extraction ratio for chemotherapy used regionally in the liver, a number of other agents hold theoretical potential, and have thus been tested. Cosimelli et al. *(69,70)* have extensively studied the use of cisplatin administered by HAI in conjunction with iv 5-FU. Significant neurotoxicity was encountered with this treatment regimen, and because the tumor response rate was only 50%, it is unlikely that cisplatin will be a useful agent for HAI. Other agents, traditionally considered to be ineffective against CRC, have also been tested, with the hope that increased drug concentration would increase response rates. Mitomycin C, which has less than a 10% response rate as a single agent, was utilized in a 6-wk schedule using HAI *(71,72)*. Despite a reasonable toxicity profile, the overall response rate of 20%, with an average median survival of 16 mo, is probably inferior to systemic 5-FU/LV and merits no further study. Mitoxantrone, an anthracycline with no activity in CRC when administered iv, had no activity when administered by a HAI route *(73)*. These studies underscore the need for a sound pharmacokinetic basis when choosing agents for regional therapy.

The use of biologic agents in HAI is very limited. Both Interleukin-2 and interferon-α have been used in HAI as biomodulators of 5-FU in small clinical trials *(74,75)*. Although response rates were average for HAI trials, they did not appear to add to hepatobiliary toxicity in these phase II trials. At present, their roles remain undefined.

Another novel combination of treatment modalities is the use of radiation therapy and HAI. Most fluoropyrimidines act as radiation sensitizers, making their use with radiation logical. One early trial treated 27 patients sequentially with HAI of 5-FU, followed by 20 Gy of external beam radiation to the dominant liver metastases. The overall response rate was less than 25%, but toxicity was limited, and the treatment was tolerable *(76)*. A more aggressive approach utilized FUDR (0.2 mg/kg/d) with nonconformal, noncoplanar radiation therapy at maximum doses (48–72 Gy). Again, toxicity was tolerable if sufficient liver was spared from radiation, but the response rate was a disappointing 50%, which is similar to the expected response rate from HAI of FUDR alone *(77)*.

9. CONCLUSION

HAI is a successful example of regional delivery of chemotherapy. HAI of FUDR generates the highest tumor response rates for patients with metastatic colon cancer, while limiting systemic toxicity. The totally implanted pump devices are the most convenient means for HAI, and are safe when installed and managed by experienced teams with expertise.

Unfortunately, HAI therapy has not realized the promise of an effective therapy, which achieves significant prolongation of survival or even cure. The personal and financial cost of the procedure may not be justified for palliation alone, and at present this technique should remain within the confines of well-designed clinical trials. Recent results and success need to be followed up with randomized trials addressing the issues of hepatotoxicity and systemic control. This is especially justified because of the continued lack of effective systemic agents to combat CRC.

REFERENCES

1. Landis SH, Murray T, Bolden S, and Wingo PA. Cancer Statistics, 1998, *CA Cancer J. Clin.,* **48** (1998) 6–30.
2. Welch JP and Donaldson GA. Clinical correlation of an autopsy study of recurrent colorectal cancer, *Ann. Surg.,* **189** (1979) 496–502.
3. Bierman HR, Byron RL, and Kelly KH. Treatment of inoperable visceral and regional metastases by intra-arterial catheterization, *Cancer Res.,* **11** (1951) 236.
4. Eckman WW, Patlak CS, and Fenstermacher JD. Critical evaluation of the principles governing the advantages of intra-arterial infusions, *J. Pharmacokinet. Biopharmacol.,* **2** (1974) 257.
5. Chen H-SG and Gross JF. Intra-arterial infusion of anticancer drugs: theoretic aspects of drug delivery and review of responses, *Cancer Treat. Rep.,* **64** (1980) 31–40.
6. Collins JM. Pharmacologic rationale for regional drug delivery, *J. Clin. Oncol.,* **2** (1984) 498–504.
7. Ensminger WD, Rosowsky A, Raso V, et al. Clinical-pharmacological evaluation of hepatic arterial infusions of 5-fluoro-2' deoxyuridine and 5-fluorouracil, *Cancer Res.,* **38** (1978) 3784–3792.
8. Hu E and Howell SB. Pharmacokinetics of intra-arterial mitomycin C in man. *Cancer Res.,* **43** (1983) 4474.
9. Kelsen DP, Hoffman J, Alcock N, et al. Pharmacokinetics of regional infusion of cisplatin, *Proc. Am. Assoc. Cancer Res.,* **21** (1980) 186.
10. Breedis C and Young G. Blood supply of neoplasms of the liver, *Am. J. Pathol.,* **30** (1954) 969–985.

11. Huberman MS. Comparison of systemic chemotherapy with hepatic arterial infusion in metastatic colorectal carcinoma, *Semin. Oncol.,* **10** (1983) 238–248.

12. Lee YT. Regional management of liver metastases, I. *Cancer Invest.,* **1** (1983) 237–257.

13. Clouse ME, Ahmed R, Ryhan RB, Oberfield RA, and McCaffrey JA. Complications of long-term transbrachial hepatic arterial infusion chemotherapy, *A.J.R.,* **129** (1977) 799–803.

14. Cady B. Hepatic arterial patency and complications after catheterization for infusion chemotherapy, *Ann. Surg.,* **178** (1973) 156–161.

15. Patt YZ and Mavligit GM. Arterial chemotherapy in the management of colorectal cancer: an overview, *Semin. Oncol.,* **18** (1991) 478–490.

16. Curley SA, Roh MS, Chase JL, and Hohn DC. Adjuvant hepatic arterial infusion chemotherapy after curative resection of colorectal liver metastases, *Am. J. Surg.,* **166** (1993) 743–748.

17. Blackshear PJ, Dorman FD, Blackshear PL Jr, et al. Permanently implantable self-recycling low flow constant rate multipurpose infusion pump of simple design, *Surg. Forum,* **21** (1970) 136–137.

18. Blackshear PJ, Dorman FD, Blackshear PL Jr, et al. Design and initial testing of an implantable infusion pump, *Surg. Gynecol Obstet.,* **134** (1972) 51–56.

19. Reed ML, Vaitkevicius VK, Al-Sarraf M, et al. Practicality of chronic hepatic artery infusion therapy of primary and metastatic hepatic malignancies: ten-year results of 124 patients in a prospective protocol, *Cancer,* **47** (1981) 402–409.

20. Oberfield RA, McCaffrey JA, Polio J, et al. Prolonged and continuous percutaneous intra-arterial hepatic infusion chemotherapy in advanced metastatic liver adenocarcinoma from colorectal primary, *Cancer,* **44** (1979) 414–423.

21. Barone RM, Byfield JE, Goldfarb PB, et al. Intra-arterial chemotherapy using an implantable infusion pump and liver irradiation for the treatment of hepatic metastases, *Cancer,* **50** (1982) 850–862.

22. Cohen AM, Greenfield A, Wood WC, et al. Treatment of hepatic metastases by transaxillary hepatic artery chemotherapy using an implanted drug pump, *Cancer,* **51** (1983) 2013–2019.

23. Patt YZ, Mavligit GM, Chuang VP, et al. Percutaneous hepatic arterial infusion (HAI) of mitomycin C and floxuridine (FUDR): an effective treatment for metastatic colorectal carcinoma in the liver, *Cancer,* **46** (1980) 261–265.

24. Balch CM, Urist M, Soong SJ, and McGregor M. Prospective phase II clinical trial of continuous FUDR regional chemotherapy for colorectal metastases to the liver using a totally implantable drug infusion pump, *Ann. Surg.,* **198** (1983) 567–573.

25. Kemeny N, Daly J, Oderman P, et al. Hepatitic artery pump infusion: toxicity and results in patients with metastatic colorectal carcinoma, *J. Clin. Oncol.,* **2** (1984) 595–600.

26. Niederhuber JE, Ensminger W, Gyves J, et al. Regional chemotherapy of colorectal cancer metastatic to the liver, *Cancer,* **53** (1984) 1336–1343.

27. Cohen AM, Kaufman SD, Wood WC, and Greenfield AJ. Regional hepatic chemotherapy using an implantable infusion pump, *Am. J. Surg.,* **145** (1983) 529–533.

28. Schwartz SI, Jones LS, and McCune CS. Assessment of treatment of intrahepatic malignancies using chemotherapy via an implantable pump, *Ann. Surg.,* **201** (1985) 560–567.

29. Shepard KV, Levin B, Karl RC, et al. Therapy for metastatic colorectal cancer with hepatic artery infusion chemotherapy using a subcutaneous implanted pump, *J. Clin. Oncol.,* **3** (1985) 161–169.

30. Curley SA, Chase JL, Roh MS, and Hohn DC. Technical considerations land complications associated with the placement of 180 implantable hepatic arterial infusion devices, *Surgery,* **114** (1993) 928–935.

31. Kemeny N and Sigurdson ER. Intra-arterial chemotherapy for liver tumours, In Blumgart LH (ed), Surgery of the Liver and Biliary Tract, 2nd ed., vol. 2. Churchill Livingstone, Edinburgh, 1994, 1473–1491.

32. Hohn DC, Stagg RJ, Price DC, and Lewis BJ. Avoidance of gastroduodenal toxicity in patients receiving hepatic arterial 5-Fluoro-2′-deoxyuridine, *J. Clin. Oncol.,* **3** (1985) 1257–1260.

33. Hohn D, Melnick J, Stagg R, et al. Biliary sclerosis in patients receiving hepatic arterial infusions of floxuridine, *J. Clin. Oncol.,* **3** (1985) 98–102.

34. Doria MI Jr, Shepard KV, Levin B, and Riddell RH. Liver pathology following hepatic arterial infusion chemotherapy. Hepatic toxicity with FUDR, *Cancer,* **58** (1986) 855–861.

35. Grage TB, Vassilopoulos PP, Shingleton WW, et al. Results of a prospective randomized study of hepatic artery infusion with 5-fluorouracil versus intravenous 5-fluorouracil in patients with hepatic metastases from colorectal cancer: a central oncology group study, *Surgery,* **86** (1979) 550–555.

36. Chang AE, Schneider PD, Sugarbaker PH, et al. Prospective randomized trial of regional versus systemic continuous 5-fluorodeoxyuridine chemotherapy in treatment of colorectal liver metastases, *Ann. Surg.,* **206** (1987) 685–693.

37. Kemeny N, Daly J, Reichman B, et al. Intrahepatic or systemic infusion of fluorodeoxyuridine in patients with liver metastases from colorectal carcinoma. A randomized trial, *Ann. Intern. Med.,* **107** (1987) 459–465.

38. Hahn DC, Stagg JR, Friedman MA, et al. Randomized trial of continuous intravenous versus hepatic intraarterial floxuridine in patients with colorectal cancer metastatic to the liver: the Northern California Oncology Group Trial, *J. Clin. Oncol.,* **7** (1989) 1646–1654.

39. Martin JK Jr, O'Connell MJ, Wieand HS, et al. Intra-arterial floxuridine vs systemic fluorouracil for hepatic metastases from colorectal cancer. A randomized trial, *Arch. Surg.,* **125** (1990) 1022–1027.

40. Rougier P, Laplanche A, Huguier M, et al. Hepatic arterial infusion of floxuridine in patients with liver metastases from colorectal carcinoma: long-term results of a prospective randomized trial, *J. Clin. Oncol.,* **10** (1992) 1112–1118.

41. Allen-Mersh TG, Earlam S, Fordy C, et al. Quality of life and survival with continuous hepatic-artery floxuridine infusion for colorectal liver metastases, *Lancet,* **344** (1994) 1255–1260.

42. Earlam S, Glover C, Davies M, et al. Effect of regional and systemic fluorinated pyrimidine chemotherapy on quality of life in colorectal liver metastasis patients, *J. Clin. Oncol.,* **15** (1997) 2022–2029.

43. Meta-Analysis Group in Cancer. Reappraisal of hepatic arterial infusion in the treatment of nonresectable liver metastases from colorectal cancer, *J. Natl. Cancer Inst.,* **88** (1996) 252–258.

44. Harmantas A, Rotstein LE, and Langer B. Regional versus systemic chemotherapy in the treatment of colorectal carcinoma metastatic to the liver. Is there a survival difference? Meta-analysis of the published literature, *Cancer,* **78** (1996) 1639–1645.

45. Durand-Zaleski I, Roche B, Buyse M, et al. Economic implications of hepatic arterial infusion chemotherapy in treatment of nonresectable colorectal liver metastases, *J. Natl. Cancer Inst.,* **89** (1997) 790–795.

46. Hohn DC, Rayner AA, and Economou JS. Toxicities and complications of implanted pump hepatic arterial and intravenous floxuridine infusion, *Cancer,* **57** (1986) 465–470.

47. Shea Jr WJ, Demas BE, Goldberg HI, et al. Sclerosing cholangitis associated with hepatic arterial FUDR chemotherapy: radiographic-histologic correlation, *A.J.R.,* **146** (1986) 717–721.

48. Brown KT, Kemeny N, and Berger MF. Obstructive jaundice in patients receiving hepatic artery infusional chemotherapy: etiology, treatment implications, and complications after transhepatic biliary drainage, *J.V.I.R.,* **8** (1997) 229–234.

49. Grem JL, Hoth D, Hamilton MJ, et al. Overview of the current status and future directions of clinical trials of 5-fluorouracil and folinic acid, *Cancer Treat. Rep.,* **71** (1987) 1249.

50. Arbuck SG. Overview of clinical trials using 5-FU and leucovorin for the treatment of colorectal cancer, *Cancer,* **63(Suppl 6)** (1989) 1036–1044.

51. Kemeny N, Cohen A, Bertino JR, et al. Continuous intrahepatic infusion of floxuridine and leucovorin through an implantable pump for the treatment of hepatic metastases from colorectal carcinoma, *Cancer,* **65** (1989) 2446–2450.

52. Kemeny N, Seiter K, Niedzwiecki D, et al. Randomized trial of intrahepatic infusion of fluorodeoxyuridine with dexamethasone versus fluorodeoxyuridine alone in the treatment of metastatic colorectal cancer, *Cancer,* **69** (1992) 327–334.

53. Kemeny N, Seiter K, Conti JA, et al. Hepatic arterial floxuridine and leucovorin for unresectable liver metastases from colorectal carcinoma, *Cancer,* **73** (1994) 1134–1142.

54. Kemeny N, Conti JA, Cohen A, et al. Phase II study of hepatic arterial floxuridine, leucovorin, and dexamethasone for unresectable liver metastases from colorectal cancer, *J. Clin. Oncol.,* **12** (1994) 2299–2295.

55. Arisawa Y, Sutanto-Ward E, Fortunato L, and Sigurdson ER. Hepatic artery dexamethasone infusion inhibits colorectal hepatic metastases: a regional antiangiogenic therapy, *Ann. Surg. Oncol.,* **2** (1995) 114–120.

56. Safi F, Bittner R, Roscher R, et al. Regional chemotherapy for hepatic metastases of colorectal carcinoma (continuous intraarterial versus continuous intraarterial/intravenous therapy): results of a controlled clinical trial, *Cancer,* **64** (1993) 379–387.

57. Stagg RJ, Venook AP, Chase JL, et al. Alternating hepatic intra-arterial floxuridine and fluorouracil: a less toxic regimen for treatment of liver metastases from colorectal cancer, *J. Natl. Cancer Inst.,* **83** (1991) 423–428.

58. Davidson BS, Izzo F, Chase JL, et al. Alternating floxuridine and 5-fluorouracil hepatic arterial chemotherapy for colorectal liver metastases minimizes biliary toxicity, *Am. J. Surg.,* **172** (1996) 244–247.

59. Kemeny N, Conti JA, Sigurdson E, et al. Pilot study of hepatic artery floxuridine combined with

systemic 5-fluorouracil and leucovorin. A potential adjuvant program after resection of colorectal hepatic metastases, *Cancer,* **71** (1993) 1964–1971.

60. Poon MA, O'Connell MJ, Wieand HS, et al. Biochemical modulation of fluorouracil with leucovorin: confirmatory evidence of improved therapeutic efficacy in advanced colorectal cancer, *J. Clin. Oncol.,* **9** (1991) 1967–1972.

61. Wagner JG, Gyves JW, Stetson PI, et al. Steady state nonlinear pharmacokinetics of 5-fluorouracil during hepatic arterial and intravenous infusions in cancer patients, *Cancer Res.,* **46** (1986) 1499–2506.

62. Warren HW, Anderson JH, O'Gorman P, et al. Phase II study of regional 5-fluorouracil infusion with intravenous folinic acid for colorectal liver metastases, *Br. J. Cancer,* **70** (1994) 677–680.

63. Anderson JH, Kerr DJ, Cooke TG, and McCarelle CS. Phase I study of regional 5-fluorouracil and systemic folinic acid for patients with colorectal liver metastases, *Br. J. Cancer,* **65** (1992) 913–915.

64. Kerr DJ, Ledermann JA, McArdle CS, et al. Phase I clinical and pharmacokinetic study of leucovorin and infusional hepatic arterial fluorouracil, *J. Clin. Oncol.,* **13** (1995) 2968–2972.

65. Sugihara K. Continuous hepatic arterial infusion of 5-fluorouracil for unresectable colorectal liver metastases: phase II study, *Surgery,* **117** (1995) 624–628.

66. Valeril A, Mini E, Tonelli P, et al. Intra-arterial hepatic chemotherapy with 5-fluorouracil and 5-methyltetrahydrofolate in the treatment of unresectable liver metastases from colorectal cancer, *Anticancer Res.,* **14** (1994) 2215–2220.

67. Boyle FM, Smith RC, and Levi JA. Continuous hepatic artery infusion of 5-fluorouracil for metastatic colorectal cancer localized to the liver, *Aust. NZ J., Med.,* **23** (1993) 32–34.

68. Patt YZ, Boddie AW Jr, Charnsangavej C, et al. Hepatic arterial infusion with floxuridine and cisplatin: overriding importance of antitumor effect versus degree of tumor burden as determinants of survival among patients with colorectal cancer, *J. Clin. Oncol.,* **4** (1986) 1356–1364.

69. Cosimelli M, Mannella E, Anza M, et al. Two consecutive clinical trials on cisplatin (CDDP), hepatic arterial infusion (HAI), and I.V. 5-fluorouracil (5-FU) chemotherapy for unresectable colorectal liver metastases: an alternative to FUDR-based regimens, *J. Surg. Oncol.,* **2(Suppl)** (1991) 63–68.

70. Cortesi E, Capussotti L, Di Tora P, et al. Bolus vs. continuous hepatic arterial infusion of cisplatin plus intravenous 5-fluorouracil chemotherapy for unresectable colorectal metastases, *Dis. Colon Rectum,* **37(Suppl)** (1994) S138–S143.

71. Preketes AP, Caplehorn JRM, King J, et al. Effect of hepatic artery chemotherapy on survival of patients with hepatic metastases from colorectal carcinoma treated with cryotherapy, *World J. Surg.,* **19** (1995) 768–771.

72. Makela J, Kantola R, Tikkakoski T, et al. Superselective intra-arterial chemotherapy with mitomycin C in hepatic metastases from colorectal cancer, *J. Surg. Oncol.,* **65** (1997) 127–131.

73. Jones DV Jr, Patt YZ, Ajani JA, et al. Phase I–II trial of mitoxantrone by hepatic arterial infusion in patients with hepatocellular carcinoma or colorectal carcinoma metastatic to the liver, *Cancer,* **72** (1993) 2560–2563.

74. Okuno K, Hirohata T, Kanamura K, et al. Hepatic arterial infusions of interleukin-2-based immuno-chemotherapy in the treatment of unresectable liver metastases from colorectal cancer, *Clin. Ther.,* **15** (1993) 672–683.

75. Patt YZ, Hoque A, Lozano R, et al. Phase II trial of hepatic arterial infusion of fluorouracil and recombinant human interferon alfa-2b for liver metastases of colorectal cancer refractory to systemic fluorouracil and leucovorin, *J. Clin. Oncol.,* **15** (1997) 1432–1438.

76. Miller RL, Bukowski RM, Andresen S, and Gahbauer R. Phase II evaluation of sequential hepatic artery infusion of 5-fluorouracil and hepatic irradiation in metastatic colorectal carcinoma, *J. Surg. Oncol.,* **37** (1988) 1–4.

77. Robertson JM, Lawrence TS, Walker S, et al. Treatment of colorectal liver metastases with conformal radiation therapy and regional chemotherapy, *Int. J. Radiat. Oncol. Biol. Phys.,* **32** (1995) 445–450.

78. Ensminger WD, Thompson M, Come S, et al. Hepatic arterial BCNU: a pilot clinical-pharmacologic study in patients with liver tumors, *Cancer Treat. Rep.,* (1978) 1509.

79. Balch CM, Urist MM, McGregor ML. Continuous regional chemotherapy for metastatic colorectal cancer using a totally implantable infusion pump. A feasibility study in 50 patients, *Am. J. Surg.,* **145** (1983) 285–290.

4 Regional Chemotherapy of Melanoma

Mary S. Brady and Daniel G. Coit

CONTENTS

1. INTRODUCTION

In 1999, an estimated 40,300 Americans will be diagnosed with cutaneous melanoma. Of these, approx 50% will have primaries that occur on the extremity *(1)*. Although most patients present with disease that can be cured with surgery alone, approx 10–15% of patients with extremity melanoma will develop local recurrence, satellitosis, or in-transit disease that is difficult to control or cure *(2)*. Indeed, the most common pattern of recurrence in patients treated for localized melanoma is local-regional *(3–6)*. Patients at highest risk for recurrent disease are those who present with deep primary melanoma or clinically positive regional nodal disease, or both.

Although these regional recurrences often precede or coincide with the appearance of systemic metastasis, an improvement in disease-free survival (DFS) can be obtained in some patients, using aggressive regional therapy in the form of isolated limb perfusion (ILP). ILP is a surgical procedure that involves intravascular delivery of high doses of antitumor agents to the affected extremity only, thereby avoiding the toxicity associated with systemic exposure. This chapter reviews the management of regionally recurrent melanoma, the history and rationale of ILP, the technical aspects of the procedure

From: *Current Clinical Oncology: Regional Chemotherapy: Clinical Research and Practice*
Edited by: M. Markman © Humana Press Inc., Totowa, NJ

itself, the published clinical experience with ILP in patients with melanoma, and future prospects for regional therapy for melanoma.

2. THERAPEUTIC OPTIONS FOR PATIENTS WITH IN-TRANSIT OR LOCALLY RECURRENT MELANOMA

Treatment options for patients with recurrent melanoma limited to an extremity fall into three categories: local therapy of individual lesions, regional therapy of the extremity, or systemic therapy. Local treatment options include surgical excision, injection therapy with immune adjuvants, and CO_2 laser ablation. Surgical excision is a reasonable procedure when the lesions are few in number, and is more effective than laser ablation or injection therapy when the lesions are subcutaneous (SC). Injection therapy with bacilles Calmette-Guérin vaccine, dinitrochlorobenzene, or interferon (IFN) can provide relief for lesions that are primarily dermal in location, but is less effective when SC tumors are present (7–10). Regional response rates are consistently greater than 50%, and transient systemic responses may also occur (9). Pain at the site of injection is a common problem, limiting the number of sites that can be treated at one time.

Laser ablation is another local technique that can be used to treat recurrent melanoma in an extremity. The procedure can be performed under local or general anesthesia, as appropriate. Again, only cutaneous lesions are amendable to treatment. A disadvantage of laser therapy, compared to injection therapy, may be a relatively higher rate of local recurrence at the treated sites (11).

Systemic chemotherapy is an option in patients who are not candidates for local-regional therapy. Single-agent therapy with dacarbazine (DTIC) will result in a 15–20% response rate, most of which is partial and transient. Multiagent therapy with DTIC, cisplatin, carmustine, and tamoxifen produces consistently higher response rates, but no convincing data that survival is prolonged (12).

Regional therapy options include ILP, isolated limb infusion (ILI), and amputation. Major amputation is uncommonly performed for recurrent melanoma, even when confined to the extremity. Most patients with advanced disease in the extremity will die of systemic disease, and more effective strategies for palliation can usually be used without limb sacrifice. In a selected group of patients with disease limited to the extremity, however, amputation can be associated with 5-yr survival of 15–35% (13–15). ILI is similar to ILP, in that it allows relatively high doses of chemotherapy to be administered to the extremity. Cannulation of the vessels is performed angiographically, resulting in less morbidity than ILP. Response rates are lower, however, and more than one treatment may be necessary to achieve the same results as ILP.

ILP holds several advantages over the local or systemic approaches discussed above. Unlike injection therapy or systemic chemotherapy, it is usually administered as a single treatment. More importantly, the entire extremity is treated, including clinical as well as subclinical disease. Response rates are higher with ILP than with systemic chemotherapy. Approximately 80% of patients will respond to ILP with melphalan, the most common agent used. Of these, half will have a complete response (CR), with no evidence of disease in the extremity following treatment. One-third of patients sustaining a CR will survive 10 yr, which is comparable to the experience of patients treated with amputation (Table 1).

ILP is accomplished by isolating the limb using venous and arterial cannulation, followed by application of a tourniquet at the root of the limb. This allows effective isolation of the limb from the systemic circulation, and delivery of high doses of

Table 1
Survival Following Therapeutic ILP

Author, year (ref.)	No. patients, presentation	Agents	Conditions	Survival DFS	OS
Stehlin, 1975 (16)	73[a]	L-PAM	Hyperthermia	NA	48
Hartley and Fletcher, 1987 (17)	22, in-transit	L-PAM	Hyperthermia	NA	58
	26, + nodes			NA	71
	17, both			NA	29
Di Filippo et al., 1989 (18)	5, local recurrence	L-PAM	Hyperthermia	80	80
	41, in-transit			44	55
	27, + nodes			27	47
	21, both			24	35
Klaase et al., 1994 (19)	31, local recurrence	L-PAM	Normothermia	NA	58
	36, satellitosis			NA	57
	71, in-transit			NA	45
	32, + node			NA	23
	46, both			NA	27
Krementz et al., 1994 (20)	36, local recurrence	[b]	Hyperthermia	NA	80
	143, in-transit			NA	36
	145, in-transit/+ nodes			NA	23
	180, + nodes			NA	45
Bryant et al., 1995 (21)	8, local recurrence	L-PAM	Hyperthermia	NA	75
	41, in-transit			NA	44
	8, + nodes			NA	56
	25, both			NA	23

L-PAM = melphalan; DFS = disease-free survival; OS = overall survival; + nodes = positive nodes; NA = not available.

[a]Local recurrence (patient no. 8), in-transit (patient no. 30), node positive (n = 17), node + and in-transit (patient no. 18).

[b]Single-agent therapy with L-PAM, nitrogen mustard, or thio-TEPA.

antitumor agents, usually melphalan, without significant systemic toxicity. Arterial infusion facilitates delivery to the tumor vasculature and regional nodes. Oxygenation of arterial inflow potentiates the effects of alkylating agents, and may be directly tumoricidal to cancer cells. Hyperthermia increases the effectiveness of the chemotherapy, essentially doubling uptake of drug by tumor cells (22), and is, itself, tumoricidal (23).

3. DEVELOPMENT OF REGIONAL CHEMOTHERAPY
FOR MELANOMA:
A HISTORICAL PERSPECTIVE

ILP was developed by Creech et al. (24) at Charity Hospital in New Orleans. The first perfusion was performed in 1957 on a 76-yr-old man with recurrent melanoma and satellitosis of the lower extremity. The patient had a CR to perfusion with nitrogen mustard, and remained free of disease until he died of other causes 16 yr later. Creech and his colleagues, particularly Edward Krementz et al. (20) continued to develop the technique of ILP, using various agents and conditions throughout the ensuing several decades. Although these original investigators used ILP on patients with a variety of regionally confined tumors, the vast majority of patients were treated for melanoma.

In 1967, Cavaliere *(23)* reported that hyperthermia itself was directly tumoricidal in vitro. Stehlin et al. *(16)* combined chemotherapy and hyperthermia in ILP, and showed increased response rates in humans. Since then, hyperthermia, in combination with chemotherapy and/or cytokine therapy, has been a standard approach to patients with advanced local or regional melanoma of the extremity.

Since its initial development, many centers have reported their experience with ILP, using a variety of techniques and agents. Until recently, few controlled clinical trials were performed. Interpretation of the large body of single-institution, retrospective reports is difficult, primarily because of the heterogeneity of patients reported (particularly adjuvant vs therapeutic perfusion), variations in surgical treatment, and poorly defined criteria for judging response to the treatment. Nonetheless, this initial experience made it clear that the technique of ILP plays an important role in the management of patients with regional melanoma. These reports are summarized in Table 1.

4. INDICATIONS FOR PERFUSION AND SELECTION OF PATIENTS

ILP can be performed as an adjuvant therapy for patients with high-risk regional disease who are currently without evidence of disease (adjuvant ILP), to treat existing regional disease in patients without systemic melanoma (therapeutic ILP), and for patients with systemic disease who require palliation of bulky regional melanoma (palliative ILP).

At Memorial Sloan-Kettering Cancer Center (MSKCC), ILP is generally reserved for patients with locally recurrent melanoma or in-transit disease of an extremity that is not amendable to surgical excision or injection therapy (therapeutic ILP). There is currently no role for adjuvant ILP, except within the confines of a clinical trial. Patients with stage IV disease who require palliation because of bulky or ulcerated lesions are also candidates for ILP.

Because isolation of the vascular circuit requires cannulation of the major arterial inflow to the limb, ILP is contraindicated in patients with significant peripheral vascular disease. In addition, patients with active infection of the leg or a biopsy wound should not undergo ILP. Relative contraindications include advanced age, severe lymphedema of the extremity, or prior radiation therapy to the extremity. In addition, patients with disease located in the proximal thigh, especially over the lateral posterior aspect of the upper thigh, are less likely to benefit from ILP, because this area is usually poorly perfused.

5. SURGICAL TECHNIQUE

Patients who undergo ILP should donate 2–3 units of blood preoperatively. This will allow pump priming with autologous blood. A certified cardiopulmonary perfusionist, experienced in regional perfusion, is essential. Experienced nuclear medicine, anesthesia, and nursing personnel are critical components of the team.

The complex procedure of ILP can be conceptualized by breaking it down into its essential components. The patient is anesthetized, and appropriate means of cardiovascular and temperature monitoring are placed. The surgeon exposes and isolates the artery and vein while the limb is warming in a pediatric warming blanket. Cannulation of the vessels is performed once a sufficient length of vessel is dissected and collaterals are ligated. Ligation of collateral vessels is critical to the success of the procedure. Once the vessels are cannulated, a tourniquet is placed at the root of the limb, and the extremity is placed on bypass. Warming is completed by the heated perfusate. When the desired temperature is reached, usually 38°C or higher, drug is added to the perfusion circuit in one bolus or divided doses. Leak rates are monitored using radioisotopes, to ensure effective isolation of the limb. Once the perfusion is complete, the limb is flushed to remove drug, and the vessels are decannulated and repaired. These individual components of the procedure are discussed in more detail below.

5.1. Intraoperative Preparation

The patient is placed on a warming blanket, and exposed areas are covered with warm blankets to maintain the core temperature. The procedure is performed under general anesthesia, with central venous and peripheral arterial monitoring. A compression boot is used on the nonperfused lower extremity, to prevent deep venous thrombosis. A Foley catheter is placed, and the extremity is prepped and draped freely. Thermistor probes are placed on the skin and within the muscle of the extremity, to ensure accurate temperature monitoring. The extremity below the groin, or beyond the elbow, is wrapped carefully in gauze, and padded, prior to wrapping it in a recirculating warming blanket.

5.2. Vascular Isolation

Perfusion of the extremity for melanoma can be performed via the external iliac, femoral, or axillary vessels. Popliteal perfusion is uncommonly performed for melanoma, because it treats only the distal leg, and is more commonly used for sarcoma of the distal extremity.

5.2.1. EXTERNAL ILIAC PERFUSION

External iliac perfusion is the most common form of extremity perfusion for melanoma. It is preferred in patients who have undergone a prior inguinal lymphadenectomy or femoral perfusion. This avoids dissection of the vessels in a previously operated field, with attendant scarring and fibrosis. The area of perfusion is the same as that of femoral perfusion, because the tip of the cannula rests in the same location, just proximal to the profunda femoris in the common femoral artery. In addition, the level of the tourniquet is identical, which is the factor that defines the proximal extent of perfusion.

A renal transplant incision is used for access to the external iliac artery and vein. This is an oblique incision midway between the anterior superior iliac spine and the pubic tubercle. Use of the Buchwalter retractor facilitates exposure of the external iliac vessels and retraction of the bladder medially. The artery and vein are mobilized and isolated by ligating and dividing all branches and tributaries between the common iliac bifurcation and the inguinal ligament (including the inferior epigastrics and the deep circumflex iliac vessels) through an extraperitoneal approach. The internal iliac artery and vein are controlled, but not divided. The obturator vessels are ligated, but not divided. The vessels are surrounded with umbilical tape and Rummel tourniquets prior to cannulation.

5.2.2. FEMORAL PERFUSION

Patients undergoing femoral perfusion require a standard lymphadenectomy incision, if this is performed at the same time. If a nodal dissection is not planned, then a standard femoral incision, allowing access to the femoral vessels, is performed. This is an axial incision overlying the femoral artery and vein beneath the inguinal ligament.

5.2.3. UPPER EXTREMITY PERFUSION

In patients undergoing upper extremity perfusion, the proximal axillary artery and vein are exposed through an incision extending from the clavicle to the anterior axillary line overlying the vessels. The vessels are exposed by retracting or dividing the pectoralis minor muscle, and retracting the pectoralis major muscle medially.

5.2.4. NODAL DISSECTION PRIOR TO ILP

Patients with clinical evidence of regional nodal involvement should undergo a node dissection at the time of ILP. This is usually not associated with increased morbidity in patients undergoing pelvic or axillary node dissection, but can be problematic in patients undergoing inguinal lymphadenectomy. In these patients, wound breakdown is common, although this will heal in the majority of patients. Patients with clinically negative nodes are unlikely to derive an additional benefit from an elective node dissection at the time of ILP, and will be at increased risk of complications related to the combined procedure, particularly lymphedema and wound infection.

5.2.5. HYPERTHERMIA

Mild hyperthermia (38–40°C) is most commonly used during ILP. True hyperthermia (40–43°C) has been advocated by some, but may be associated with increased toxicity, without convincing evidence that response rates are increased *(25)*. Hyperthermia is achieved by wrapping the leg in a warming blanket, and heating the perfusion circuit. The latter is primarily responsible for establishing and maintaining the increased temperature of the extremity, although the recirculating warming blanket helps to maintain the correct temperature of the skin, and to minimize evaporative heat loss. It is important to remember that an increased room temperature, as well as warm intravenous fluids, also contribute to maintaining the patient's temperature during the procedure.

5.2.6. CANNULATION

Selection of the appropriate arterial and venous cannulas is essential to the success of the perfusion. The largest venous cannula that can be accommodated by the vein should be employed because the venous outflow from the limb is the critical determinant of the flow rate, which determines the amount of drug that can be delivered to the extremity.

Heparin is given systemically prior to arterial cannulation (300 U/kg). The artery is occluded with a Rummel tourniquet, and the time is recorded. A transverse arteriotomy is used, and the cannula, filled with perfusate, is passed so that the tip is below the proposed level of the tourniquet. Marking this distance with a silk tie, prior to passing the cannula, will facilitate accurate placement of the tip of the cannula just proximal to the profunda femoris during external iliac perfusion. The Rummel tourniquets are snugged, and the cannulas are secured to the Rummel tourniquets to prevent accidental dislodgement. The vein is then cannulated in a similar fashion. Two Steinman pins are placed in the anterior superior iliac spine, and angled cephalad, posterior, and lateral. The root of the limb is wrapped in a sterile Esmarch's bandage. For upper extremity perfusions, Steinman pins are placed in the scapula in the midaxillary line. At this point, all air is excluded from the circuit, and the extremity is placed on bypass. The extremity begins to warm more rapidly when warm perfusate is infusing. The temperature should reach 38°C prior to adding drug. The rate of arterial inflow is determined by gravity drainage from the venous line to the reservoir in the pump oxygenator.

5.3. Perfusion Circuit

The extracorporeal circuit consists of a roller pump, membrane oxygenator, and heat exchanger. The circuit is primed prior to cannulation with a balanced salt solution and autologous blood. Flow rates should be between 600 and 1200 mL/min for iliac/femoral perfusion, and 300–600 mL/min for axillary perfusion. The systemic arterial pressure is monitored and adjusted pharmacologically by the anesthesiologist, as necessary, based on leak monitoring.

5.4. Cardiovascular Monitoring

Maintaining a mean systemic arterial pressure, greater than or equal to 20 mmHg of the perfusion pressure, is important to minimize leak. Phenylephrine is generally used for this purpose. The perfusion pressure invariably rises slowly as the perfusion progresses. A high flow rate should be maintained, because this facilitates rapid and effective warming of the limb, with vasodilation and optimal tumor perfusion. In addition, oxygen delivery to the tissues is maintained, thereby avoiding the increased toxicity associated with hypoxia.

5.5. Leak Monitoring Using Radioisotopes

Accurate monitoring of systemic leak is essential during ILP. The leak monitoring system is based on determining deviation from background radioactivity present in a defined circulating blood volume. This is established prior to perfusion by injecting a small amount of radioisotope (a calibration dose) into the systemic circulation. The calibration dose is injected once the extremity is isolated and stable flow rates and reservoir volumes are established.

At MSKCC, a calibration dose of 500 μCi of technetium (Tc)-labeled albumin is injected into the central venous pressure line, to determine background counts. Once the limb is isolated and warm, prior to adding drug, 5000 μCi is injected into the perfusate. Because a much larger dose is given into the perfusate (10-fold), a doubling of the baseline counts in the systemic circulation signifies a 10% leak. Leak rates are continuously monitored by a gamma counter placed over the precordium. Leak should not exceed 5% with chemotherapeutic agents, or 1% (over 10 min) with tumor necrosis factor-α (TNF-α). Patients with leak rates exceeding 1% with TNF-α require vasopressor support.

An alternative to Tc-labeled albumin is radiolabeled red blood cells. The advantage of using tagged red blood cells, instead of Tc-labeled albumin, is that there is less decay with time. Five mL of the patient's blood is drawn 30 min before the perfusion, and labeled with Tc-99.

The surgeon requires a continuous assessment of both leak rate and reservoir volume throughout the procedure, in order to adjust the perfusion circuit, and to minimize potential morbidity to the patient. Large shifts in reservoir volume or dramatic initial leak rates suggest a missed collateral vessel or a cannula that is positioned too proximally, with side holes above the tourniquet. Less dramatic changes that occur are usually addressed by adjusting the flow rate, tourniquet, or systemic arterial pressure. Mean arterial pressure should be maintained at least 20 mmHg above mean perfusion pressure. An increasing reservoir volume indicates a systemic to perfusate leak, and can usually be addressed by increasing the flow rate. Common problems requiring adjustment and corrective measures are listed in Table 2.

5.6. Washout and Decannulation

At the end of the procedure, the extremity is flushed with low-mol-wt dextran or crystalloid, to remove unbound drug and toxic end products. Careful monitoring of intake and output is important to prevent unnecessary blood loss. Massaging the extremity during washout will facilitate clearing. When the effluent is clear, the limb is filled

Table 2
Adjustments Required During ILP

Indicator	Problem	Correction
Increased counts (gradual)	Circuit to patient leak	Increase arterial pressure Decrease flow rate Adjust tourniquet
Increased reservoir volume	Patient to circuit leak	Ligate collaterals Increase flow rate Increase venous outflow pressure
Dramatic initial leak	Misplaced cannula	Adjust
Increased counts and reservoir volume	Two-way leak	Priority: decrease circuit to patient leak

Modified with permission from ref. 2.

with autologous blood, the pump is turned off, the perfusion tubing is clamped, the tourniquet is removed, and the vessels are decannulated and repaired. The venous cannula is removed first, and the venotomy is closed with a 5-0 prolene. The arteriotomy is then repaired with a 4-0 or 5-0 prolene. Protamine may be given after the arterial clamp is removed, if necessary.

5.7. Temperature During ILP

ILP can be performed under normothermic conditions (≤38°C), mild hyperthermia (38–40°C), or true hyperthermia (>40°C). Because a high temperature (≥41.5°C) is, in itself, tumoricidal, and because mild-to-moderate increases in temperature can increase the activity of alkylating agents, one might assume that hotter is better. In addition, warming the limb potentially increases blood flow to tumor. It is not clear whether true hyperthermia is superior to mild hyperthermia in producing a clinical response. Increased toxicity with increased temperatures, however, is commonly reported (16,26,27).

Klaase et al. (28) reported a retrospective analysis comparing normothermic and mildly hyperthermic conditions in patients undergoing adjuvant ILP. They reported no difference in DFS or overall survival (OS) between 166 patients with recurrent extremity melanoma undergoing normothermic ILP and 218 patients undergoing ILP with mild hyperthermia. Although patients undergoing hyperthermic ILP had somewhat more acute regional toxicity, long-term morbidity was comparable between the two groups. Kroon et al. (29,30) have reported excellent response rates for patients undergoing normothermic ILP with melphalan, comparable to those reported at centers using mild hyperthermia. It should be noted, however, that, in his larger series, most patients underwent a planned double perfusion, making it difficult to determine whether this was responsible for the higher response rates (Table 3).

5.8. Length of Perfusion

Most perfusions with melphalan are performed for 45 min to 1 h. This is somewhat arbitrary, however, because, when the drug is given as a bolus, most of the area under the curve (the effective drug exposure time) occurs in the first 30 min. Perfusion with

Table 3
Response Rates Following Therapeutic ILP for Melanoma

Author, year (ref.)	No. patients	Agents	Conditions	CR (%)	PR (%)	OR (%)
Di Filippo et al., 1989 (18)	69	L-PAM	Hyperthermia	39	43	82
Storm and Morton, 1985 (31)	26	L-PAM	Hyperthermia	62	19	81
Kroon et al., 1987 (29)	18	L-PAM	Normothermia	40	44	84
Kroon et al., 1993 (30)[a]	43	L-PAM	Normothermia Double perfusion	77	2	79
Klaase et al., 1994 (19)[b]	120	L-PAM	Normothermia	54	25	79
Bulman and Jamieson, 1980 (32)	29	L-PAM	Normothermia	NA	NA	48
Skene et al., 1990 (33)	67	L-PAM	Hyperthermia	NA	NA	74
Minor et al., 1985 (34)	18	L-PAM	Hyperthermia	82	18	100
Lienard et al., 1992 (35)	29	TNF, IFN, L-PAM	Hyperthermia	90	10	100
Fraker et al., 1996 (36)	25[c]	TNF, IFN, L-PAM	Hyperthermia	76	16	92
Fraker et al., 1996 (36)	11	TNF, IFN, L-PAM	Hyperthermia	36	64	100
Thompson et al., 1997 (37)	111	[e]	Hyperthermia	73	13	86

[a]Patients were reperfused 6 wk after initial ILP.
[b]Normo and hyperthermic.
[c]4 mg TNF.
[d]6 mg TNF.
[e]L-PAM (18%), L-PAM and dactinomycin (77%), cisplatin (5%).
L-PAM = melphalan; TNF = tumor necrosis factor α; IFN = interferon γ; CR = complete response; PR = partial response; OR = overall response; NA = not available.

melphalan and TNF-α is generally a 90-min perfusion. Again, this is somewhat arbitrary. The TNF-α is given for 30 min, followed by melphalan for 60 min.

5.9. Postoperative Care

Antiemetic medications should be readily available postoperatively, because patients nearly always experience significant nausea. The average inpatient stay is 5–7 d. Heparin may be given subcutaneously to prevent deep venous thrombosis. Patients who undergo regional nodal dissection at the time of ILP almost invariably develop wound-edge necrosis requiring debridement. The extremity must be monitored for early signs of compartment syndrome, which would necessitate fasciotomy to prevent permanent neurologic damage or limb loss. This is usually apparent on postperfusion d 4–7 and is manifested as increased pain in the extremity, a rise in creatinine phosphokinase levels in the blood, and tense swelling of the extremity. The presentation of compartment syndrome can be quite subtle, however, and must be carefully considered in the postoperative period. Hemoglobin and hematocrit must be monitored postoperatively because significant anemia can occur secondary to blood loss during washout and/or systemic leak of chemotherapeutic agents. This is most likely to reach a nadir at d 7–10.

6. AGENTS USED IN ILP

6.1. Melphalan (L-Phenlyalanine Mustard, L-PAM)

Melphalan remains the best single agent for ILP, and the gold standard against which other agents or combinations must be compared. It is an alkylating agent that is a nitrogen mustard derivative of phenylalanine. Melphalan was initially used for patients with melanoma, because it is cytotoxic to tumors that take up phenylalanine or tyrosine *(38)*. The drug is made up no more than 1 h prior to delivery into the perfusion circuit, in order to minimize breakdown. Melphalan retains approx 90% potency for 3 h at room temperature, but has a much shorter half-life under hyperthermic conditions.

Different methods of determining the dose of melphalan to be given during ILP have been used. These include calculations based on body surface area, body wt, limb volume, and blood volume in the circuit. The two most commonly used methods are based on the patient's weight or limb volume *(39)*. Estimates based on patient weight are easy, and require relatively high doses of drug with acceptable toxicity. The standard dose based on patient weight is 3 mg/kg (with a maximum of 200 mg) for the lower extremity and 1.5 mg/kg for the upper extremity. Estimates based on limb volume require immersion of the limb in water, which can be awkward and even dangerous in patients with limited mobility. Dosages based on limb volume are 10 mg/L (L = liters of limb volume) for the lower extremity and 13 mg/L for the upper extremity.

There have been several strategies employed to improve the efficacy of ILP with melphalan. Klasse et al. *(40)* evaluated dose fractionation by treating 42 patients with a double normothermic perfusion. They compared the response of these patients to that of 45 historical control patients undergoing a single normothermic ILP. Doses of 6 mg/L and 9 mg/L in two separate perfusions were used for the double-perfusion group. Patients with single perfusions received melphalan at a dose of 10 mg/L. Although there was a higher CR rate in the double-perfusion group, this did not translate into a difference in DFS or OS, compared to patients who underwent a single perfusion only. The median follow-up of both groups was relatively short, however, making it difficult to conclude that there is no advantage to a double-perfusion schedule. For those in the double-perfusion group, the median follow-up was 21 mo (24 mo for historical controls). In addition, relatively small numbers of patients were compared *(40)*.

6.2. Other Chemotherapeutic Agents in ILP

Other chemotherapeutic agents have been tried in ILP for patients with melanoma. In general, these other agents are less efficacious or equally efficacious as melphalan, and have greater toxicity. These include cisplatin, nitrogen mustard, DTIC, actinomycin D, and thio-TEPA.

Most experience with a single agent other than melphalan has been reported with cisplatin. Cisplatin is a non-cell, cycle-dependent drug that functions by inhibiting DNA synthesis. It has activity against melanoma that may be dose-related. The systemic dose-limiting toxicity is renal. Cisplatin remains bound to tissues up to 1 mo following ILP. Fletcher et al. *(41)* reported their experience with 145 patients with stage IIIA and IIIB melanoma undergoing adjuvant hyperthermic ILP with cisplatin. They reported an overall survival of 47% at 5 yr. Coit et al. *(42)* reported response rates for cisplatin similar to those seen with melphalan, but substantially increased local-regional morbidity. Others have reported modest response rates, but increased toxicity *(43–45)*.

The most effective single agent for the systemic treatment of patients with metastatic melanoma is DTIC. Used systemically, response rates of up to 20% can be obtained. Unfortunately, less than 5% of patients sustain a CR *(46)*. It would seem, therefore, to be a logical choice for use in ILP. The problem is that it is converted to its active metabolite in the liver, making it a theoretically poor choice. Although initial reports suggested only modest response rates *(47,48)*. Didolkar et al. *(49)* reported a CR in 6 of 10 patients undergoing hyperthermic ILP with DTIC. This favorable experience has not been confirmed by other investigators, or published in full.

Several investigators have evaluated multiagent chemotherapy, usually including other agents in combination with melphalan. The most common combination is melphalan and actinomycin D. Martijn et al. *(50)* evaluated response rates in patients undergoing perfusion with melphalan and actinomycin D, compared to melphalan alone, and found no advantage to combination therapy. There is currently no convincing data to support the use of combinations of drugs over single-agent perfusion with melphalan.

6.3. Combinations of Melphalan and Cytokines in ILP:
Tumor Necrosis Factor α in ILP

Significant progress in the treatment of patients with extremity melanoma was made by investigators in Europe, who somewhat empirically combined TNF-α, interferon-γ (IFN-γ) and melphalan in hyperthermic ILP, and demonstrated significantly increased CR rates over those seen in historical experience with melphalan alone *(51,52)*. TNF-α is a cytokine that has significant tumoricidal activity in animals, primarily by destroying tumor microvasculature *(53)*. It increases procoagulant activity, causing thrombosis and coagulative necrosis of the tumor. Despite exciting preclinical results in murine models, clinical trials evaluating systemic TNF-α as single-agent therapy in phase I and II trials, for patients with a wide variety of solid tumors, have been disappointing, with response rates consistently less than 5% *(54)*. The reason for the discrepancy between experimental and clinical experience is that the dose required to achieve a response in the mouse is 10× higher than that tolerated by man. Use of effective doses of TNF-α in man results in severe toxicity, primarily hypotension, renal failure, hepatic and pulmonary failure, and death.

Posner et al. *(55)* evaluated the efficacy of TNF-α alone in ILP, and the results were discouraging. Investigators in Europe used TNF-α in combination with IFN-γ and melphalan in patients with recurrent melanoma of the extremity and unresectable soft tissue sarcoma. They reported a striking increase in CR rates with the combination therapy *(56)*. Although the combination was somewhat empiric, it had been previously demonstrated that synergism occurred when TNF-α was used in combination with alkylating agents; in vitro and in vivo evidence also showed that hyperthermia enhances the antitumor efficacy of TNF-α *(57,58)*. In addition, INF-γ upregulates TNF-α receptors, and is synergistic with TNF-α in animal models *(59,60)*.

In 1992, Liernard et al. *(35)* reported the European experience using ILP with TNF–melphalan–IFN-γ for patients with in-transit melanoma. Eighteen of the 29 patients in the trial had previously undergone an ILP and failed. The perfusions were carried out under hyperthermic conditions (40–40.5°C) for 90 min. Four mg of TNF-α was injected as a bolus into the arterial line. IFN-γ was given subcutaneously before the perfusion for 2 d, and in the perfusate at a dose of 2 mg. Melphalan was used in the perfusate at 40 µg/mL limb volume.

Hypotension and chills were mild and transient, mostly because the patients were treated with a continuous dopamine infusion and aggressive hydration from onset of the perfusion, and subsequently for 48 h. Hematologic toxicity was the most common morbidity, occurring in 55% of the patients, but this was usually mild (14 of 16 patients). Regional toxicity was acceptable.

The authors reported a surprising 100% response rate, 90% of which were CRs. These response rates were markedly improved over historical data using melphalan alone. DFS was 63% at 12 mo from perfusion. Unfortunately, long-term durability of these responses has not been reported.

Lejeune et al. *(52)* reported the results of a phase II trial, which indicated no significant difference in patients undergoing perfusion with TNF-α and melphalan, compared to those undergoing perfusion with TNF-α, IFN-γ, and melphalan. A phase III trial comparing these two approaches is currently under way *(52)*.

Systemic levels of TNF-α are documented in patients undergoing ILP with the agent that are higher than the picogram quantities found in patients dying of septic shock *(61)*. This results from the absence of endotoxin in the perfused patients. The physiologic effects of pure TNF-α are well managed with vasopressors and fluid *(62)*. The distinction between septic shock and the systemic manifestations of TNF-α is facilitated by the use of "systemic inflammatory response" to describe the physiologic manifestations of TNF-α in the absence of endotoxin *(63)*. Because of the potential for shock, infection of tumor on the extremity is an absolute contraindication to perfusion with TNF-α.

No formal phase I studies were conducted to evaluate the optimal dose of TNF-α to be used in ILP, before phase II studies were conducted. The original reports from Europe suggested that a dose of between 2 and 4 mg TNF-α was efficacious *(35,51,56)*. Investigators at the National Cancer Institute (NCI) compared 4 to 6 mg TNF in ILP in a phase II/III trial, and demonstrated that 4 mg TNF was more efficacious than 6 mg, and was associated with significantly less toxicity. The toxicity observed in the patients receiving 6 mg was mostly secondary to neuropathy and myopathy *(36)*. These investigators also demonstrated that the combination of TNF-α and melphalan may be particularly useful in patients with bulky disease, and in those who have failed prior perfusion with other agents. Bartlett et al. *(64)* demonstrated that 16 of 17 patients who had failed a prior perfusion responded to the combination treatment, and of these, 12 sustained a CR.

A phase III trial conducted by investigators at the NCI randomized patients to receive either hyperthermic ILP with melphalan alone or melphalan, TNF-α, and IFN-γ. A trend toward higher CR rates was found in the three-drug arm, compared to melphalan alone (81 vs 65%, respectively), but this was not statistically significant *(65)*. A very significant improvement in the rate of CRs was observed in patients with extensive disease (60 vs 17% for the three-drug arm vs melphalan alone). Patients with a relatively low tumor burden had an excellent chance of responding to either melphalan alone (81%) or combination treatment (87%). Low tumor burden was defined as 10 or fewer tumor nodules and no nodule >3 cm in size.

The issue of duration of response is important when considering therapeutic ILP. Improved CR rates do not necessarily translate into improved survival. There is little question that adding TNF-α to the perfusion will increase the likelihood of a CR, especially in patients with extensive disease. In addition, a double-perfusion schedule with melphalan may also increase CR rates. It remains to be determined whether these responses are more durable. This is despite the fact that a CR to perfusion is a consistent

Table 4
Adjuvant ILP for Patients
with High-Risk Primary Melanoma, Case-Controlled Studies

Author, year (ref.)	Patients	WE	WE + ILP	5-yr DFS	5-yr OS (%)
McBride et al., 1975 (66)	≥Clark III, primary	71	92	NA	44 vs 67, P <.05[a]
Franklin et al., 1988 (68)	≥1.5 mm	238	227	NA	73 vs 77[a], P = .9[a]
Edwards et al., 1990 (67)	Primary melanoma	151	149	NS	77 vs 84, P = .33
	Subset >2 mm	25	25	P = .06	44 vs 85, P <.01

[a]10-yr overall survival.
WE = wide excision; WE + ILP = wide excision and isolated limb perfusion; DFS = disease-free survival; OS = overall survival; NS = not significant; NA = not available.

predictor of survival following ILP *(18,19,21)*. Significant improvements in a patient's quality of life may be justification enough.

7. CLINICAL EXPERIENCE WITH ILP WITH MELPHALAN

7.1. Adjuvant ILP with Melphalan

Several case control studies evaluating adjuvant ILP with melphalan, in patients with high-risk primary melanoma of the extremity, have been reported. In these studies, patients with localized primary disease were treated with excision and adjuvant perfusion, and compared with historical or concurrent control patients treated with excision only. The first report of these demonstrated a significant improvement in OS for patients undergoing adjuvant ILP, particularly at 10-yr follow-up (83 vs 57% OS, $P < .005$). In this study, 92 patients undergoing adjuvant perfusion were compared to historical controls. Patients had primary melanoma that was invasive to the reticular dermis (Clark level III) or beyond. Unfortunately, patients were not matched with controls for depth of the lesion, which is the most important clinical predictor of survival. In addition, females were overrepresented in the perfused group *(66)*.

Two case-matched studies, one from the Netherlands and one from Houston, demonstrated no difference in survival between patients undergoing wide excision (WE) alone vs those undergoing WE and ILP *(67,68)*. The study from the Netherlands is the largest of these, with 238 patients in the excision-alone group and 227 in the adjuvant perfusion group *(68)*. These case-matched retrospective reports are summarized in Table 4.

7.2. Adjuvant Perfusion for High-Risk Primary Melanoma: Prospective Randomized Trials

There are three prospective randomized trials evaluating the efficacy of adjuvant ILP in patients with high-risk primary melanoma (Table 5). In general, these are patients with primary melanoma >1.5 mm in depth. The first trial was reported by Ghussen et al. *(69)* who compared the outcome of patients randomized to WE and regional node dissection, or to WE, regional node dissection, and adjuvant hyperthermic ILP with melphalan. Although the trial included patients with stages I–III melanoma, a subgroup of patients had localized primary melanoma (>1.5 mm or Clark IV, $n = 37$). At 5-yr

Table 5
Adjuvant ILP for High-Risk Primary Melanoma: Prospective Randomized Trials

Authors, yr (ref.)	Patients	WE	WE + ILP	5-yr DFS %	OS
Ghussen et al., 1988 (69)	≥1.5 or ≥Clark IV	18	19	61 vs 95, P <.02	NS
Fenn et al., 1997 (70)	≥1.7 mm	14	16	36 vs 88, P <.004[a]	50 vs 88, p <.03[a]
Schraffordt et al., 1997 (71)	≥1.5 mm	412	420	NS[b]	NS[b]

[a]Median follow-up 63 mo in control group (WE) and 80 mo in the ILP group (WE + ILP).
[b]Median follow-up 6.4 yr.
WE = wide excision; WE + ILP = wide excision and isolated limb perfusion; DFS = disease-free survival; OS = overall survival; NS = not significant.

follow-up, there was a significant survival advantage in patients treated with perfusion ($n = 19$), compared to those treated with WE only ($n = 18$). The major problem with this study, however, is the 95% survival found in the patients undergoing ILP, which is so much more favorable than any previous or subsequent reports that the trials must be interpreted with caution. In addition, the 61% survival for the patients treated with operation only is lower than what would be expected, based on data from other institutions.

Fenn et al. (70) recently reported the results of a small trial conducted in the United Kingdom, evaluating adjuvant ILP in patients with primary melanoma of the extremity ≥1.7 mm in depth. Fourteen patients underwent WE only, and 16 underwent WE and hyperthermic ILP with melphalan. As has been reported by other investigators, patients undergoing ILP had a lower nodal failure rate. With a median follow-up of ≥63 mo, they found that patients in the perfusion group were significantly more likely to survive than those in the excision-alone group (88 vs 50%, respectively; $P <.03$). The extremely poor survival in the control group makes it difficult to draw conclusions from this trial.

The most important of these trials is the large World Health Organization (WHO) phase III trial, which evaluated the value of adjuvant ILP in 852 patients with primary extremity melanoma ≥1.5 mm (71). Patients were randomized to WE or to WE and adjuvant ILP with melphalan and mild hyperthermia. Prophylactic regional node dissection was performed at the discretion of the investigator, but the policy of the center participating had to be consistently applied. As a result, 47% of the WE and ILP group received an elective node dissection, compared to 38% of the WE only group.

The trial results at preliminary analysis demonstrate no advantage to adjuvant perfusion in the group as a whole. Among the 412 evaluable patients (median follow-up 6.4 yr), there is a trend toward a longer DFS in the ILP group. This is only significant, however, in the patients who did not undergo an elective node dissection. Within this group, the difference is highly significant in patients with primary melanoma 1.5–3 mm in depth. In all patients who did not undergo an elective node dissection, the incidence of in-transit disease was reduced in the patients undergoing adjuvant ILP, from 6.6% (WE) to 2.2% (WE + ILP), as was the incidence of regional nodal failure (in those who did not undergo elective node dissection), from 16.7 to 12.6%. At last analysis, however, there is no OS difference between the two groups. Based on this important and well-conducted trial, there is currently no role for adjuvant perfusion in patients with high-risk primary melanoma, outside of the context of a clinical trial.

Table 6
Adjuvant ILP for Advanced[a] Extremity Melanoma: Prospective Randomized Trials

Authors	Resection	Resection + ILP	DFS %	OS
Ghussen et al., 1988 (69)	36	34	47 vs 85, P <.02	78 vs 97, P <.03
Hafstrom et al., 1991 (72)	36	33	17 vs 30, P = .044	NS

[a]Advanced = satellitosis, local recurrence, in-transit disease, or a combination of these.
ILP = isolated limb perfusion; NS = not significant; DFS = disease-free survival; OS = overall survival.

7.3. Adjuvant Perfusion for Regional Melanoma: Prospective Randomized Trials

There are two prospective randomized trials evaluating the efficacy of adjuvant ILP in patients with advanced melanoma of the extremity in the form of in-transit disease, satellitosis, local recurrence, or a combination of these (Table 6). The first trial was reported by Ghussen et al. (69), and included 70 patients with advanced melanoma of the extremity, in whom all disease could be resected. An interim analysis demonstrated a highly significant difference in recurrence rate between the 34 patients randomized to perfusion and the 36 patients treated with resection only. At a median follow-up of 554 d, the DFS was 47% in the resection-only patients and 85% in the patients treated with adjuvant ILP ($P <.02$). Again, as in the subgroup of patients with primary melanoma in this trial, the 85% survival for patients in the ILP group is much more favorable than that reported for similar patients in other trials, which makes it difficult to recommend adjuvant perfusion in these patients, based on this trial.

The second trial was published by Hafstrom et al. (72), who compared WE alone (36 patients) to WE and adjuvant ILP (33 patients) in patients with advanced, completely resected melanoma of the extremity. Patients were stratified according to whether the disease was located on the upper or lower extremity. They found that although there was an improvement in DFS in the 33 patients in the ILP group (33 vs 17%, respectively, $P <.05$), OS was not significantly different (55 vs 44%, respectively, P = not significant). These data are much more consistent with the survival experience from other centers in similar patients. Currently no data support adjuvant perfusion for advanced, but complete resected, melanoma of the extremity, outside the confines of a clinical trial.

8. THERAPEUTIC ILP

There are two important ways to gage the efficacy of ILP in patients undergoing therapeutic ILP. The most immediately available data are the percentage of patients who experience a clinical response to the treatment, either partial or complete. A partial response (PR) is defined as a 50% or greater decrease in the sum of the products of perpendicular diameters of all measurable lesions, without the appearance of new lesions. A CR is defined as the disappearance of all clinical evidence of disease. Most reports suggest that about 80% of patients undergoing therapeutic ILP with melphalan as a single agent will have a significant clinical response (CR + PR), with at least half of these responses complete (Table 3). The other parameter of importance is duration of response. Although newer combinations of drugs may result in an increase in the percentage of patients sustaining a clinical response, if this is not durable, then little progress has been made. Duration of response can be measured by DFS and/or median duration of response. Data on the duration of response are sparse, but several reports suggest that approx one-third to one-half of all CRs to therapeutic ILP with melphalan are durable *(18,37)*.

In a large, multi-institutional study from the Netherlands, 54% of patients had a CR to therapeutic ILP with melphalan, with an overall response rate of 79% *(19)*. The median duration of CR was 9 mo *(19)*. The highest reported CR, using melphalan alone, is 82%, reported by Minor et al. *(34)*, which was a small study involving 18 patients undergoing hyperthermic ILP with melphalan.

Several investigators have reported clinical features associated with a CR to therapeutic ILP. In the large, multiinstitutional experience from the Netherlands, Klaase et al. *(19)* found that patients with pathologically or clinically negative regional lymph nodes, leg-as-opposed-to-arm disease, and multiple-as-opposed-to-single perfusions, were more likely to have a CR to ILP. Similarly, Bryant et al. *(21)* observed that disease stage was associated with a CR, i.e., patients with a lesser tumor burden were more likely to respond than those with bulky regional disease. De Filippo et al. *(18)* also noted that patients with a smaller tumor burden (fewer tumor nodules) were more likely to experience a CR to perfusion, and that a minimum intratumoral temperature of 41.5°C and higher-than-standard doses of chemotherapy were associated with more CRs.

Krementz et al. *(20)* reported that, in their large retrospective experience with ILP in over 1000 patients with melanoma, stage was the most important predictor of outcome. Survival at 10 yr was 70% for patients with localized disease, 61% for patients with local recurrence or satellitosis, 30% for patients with in-transit melanoma, 38% for patients with nodal disease, 16% for patients with both in-transit and nodal disease, and 7% for patients with systemic disease.

The most important predictor of survival following therapeutic ILP is a CR to perfusion. Fewer lesions, a lower number of prior relapses, and female sex were also found to be associated with survival following ILP *(18)*. Gohl et al. *(73)* reported their experience in 163 patients undergoing therapeutic ILP with melphalan and actinomycin D. All patients underwent a regional node dissection as well. Gohl et al. reported a 10-yr survival of 37% for the entire group. When evaluated by stage, those with in-transit disease ($n = 51$), or lymph nodes metastasis ($n = 79$) exclusively, did best, with 10-yr survival of 41 and 40%, respectively. Patients with both did more poorly: 26% survival at 10 yr *(73)*.

8.1. Palliative Perfusion: Stage IV Patients

ILP is occasionally beneficial in the patient with stage IV disease, in order to maintain a functional extremity. Effective palliation can be achieved in 49–63% of patients for a mean period of 2–23 mo *(32,74,75)*. Five-yr survival is poor (7%), as reported by Krementz et al. *(20)*.

9. MORBIDITY OF ILP

When considering the complications of ILP, it is useful to distinguish between those that are short- or long-term, and those that are regional or systemic. The acute morbidity of ILP with melphalan alone, or melphalan and TNF-α is significant, but generally well tolerated. The most common systemic effects are hematologic toxicity, mostly related to leakage of chemotherapy or TNF-α into the systemic circulation, resulting in thrombocytopenia and leukopenia. In most patients, this is mild. The most common

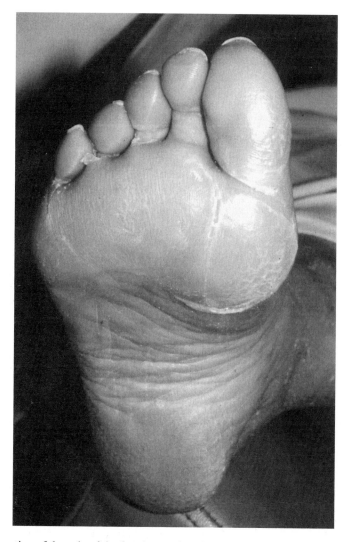

Fig. 1. Desquamation of the sole of the foot in a patient 8 wk after hyperthermic ILP with melphalan.

acute regional complications are muscle edema, which may (rarely) necessitate fasciotomy, thromboembolic events, and local wound complications. Amputation necessitated by complications of ILP is rare, occurring in less than 1% of patients *(76)*. In the largest single-institution experience reported (comprising over 1000 patients with melanoma, from 1957 to 1992) by Krementz et al. *(20)*, only eight amputations were performed, all prior to 1966. Mortality is uncommon, and is usually related to systemic leak and subsequent leukopenia or cardiovascular complications *(76)*. Nail loss and desquamation of the skin of the palms (for upper extremity ILP) or soles of the feet (lower extremity ILP) is not uncommon (Fig. 1).

When considering the long-term morbidity of ILP, it is important to remember that many patients will have significant discomfort prior to therapeutic perfusion, because of repeated operative resection or unresectable local disease. Nonetheless, ILP has distinct long-term morbidity for patients. In a review of the experience from the Netherlands, Vrouenraets et al. *(77)* reported that 44% of 367 patients had some degree of objective or subjective morbidity at least 1 yr following ILP. The most common

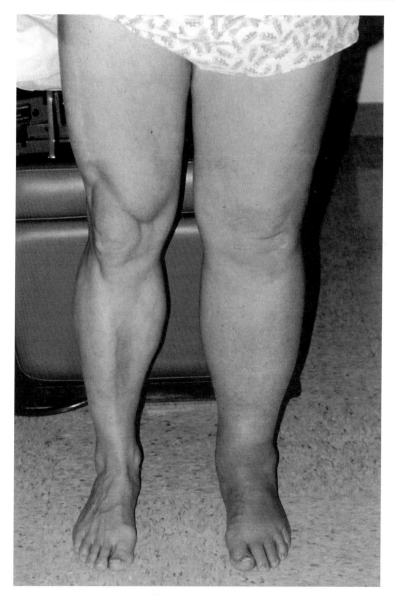

Fig. 2. Lymphedema of the left lower extremity in a 55-yr-old male treated with inguinal node dissection and hyperthermic ILP 15 yr previously.

problem was lymphedema, which occurred in 28% of patients undergoing perfusion (Fig. 2). Other concerns were neuropathy or pain (12%), muscle atrophy (11%), and recurrent infection (3%). Acute regional toxicity following perfusion, and concurrent lymphadenectomy, predicted long-term morbidity. Neuropathy was more common following an axillary perfusion. Women and young patients were more likely to sustain long-term morbidity.

In 1972, Schraffordt Koops (78) observed that hyperthermia increased the complications of ILP with melphalan. In particular, foot drop secondary to peroneal nerve dysfunction was a common complication, caused by the development of compartment syndrome in the perfused extremity. He advocated fasciotomy in the presence of inflammatory edema of the perfused limb, to prevent this complication. Most modern series report a less-common incidence of compartment syndrome, although patients must be monitored carefully, so that a prompt fasciotomy can be performed, if necessary, to circumvent neuromuscular damage. In a small prospective evaluation of morbidity following ILP from the Netherlands, Olieman et al. *(79)* reported no difference in function of the extremity between 46 patients with stage I melanoma undergoing WE and ILP and 37 patients undergoing WE only. They routinely perform fasciotomy in patients to avoid compartment syndrome/fibrosis postperfusion, and argue that this prevents functional morbidity *(79)*.

A subset of patients, accrued to the prospective WHO trial of adjuvant perfusion, were evaluated to determine functional morbidity at 2 yr. Patients treated with adjuvant ILP (*n* = 36) were compared to those undergoing excision only (*n* = 29). The most common morbidity in the ILP group was decreased ankle extension (40% of those undergoing lower-extremity perfusion). Patients undergoing upper-extremity perfusion had diminished shoulder abduction. No patients had functional morbidity that was considered severe *(80)*. Similar results were reported by van Geel et al. *(81)* who found that only 1 of 57 patients had severe symptoms related to the perfused extremity. The most common functional morbidity was decreased ankle mobility, occurring in over 25% of patients undergoing lower-extremity perfusion *(81)*.

10. NEW STRATEGIES: ILI

A promising alternative to the technical complexity of ILP is ILI. A large experience with this technique was recently reported by Harman *(82)* and Thompson *(83)* from the Sydney Melanoma Unit. ILI involves percutaneous placement of arterial and venous catheters in the radiology suite. The patient is then taken to the operating room, where general anesthesia is performed, pneumatic tourniquets are inflated at the root of the extremity, and the patient is fully heparinized. Infusion of chemotherapy commences under normothermic, hypoxic conditions. A pneumatic tourniquet is used to isolate the limb, once the arterial and venous catheters have been placed. The limb is then infused for 20 min using a syringe and 3-way tap, followed by a flush with saline.

Harman et al. *(82)* reported their results in 120 patients, using melphalan and actinomycin D in ILP. They reported 39% CRs and 52% PRs (overall response 91%) following single perfusions and 45% CRs and 42% PRs (overall response 87%) following double perfusions *(82,83)*. The advantage of ILI is that it does not require surgical placement of the catheters, and can be used in patients who are not good candidates for ILP, because of advanced age or co-morbid conditions, which increase their risk of complications or mortality from ILP. In addition, ILI can be repeated with much less morbidity than ILP. It remains to be seen whether the durability of responses observed by Harman et al. *(82)* is comparable to that seen with ILP.

11. CONCLUSIONS

ILP remains a useful therapeutic modality in a subset of patients with recurrent melanoma limited to the extremity. Because of its complexity, it should be performed by surgeons experienced with the technical aspects of the procedure, as well as with management of the patient following ILP. Although there is currently no role for adjuvant ILP in the therapy of patients with extremity melanoma, outside of a clinical trial, it remains to be seen whether newer agents or combinations will expand the role of the procedure in patients with extremity melanoma.

The history of the development and use of ILP over the past 40 yr has been one of retrospective analysis of an uncontrolled clinical experience. It is clear that, in order to define the role of ILP in patients with melanoma for the future, carefully designed and controlled trials are essential.

REFERENCES

1. Balch CM, Houghton AN, and Peters LJ. Cutaneous melanoma, In DeVita VT, Hellman S, Rosenberg SA, (eds), *Cancer: Principles and Practice of Oncology*, 4th ed. Lippincott, Philadelphia, 1993, 1612– .
2. Fraker DL. Hyperthermic regional perfusion for melanoma of the limbs, In Balch CM, et al. (eds), *Cutaneous Melanoma,* 3rd ed. Quality Medical, St. Louis, (1998) pp. 281–300.
3. Reintgen DS, Cox C, Singluff CL Jr, and Seigler HR. Recurrent malignant melanoma: the identification of prognostic factors to predict survival, *Ann. Plast. Surg.,* **28** (1992) 45–49.
4. Fusi S, Ariyan S, and Sternlicht A. Data on first recurrence after treatment for malignant melanoma in a large patient population, *Plast. Reconstr. Surg.,* **91** (1993) 94–98.
5. Milton GW, Shaw HM, Farago GA, and McCarthy WH. Tumor thickness and the site and time of first recurrence in cutaneous malignant melanoma (stage I), *Br. J. Surg.,* **67** (1980) 543–546.
6. McCarthy WH, Shaw HM, Thompson JF, and Milton GW. Time and frequency of recurrence of cutaneous stage I malignant melanoma with guidelines for follow-up study, *Surg. Gynecol. Obstet.,* **166** (1988) 497–502.
7. Cohen MH, Jessup JM, Felix EL, Weese JL, and Herberman RB. Intralesional treatment of recurrent metastatic cutaneous malignant melanoma: a randomized prospective study of intralesional bacillus Calmette-Guérin versus intralesional dinitrochlorobenzene, *Cancer,* **41** (1978) 2456–2463.
8. Bauer R, Kopald K, Lee J, et al. Long term results of intralesional BCG for locally advanced recurrent melanoma, *Proc. Am. Soc. Clin. Oncol.,* **9** (1990) 276.
9. von Wussow P, Block B, Hartmann F, and Deicher H. Intralesional interferon-alpha in advanced malignant melanoma, *Cancer,* **61** (1988) 1071–1974.
10. Si Z, Hersey P, and Coates AS. Clinical responses and lymphoid infiltrates in metastatic melanoma following treatment with intralesional GM-CSF, *Melanoma Res.,* **6** (1966) 247–255.
11. Strobbe LJ, Nieweg OE, and Kroon BB. Carbon dioxide laser for cutaneous melanoma metastases: indications and limitations, *Eur. J. Surg. Oncol.,* **23** (1997) 435–438.
12. Buzaid AC, Bedikian A, and Houghton AN. Systemic chemotherapy and biochemotherapy, In Balch CM, et al., (eds), *Cutaneous Melanoma,* 3rd ed. Quality Medical, St. Louis, (1998) pp. 405–418.
13. Jaques DP, Coit DG, and Brennan MF. Major amputation for advanced malignant melanoma, *Surg. Gynecol. Obset.,* **196** (1989) 1–6.
14. Turnbull A, Shah J, and Fortner J. Recurrent melanoma of an extremity treated by major amputation, *Arch Surg,* **106** (1973) 496–498.
15. Kourtesis GJ, McCarthy WH, and Milton GW. Major amputations for melanoma, *Aust. NZ J. Surg.,* **53** (1983) 241–244.
16. Stehlin JS Jr, Giovanella BC, De Ipolyi PD, Muenz LR, and Anderson RF. Results of hyperthermic perfusion for melanoma of the extremities, *Surg. Gynecol. Obstet.,* **140** (1975) 339–348.
17. Hartley JW and Fletcher WS. Improved survival of patients with stage II melanoma of the extremity using hyperthermic isolation perfusion with 1-phenylalanine mustard, *J. Surg. Oncol.,* **36** (1987) 170–174.
18. Di Filippo F, Calabro A, Giannarelli D, et al. Prognostic variables in recurrent limb melanoma treated with hyperthermic antiblastic perfusion, *Cancer,* **63** (1989) 2551–2561.
19. Klaase JM, Kroon BBR, van Geel AN, et al. Limb recurrence-free interval and survival in patients with recurrent melanoma of the extremities treated with normothermic isolated perfusion, *J. Am. Coll. Surg.,* **178** (1994) 564–572.
20. Krementz ET, Carter RD, Sutherland CM, Muchmore JH, Ryan RF, and Creech O. Regional chemotherapy for melanoma. A 35-year experience, *Ann. Surg.,* **220** (1994) 520–535.
21. Bryant PJ, Balderson GA, Mead P, and Egerton WS. Hyperthermic isolated limb perfusion for malignant melanoma: response and survival, *World J. Surg.,* **19** (1995) 363–368.

22. Omlor G, Gross G, Ecker KW, Burger I, and Feifel G. Optimization of isolated hyperthermic limb perfusion, *World J. Surg.,* **16** (1992) 1117–1119.
23. Cavaliere R, Ciocatto EC, Giovanella BC, et al. Selective heat sensitivity of cancer cells: biochemical and clinical studies, *Cancer,* **20** (1967) 1351–1381.
24. Creech O, Krementz ET, Ryan RF, and Winblad JN. Chemotherapy of cancer: regional perfusion utilizing an extracorporeal circuit, *Ann. Surg.,* **148** (1958) 616–632.
25. Eggermont AMM. Treatment of melanoma in-transit metastases confined to the limb, *Cancer Surveys,* **26** (1996) 335–349.
26. Stehlin JS Jr, Giovanella BC, de Ipolyi PD, and Anderson RF. Eleven years' experience with hyperthermic perfusion for melanoma of the extremities, *World J. Surg.,* **3** (1979) 305–307.
27. Vaglini M, Ammatuna M, Nava M, et al. Regional perfusion at high temperature in the treatment of stage IIIA-IIIAB melanoma patients, *Tumori,* **69** (1983) 585–588.
28. Klaase JM, Kroon BBR, Eggermont AMM, et al. Retrospective comparative study evaluating the results of mild hyperthermic versus controlled normothermic perfusion for recurrent melanoma of the extremities, *Eur. J. Cancer,* **31A** (1995) 58–63.
29. Kroon BBR, van Geel AN, Benckhuijsen C, and Wieberdink J. Normothermic isolation perfusion with melphalan for advanced melanoma of the limbs, *Anticancer Res.,* **7** (1987) 441–442.
30. Kroon BB, Klaase JM, van Geel BN, Eggermont AM, Franklin HR, and van Dongen JA. Results of a double perfusion schedule with melphalan in patients with melanoma of the lower limb, *Eur. J. Cancer,* **29A** (1993) 325–328.
31. Storm FK and Morton DL. Value of hyperthermic limb perfusion in advanced recurrent melanoma of the lower extremity, *Am. J. Surg.,* **150** (1985) 32–35.
32. Bulman AS and Jamieson CW. Isolated limb perfusion with melphalan in the treatment of malignant melanoma, *Br. J. Surg.,* **67** (1980) 660–662.
33. Skene AI, Bulman AS, Williams TR, Meirion Thomas J, and Westbury G. Hyperthermic isolated perfusion with melphalan in the treatment of advanced malignant melanoma of the lower limb, *Br. J. Surg.,* **77** (1990) 765–767.
34. Minor DR, Allen RE, Alberts D, Peng Y-M, Tardelli G, and Hutchinson J. Clinical and pharmacokinetic study of isolated limb perfusion with heat and melphalan for melanoma, *Cancer,* **55** (1985) 2638–2644.
35. Lienard D, Lejeune FJ, and Ewalenko P. In transit metastases of malignant melanoma treated by high dose rTNF alpha in combination with interferon gamma and melphalan in isolation perfusion, *World J. Surg.,* **16** (1992) 234–240.
36. Fraker DL, Alexander HR, Andrich M, and Rosenberg SA. Treatment of patients with melanoma of the extremity using hyperthermic isolated limb perfusion with melphalan, tumor necrosis factor, and interferon gamma: results of a tumor necrosis factor dose-escalation study, *J. Clin. Oncol.,* **14** (1996) 479–489.
37. Thompson JF, Hunt JA, Shannon KF, Colman MH, and Kam PCA. Frequency and duration of complete remission after therapeutic isolated limb perfusion for melanoma, *Melanoma Res.,* **7(Suppl 1)** (1997) S33.
38. Luck JM. Action of p[Di(2-chlorethyl)]-amino-L-phenylalanine on Harding-Passey mouse melanoma, *Science,* **123** (1956) 984–983.
39. Byrne DS, McKay AJ, Blackie R, and MacKie RM. Comparison of dosimetric methods in isolated limb perfusion with melphalan for malignant melanoma of the lower extremity, *Eur. J. Cancer,* **32A** (1996) 2082–2087.
40. Klaase JM, Kroon BBR, van Geel AN, Eggermont AMM, Franklin HR, and van Dongen JA. Retrospective comparative study evaluating the results of a single-perfusion versus double-perfusion schedule with melphalan in patients with recurrent melanoma of the lower limb, *Cancer,* **71** (1993) 2990–2994.
41. Fletcher WS, Pommier R, and Small K. Results of cisplatin hyperthermic isolation perfusion for stage IIIA and IIIAB extremity melanoma, *Melanoma Res.,* **4** (1994) 17–19.
42. Coit DG, Bajoran DF, and Menendez-Botet C. Phase I trial of hyperthermic isolation limb perfusion (HILP) using cisplatin (CDDP) for metastatic melanoma, *Proc. Am. Soc. Clin. Oncol.,* **10** (1991) 294.
43. Hoekstra HJ, Schraffordt Koops HS, de Vries LG, van Weerden TW, and Oldhoff J. Toxicity of hyperthermic isolated limb perfusion with cisplatin for recurrent melanoma of the lower extremity after previous perfusion treatment, *Cancer,* **72** (1993) 1224–1229.
44. Thompson JF and Gianoutsos MP. Isolated limb perfusion for melanoma: effectiveness and toxicity of cisplatin compared with that of melphalan and other drugs, *World J. Surg.,* **16** (1992) 227–233.
45. Santinami M, Belli F, Cascinelli N, et al. Seven years experience with hyperthermic perfusions in extracorporeal circulation for melanoma of the extremities, *J. Surg. Oncol.,* **42** (1989) 201–208.

46. Anderson CM, Buzaid AC, and Legha SS. Systemic treatments for advanced cutaneous melanoma, *Oncology* 9 (1995) 1149–1158.

47. Vaglini M, Belli F, Marolda R, Prada A, Santinami M, and Cascinelli N. Hyperthermic antiblastic perfusion with DTIC in stage IIIA-IIIAB melanoma of the extremities, *Eur. J. Surg. Oncol.*, **13** (1987) 127–129.

48. Aigner K, Hild P, Henneking K, Paul E, and Hundeiker M. Regional perfusion with cis-platinum and dacarbzine, *Recent Res. Cancer Res.*, **86** (1983) 239–245.

49. Didolkar MS, Viens ML, Suter CM, and Buda B. Phase II study on isolation perfusion with DTIC (imidazole carboxamide) in stage IIIA-IIIAB melanoma of the extremity, *Proc. Am. Soc. Clin. Oncol.*, **9** (1990) 276.

50. Martijn H, Oldhoff J, and Koops HS. Hyperthermic regional perfusion with melphalan and a combination of melphalan and actinomycin D in the treatment of locally metastasized malignant melanomas of the extremities, *J. Surg. Oncol.*, **20** (1982) 9–13.

51. Lejeune FJ. High dose recombinant tumour necrosis factor (rTNFα) administered by isolation perfusion for advanced tumours of the limbs: a model for biochemotherapy of cancer, *Eur. J. Cancer*, **31A** (1995) 1009–1016.

52. Lejeune F, Lienard D, Schraffordt Koops H, Kroon B, and Eggermont A. Treatment of in-transit melanoma metastases with tumour necrosis factor (TNF-α) and chemotherapy administered in isolated limb perfusion (ILP), *Melanoma Res.*, **7** (1997) S48.

53. Old LJ. Tumor necrosis factor (TNF), *Science*, **230** (1985) 630–632.

54. Alexander RB and Rosenberg SA. Tumor necrosis factor: clinical implications, In DeVita VT, Hellman S, and Rosenberg SA, (eds), *Biologic Therapy of Cancer*, Lippincott, Philadelphia, 1991, pp. 378–392.

55. Posner M, Lienard D, Lejeune F, Rosenfelder D, and Kirkwood J. Hyperthermic isolated limb perfusion (HILP) with tumor necrosis factor (TNF) alone for metastatic in transit melanoma, *Proc. Am. Soc. Clin. Oncol.*, **13** (1994) 396.

56. Lienard D, Ewalenko P, Delmotte JJ, Renard N, and Lejeune FJ. High doses recombinant tumor necrosis factor alpha in combination with interferon gamma and melphalan in isolation perfusion of the limbs for melanoma and sarcoma, *J. Clin. Oncol.*, **10** (1992) 52–60.

57. Niitsu Y, Watanabe N, Umeno H, et al. Synergistic effects of recombinant human tumor necrosis factor and hyperthermia on *in vitro* cytotoxicity and artificial metastasis, *Cancer Res.*, **48** (1988) 654–657.

58. Watanabe N, Niitsu Y, Umeno H, et al. Synergistic cytotoxic and antitumor effects of recombinant human tumor necrosis factor and hyperthermia, *Cancer Res.*, **48** (1988) 650–653.

59. Balkwill F, Lee A, Aklom G, et al. Human tumor xenografts treated with recombinant human tumor necrosis factor alone or in combination with interferons, *Cancer Res.*, **46** (1986) 3990–3993.

60. Fiers W, Brouckaert P, and Guisez Y. Recombinant interferon gamma and its synergism with tumor necrosis factor in the human and mouse systems, In Schellekens H, Stewart WE, (eds), *Biology of the Interferon System*, Elsevier, Amsterdam, (1986) 241–248.

61. Gerain J, Lienard D, Ewalenko P, and Lejeune FJ. High serum levels of the TNF-alpha after its administration for isolation perfusion of the limb, *Cytokine*, **4** (1992) 585–591.

62. Eggimann P, Chiolero R, Chassot PG, Lienard D, Gerain J, and Lejeune F. Systemic and hemodynamic effects of recombinant tumor necrosis factor alpha in isolation perfusion of the limbs, *Chest*, **107** (1995) 1074–1082.

63. Bone RC, Balk RA, Cerra FB, et al. Definitions for sepsis and organ failure and guidelines for the use of innovative therapies in sepsis, *Chest*, **101** (1992) 1644–1655.

64. Bartlett DL, Ma G, Alexander HR, Libutti SK, and Fraker DL. Isolated limb reperfusion with tumor necrosis factor and melphalan in patients with extremity melanoma after failure of isolated limb perfusion with chemotherapeutics, *Cancer*, **80** (1997) 2084–2090.

65. Fraker DL. What is the best regional therapy? *Melanoma Res.*, **7** (1997) S42.

66. McBride CM, Sugarbaker EV, and Hickey RC. Prophylactic isolation-perfusion as the primary therapy for invasive malignant melanoma of the limbs, *Ann. Surg.*, **182** (1975) 316–324.

67. Edwards MJ, Soong SJ, Boddie AW, Balch CM, and McBride CM. Isolated limb perfusion for localized melanoma of the extremity, *Arch. Surg.*, **125** (1990) 317–321.

68. Franklin HR, Koops HS, Oldhoff J, et al. To perfuse or not to perfuse? A retrospective comparative study to evaluate the effect of adjuvant isolated regional perfusion in patients with stage I extremity melanoma with a thickness of 1.5 mm or greater, *J. Clin. Oncol.*, **6** (1988) 701.

69. Ghussen F, Kruger I, Groth W, and Stutzer H. Role of regional hyperthermic cytostatic perfusion in the treatment of extremity melanoma, *Cancer*, **61** (1988) 654–659.

70. Fenn NJ, Horgan K, Johnson RC, Hughes LE, and Mansel RE. Randomized controlled trial of prophylactic isolated cytotoxic perfusion for poor-prognosis primary melanoma of the lower limb, *Eur. J. Surg. Oncol.,* **23** (1997) 6–9.

71. Schraffordt Koops H, Vaglini M, Kroon BBR, et al. Value of prophylactic isolated limb perfusion (ILP) for stage I high risk malignant melanoma: a randomized phase III trial, *Melanoma Res.,* **7(Suppl 1)** (1997) S34.

72. Hafstrom L, Rudenstam CM, Blomquist E, et al. Regional hyperthermic perfusion with melphalan after surgery for recurrent malignant melanoma of the extremities, *J. Clin. Oncol.,* **9** (1991) 2091–2094.

73. Gohl J, Meyer TH, and Hohenberger W. Hyperthermic isolated limb perfusion (HILP): a therapeutic concept in locoregional metastasized malignant melanoma. Experiences over 20 years, *Melanoma Res.,* **7(Suppl 1)** (1997) S101.

74. Krementz ET and Ryan RF. Chemotherapy of melanoma of the extremities by perfusion: fourteen years of clinical experience, *Ann. Surg.,* **175** (1972) 900–917.

75. Rosin RD and Westbury G. Isolated limb perfusion for malignant melanoma, *Practitioner,* **224** (1980) 1031–1036.

76. Taber SW and Polk HC. Mortality, major amputation rates, and leukopenia after isolated limb perfusion with phenylalanine mustard for the treatment of melanoma, *Ann. Surg. Oncol.,* **4** (1997) 440–445.

77. Vrouenraets BC, Klaase JM, Kroon BBR, van Geel BN, Eggermont AMM, and Franklin HR. Long-term morbidity after regional isolated perfusion with melphalan for melanoma of the limbs, *Arch. Surg.,* **130** (1995) 43–47.

78. Schraffordt Koops H. Prevention of neural and muscular lesions during hyperthermic regional perfusion, *Surg. Gynecol. Obstet.,* **135** (1972) 401–403.

79. Olieman AF, Schraffordt Koops H, Geertzen JH, Kingma H, Hoekstra HJ, and Oldhoff J. Functional morbidity of hyperthermic isolated regional perfusion of the extremities, *Ann. Surg. Oncol.,* **1** (1994) 382–388.

80. Vrouenraets BC, in't Veld GJ, Nieweg OE, van Slooten GW, van Dongen JA, and Kroon BBR. Long-term functional morbidity after mild hyperthermic isolated limb perfusion (ILP) with melphalan, *Melanoma Res.,* **7(Suppl 1)** (1997) S122.

81. van Geel AN, van Wijk J, and Wieberdink J. Functional morbidity after regional isolated perfusion of the limb for melanoma, *Cancer,* **63** (1989) 1092–1096.

82. Harman CR, Thompson JF, Hunt JA, Waugh RC, and Kam PC. Isolated limb infusion with cytotoxic agents for recurrent limb melanoma: results of 120 procedures, *Melanoma Res.,* **7(Suppl 1)** (1997) S111.

83. Thompson JF, Kam PCA, Waugh RC, and Harman CR. Isolated limb infusion with cytotoxic agents: a simple alternative to isolated limb perfusion, *Sem. Surg. Oncol.,* **14** (1998) 238–247.

5 Isolated Limb Perfusion for Malignant Melanoma and Soft Tissue Sarcoma

Joseph M. Klausner, Dina Lev-Chelouche, Subhi Abu-Abeid, and Mordechai Gutman

CONTENTS

1. INTRODUCTION

In 1958, Creech et al. *(1)* introduced a novel method of drug delivery in advanced cancer, and named it isolated limb perfusion (ILP). The idea was to use the newly invented technique of cardiopulmonary bypass, which at that time had paved the way for open-heart surgery, in regional chemotherapy. They described a surgical method of exposing the major blood vessels of an extremity, providing its temporary isolation, and permitting perfusion of that extremity via the heart–lung machine, utilizing high doses of chemotherapeutic drugs. It would be possible to obtain high tissue concentrations of the drug with minimal systemic exposure and complications. Following the observation that heat on its own has antineoplastic properties *(2)*, in 1969, Stehlin *(3)* modified the technique to include hyperthermia. Since then, ILP with melphalan, more than any other drug, has been widely recognized as the standard treatment strategy for advanced extremity melanoma.

Because almost half of melanomas originate in the extremities, and 10–20% of recurrences or metastases are local-regional and confined to the limb, a large number of patients become candidates for ILP. The high response rates observed, far better than with any other known modality besides amputation, and the fact that about 25% of complete responders have a 10-yr disease-free interval, promoted the use of ILP with melphalan. However, ILP did not become a widely used procedure, and several major cancer centers did not include it in their therapeutic arsenal. There are several reasons for this: ILP is a multidisciplinary procedure that is surgically demanding,

From: *Current Clinical Oncology: Regional Chemotherapy: Clinical Research and Practice*
Edited by: M. Markman © Humana Press Inc., Totowa, NJ

rather long (3–4 h), necessitating a heart–lung machine (and related technician and equipment) isotopic monitoring, and, of course, valuable operating room time. Unlike the reasonable ease with which new operative techniques are implemented through the acquisition of knowledge and skills, ILP requires knowledge of vascular surgery, a field with which most surgical oncologists are unfamiliar, and a large degree of coordination and dependence on other disciplines outside the realm of general surgery. In addition, the available literature on ILP showed great variability in surgical technique, drugs administered, degree of hyperthermia, indications, and response evaluation. Coupled with the retrospective nature of most reported patient series, it was not easy to reach valid conclusions as to when and how to implement ILP. Its wide application was therefore withheld by some major cancer centers.

The situation has gradually changed, chiefly because of two advances. The standardization of ILP and the organization of multicenter studies, with results according to modern surgical oncology and National Cancer Institute (NCI) principles, from dose-escalation to phase III studies, allowed valid result evaluation, and hence better definition of the indications for ILP. The second advance was the addition of tumor necrosis factor (TNF) to the treatment protocols *(4)*. Not only is TNF a new drug, but its potentially serious side effects necessitated modifications to the ILP technique, in order to effect better isolation. All centers introduced routine isotopic leakage monitoring. Being an exciting new cytokine, TNF therapy caused worldwide interest and inspired numerous preclinical research projects.

2. TECHNICAL CONSIDERATIONS FOR ILP

2.1. Preparations

The patient must be a suitable candidate for ILP. When the perfusion is planned for curative intent, a metastatic workup, to rule out evidence of disease outside the extremity, is indicated. When planned for palliation, a metastatic tumor outside the perfusion field is acceptable, as long as the extent of disease and patient condition did not preclude reasonable survival.

The tumor to be perfused should be confined to the limb, and not extend to the groin or axillary areas. These areas, as well as the proximal posterior thigh, the buttocks, and the upper posterior arm, are relatively poorly perfused, even with proximal vessel cannulation.

Ulcerated or infected tumors should be recognized as a septic risk. The existing bacterial colonization may turn into overt sepsis or abscess formation, following the induction of rapid necrosis with TNF or chemotherapy. Repeat cultures and preoperative antibiotics are routinely required.

Irradiated tissues at the root of the limb may impair the adequacy of complete isolation, because these tissues are less flexible and compressible, and the surgeon may find it difficult to apply an Esmark (Esmark, Degania Silicon, Israel) rubber band under such conditions.

Patient evaluation and preparation should be as for any major surgical procedure. Specific attention must be given to the peripheral vascular system. Complaints, or findings suggestive of peripheral vascular disease, may require further evaluation by angiography. Patients with severe arteriosclerotic disease, especially those with nonpalpable distal pulses, are usually not suitable candidates for ILP *(5)*.

Evaluation of the venous system for deep vein thrombosis (DVT) by ultrasound Doppler is also important. It is mandatory if there is unexplained limb edema, particularly in patients who have undergone prior surgery or ILP to the affected limb. Because the

Table 1
Site Distribution of 228 Limb Perfusions[*a]

Perfusion site	Melanoma (122)	Sarcoma (106)
Lower limb	89	88
Iliac	61	47
Femoral	18	22
Popliteal	10	19
Upper limb	33	18
Subclavian	24	11
Brachial	9	7

[a]Author series 1990–1998.

adequacy of perfusion depends on the patency and return of the venous system, patients with DVT are poor candidates for ILP. Patients with severe lymphedema of the limb are also considered unsuitable candidates for ILP.

Finally, the neurological status of the limb should be carefully recorded, particularly in patients with prior surgery, radiotherapy (RT), or tumors adjacent to nerves. Limb volume should be measured or calculated, because the drug dosage used during ILP is based on the volume of the extremity *(6)*. Limb volume can be measured using the water displacement method, in which the extremity is immersed in a calibrated cylinder filled with water. Alternatively, it can be calculated by measuring limb length and circumference at multiple points, and incorporating them into a mathematical formula used for calculating the volume of a cylinder. Finally, the patient should be informed of the procedure, and the short- and particularly the long-term related complications.

2.2. Selection of Procedure

ILP can be performed through various sites (Table 1): for the lower limb, via the external iliac, common femoral, or popliteal vessels; for the upper limb, via the brachial, axillary, and subclavian vessels. The level of perfusion should be based on the nature and extent of the tumor, and on technical considerations, such as prior surgery or RT. A principal decision prior to ILP is, therefore, the level at which the vessels are to be cannulated.

The most common perfusion is via the external iliac vessels, because the majority of candidates are melanoma patients in whom the lower limb is more commonly affected. As a rule, for melanoma patients, the most proximal vessels are selected, because the entire limb is at risk, not only the overt in-transit metastases. External iliac and axillary perfusions are therefore the preferred sites. More distal vessels for ILP may be selected for melanoma patients, only when dissection of the proximal vessels is hazardous, such as for patients requiring a second or third ILP, or for those who have undergone extensive surgery or irradiation at the root of the limb.

For soft tissue sarcoma (STS) patients undergoing ILP, more distal sites for cannulation are chosen, just proximal to the tumor mass. Perfusions via the popliteal or brachial vessels are considered simpler, despite the smaller diameter of the vessels, because these vessels are usually accessible with less dissection, and facilitate the use of a tourniquet applied proximally on the thigh or arm, to ascertain complete isolation, with no systemic leakage.

2.2.1. Surgery

ILP entails major surgery, and is performed under endotracheal general anesthesia. Given the need for systemic heparinization, epidural or regional anesthesia are not recommended. The entire extremity is made sterile. Four thermistor probes are inserted, two into the subcutaneous (SC) tissue and two into the muscles, in the distal and proximal parts of the extremity, respectively, and hooked up to a multichannel temperature module, to measure limb temperature during the procedure. A heating blanket, with controlled, recirculating hot water, is wrapped around the whole limb to maintain temperature, and sterile draping is applied on top of it. It is important that the limb can be manipulated and positioned during the procedure, to permit the application and wrapping of the Esmark band on its root. For distal cannulations (popliteal/brachial), a pneumatic tourniquet is applied proximal to the operative site.

2.2.2. Lower Limb Perfusion (Fig. 1)

2.2.2.1. Iliac Perfusion. An oblique incision is made in the iliac region. The fascia and muscles are sectioned, and the retroperitoneum is entered. The peritoneum is retracted medially. After dissecting the external iliac vessels from their origin to the inguinal ligament, the vessels are dissected circumferentially, and all side branches, including collaterals situated behind the inguinal ligament, are sectioned and ligated— the epigastric, obturates, deep internal and external circumflex vessels. The origin of the internal iliac artery is dissected, in case clamping is necessary. The internal iliac vein site, and all branches, especially from the posterior aspect of the external iliac vein, should be ligated. These deep collaterals are not affected by external Esmark banding, and their control is crucial for minimizing leakage during perfusion. The patient is systematically heparinized (200 U/kg), and the vessels are cannulated. The external iliac vein is dealt with first. It is clamped proximally and distally, and a 16–24 French-long, straight venous cannula is inserted through a venotomy, with the tip in the proximal portion of the femoral vein, and its side holes well below the level of the Esmark band. A 12–18 French straight cannula is then inserted via a transverse arterioectomy in the external iliac artery, with the tip in the common femoral artery. The cannulae are fixed with laces, and connected to the extracorporeal pump.

To complete vascular isolation of the limb, a tourniquet made of an Esmark rubber band is tightened snugly around the root of the thigh. It is anchored laterally with the aid of Steinman (Steinman Pins, GmbH, Germany) pins inserted into the anterior superior iliac spine, and the inguinal crease secures the tourniquet medially. The tourniquet's role in blocking flow leakage through collaterals in the skin, sc tissues, and muscles is of major significance.

2.2.2.2. Femoral Perfusion. Through a groin incision, the common femoral artery and vein are dissected. The branches of the superficial epigastric, superficial, and deep circumflex iliac, and superficial external pudendal vessels should be divided and clamped, as should the lateral circumflex vessels originating from the proximal profunda. Cannulation of the vessels is performed just below the level of the inguinal ligament, so that both superficial and deep femoral systems are included in the perfusion. Tourniquet application is identical to the external iliac approach.

2.2.2.3. Popliteal Perfusion. Though a vertical incision in the medial aspect of the lower third of the thigh, the vessels are dissected and isolated at the point of which they emerge from the Hunter's canal. A proximal circumferential pneumatic tourniquet is applied proximally on the thigh, and inflated to 300–400 mmHg, to achieve complete isolation.

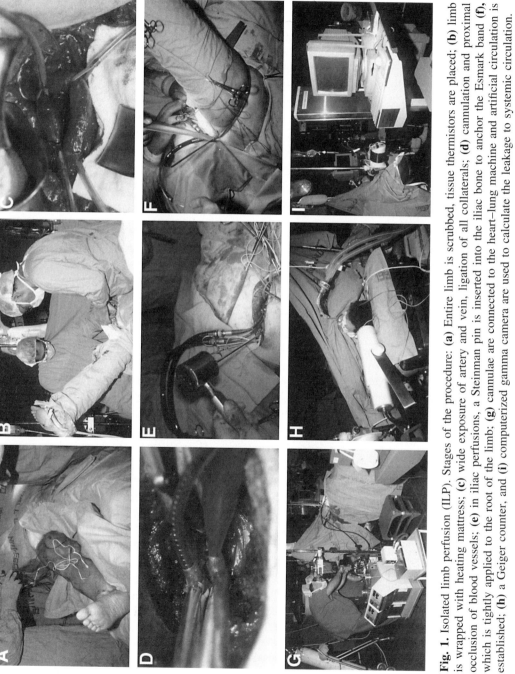

Fig. 1. Isolated limb perfusion (ILP). Stages of the procedure: **(a)** Entire limb is scrubbed, tissue thermistors are placed; **(b)** limb is wrapped with heating mattress; **(c)** wide exposure of artery and vein, ligation of all collaterals; **(d)** cannulation and proximal occlusion of blood vessels; **(e)** in iliac perfusions, a Steinman pin is inserted into the iliac bone to anchor the Esmark band **(f)**, which is tightly applied to the root of the limb; **(g)** cannulae are connected to the heart–lung machine and artificial circulation is established; **(h)** a Geiger counter, and **(i)** computerized gamma camera are used to calculate the leakage to systemic circulation.

61

2.2.3. UPPER LIMB PERFUSION

2.2.3.1. Axillary/Subclavian Perfusion. Through a subclavicular incision, the sternal and clavicular insertions of the pectoralis major are separated. The insertion of the pectoralis minor to the coracoid process is sectioned, exposing levels II and III of the axilla. The vessels are dissected circumferentially, and all collaterals are ligated and divided. The artery and vein are then clamped proximally, and cannulated (8–14 F). The tips of the cannulae are directed toward the proximal portion of the arm. An Esmark tourniquet is tightly wrapped around the root of the shoulder, and anchored with Steinman pins inserted in the humerus epiphysis. The smaller size of the shoulder, compared to the root of the lower limb, enables isolation and control to be achieved more easily.

2.2.3.2. Brachial Perfusion. This is performed through a vertical incision in the medial aspect of the arm. Smaller-sized cannulae, adjusted to the vessel size, are chosen. Minimal dissection and collateral ligation is required, because complete isolation is easily achieved with the aid of a small pneumatic (blood pressure) tourniquet applied proximally around the arm and inflated to 300 mmHg.

2.2.4. EXTRACORPOREAL CIRCULATION

The extracorporeal system consists of a roller pump, as used for cardiopulmonary bypass in cardiac surgery. Optimally, a single-head pump is necessary for ILP. The pediatric cardiac surgery disposable pack, with its smaller-sized oxygenator, venous reservoir, and tubing, is most suitable for ILP. A heat exchanger is required, to heat the perfusate to 42°C. Priming is with 700–1000 mL balanced electrolyte solution, 1 U packed red blood cells, and 1500 U heparin. Haemacel® (Hemacel, Hoechst, Switzerland) can be used to replace blood. The perfusion starts with flow rates of 30–50 mL/ L limb vol/min. This priming results in a hematocrit of ~25%, which provides adequate oxygenation. Mild hyperthermia (39–40°C) is usually used; true hyperthermia (41–42°C) is rarely used, because of severe limb toxicity. Limb temperature is increased both by heating the perfusate to 42°C, and by the application of the heated blanket draped around the limb. The temperature probes enable close monitoring.

The first stage of the ILP is devoted to heating and assessment of leakage. Significant time may be required to warm skin temperature to 39°C. Leakage from the isolated perfused limb is dependent on perfusion flow rate (7). The experience with traditional high perfusion flow rates of 700–1300 and 300–600 mL/min, for the lower and upper limbs, respectively, resulted in relatively high systemic leakage rates (12.5 ± 2.9%), and, consequently severe systemic toxicity. Decreasing the perfusion flow rate to 400–500 and 150–300 mL/min for the lower and upper limbs, respectively, reduced leakage, and, thus, the systemic toxic effects of TNF. Increased pressure may contribute to leakage by opening up and forcing blood flow through small collaterals in sc tissues, muscles, and vessels along the periosteum between the limb and systemic circulation. This is likely, with high flow rates inducing venous pressure in the perfused limb exceeding that of the sytemic pressure.

2.2.5. LEAKAGE MONITORING AND ADJUSTMENT

Perfusate leakage into the systemic circulation is continuously monitored. This was not considered routine prior to the TNF era, and surgeons tended to rely on stable reservoir volume and personal experience to estimate leakage. With the immediate threatening complications of TNF, leakage monitoring became crucial and mandatory. Protocols using microlabeled albumin on technicium-labeled red blood cells are used for monitoring leakage during ILP *(8,9)*. After establishing a stabilized perfusion, with stable flow rate and venous reservoir volume, the isotope is injected into the perfusate. A gamma camera is positioned over the precordial area or the head. Any increase in isotopic count against a stable background over the heart signifies a leak of perfusate to the systemic circulation. A leak of less than 1% can be detected, allowing rapid adjustments to limit side effects. Indications of leakage also include alterations in the calibrated venous reservoir volume, which drains the venous effluent by gravity. A decrease in reservoir volume indicates a leak from the perfused limb into the sytemic circulation; an increase in venous reservoir volume signifies a reverse leak from the systemic circulation into the limb.

With the information provided from continuous leakage monitoring and the volume of the venous reservoir, it is possible to manipulate the perfusion and minimize leakage. Rapid shifts in reservoir volume indicate a missed collateral. Rapid leakage also occurs when the cannula or its side holes are placed above the level of tourniquet. Under such circumstances, the pump should be turned off, and the operative field reexplored for identification and ligation of a missed collateral, respositioning of the cannulae, and readjustment of the tourniquet. Less-dramatic leakage can be manipulated by reapplication of the tourniquet or adjustment of the circuit flow pressure.

Leakage from the systemic circulation to the limb is less frequent, and can usually be dealt with by increasing flow rate or pressure. Systemic leaks of less than 2% can be achieved in almost 95% of patients *(7,9–10)*. This improvement in isolation techniques has made ILP a safe procedure. There is no longer a need for sophisticated, invasive systemic monitoring or intensive care, and patients are routinely transferred to the surgical ward 2–3 h following the procedure.

2.2.5. TERMINATION OF ILP

After drug administration and perfusion treatment, the circuit is interrupted, and the perfusate washed from the limb with 2 L saline and 1 L dextran polymer, or with blood. Following the washout, the pump is turned off, the tourniquet cuff is deflated, and the cannulae are removed. The vein is first repaired, then the arteriotomy is sutured, reestablishing blood flow to the limb.

3. DRUGS

3.1. Melphalan

This alkylating agent, a phenylalanine mustard, was originally selected for melanoma perfusion because phenylalanine is an essential precursor in melanin synthesis, and is taken up preferentially by melanocytes.

Melphalan is an ideal drug for ILP, possessing short half-life, low endothelial toxicity, limited cell-cycle specificity, and a relatively linear dose–response relationship for cytotoxicity *(11)*. Based on their experimental work in dogs, Creech et al. *(1)* initially used melphalan in ILP at a dose of 2 mg/kg body wt. After the addition of hyperthermia, the dose was reduced to 1–1.5 mg/kg for lower limb and 0.4–1 mg/kg for upper limb perfusion *(12)*. Currently, most centers administer melphalan adjusted to the volume of the extremity to be perfused *(13)*. Based on this dosing regimen, the optimal dose of melphalan, resulting in reversible grades 2–3 limb toxicity, is 10 mg/L limb vol for the lower extremity. A higher melphalan concentration of 13 mL/L limb vol is tolerated by, and routinely used for, upper limb perfusion. At such dosages, perfusate concentrations of melphalan are 50–100-fold higher than systemic levels, which remain less than 1 µg/mL *(14)*.

The pharmokinetics of melphalan in the perfusion circuit show it to have a biphasic disappearance curve, with a half-life in the range of 5–12 min for the first phase and 20–50 min for the second *(15)*. The initial disappearance is probably caused by its rapid uptake by the extremity's tissues, and the latter from its hydrolysis. Because of the rapid distribution of melphalan into tissue, it has been suggested that the usual perfusion time of 60 min could be reduced without hampering its therapeutic effect. However, this does not take into consideration the time needed for melphalan transportation from the extra- to intracellular compartments prior to washout at the end of ILP *(13)*. It is estimated that approx 25–40% of the administered dose of melphalan is distributed into the tissues.

Given its high response rate (60–80%), with a complete response (CR) of 30–55% in melanoma patients undergoing ILP *(16–19)*, and given the chemoresistant nature of melanoma, it is not surprising that melphalan is considered the drug of choice for this procedure.

3.2. Other Cytotoxic Drugs

Other chemotherapeutic agents, including cisplatin, cisplatin and ethopuside, melphalan and actinomycin, and dacarbazine (DTIC), have been tested in the ILP setup, but none have demonstrated better results than melphalan in animal models or humans *(3,20,21,25)*. Cisplatin appears to be a suitable agent for isolated perfusion, because its concentration in tumor tissue seems to be selectively increased in the presence of mild hyperthermia, and significant tumor levels can be achieved with relatively short exposure. Although cisplatin ILP can result in overall response rates greater than 50% in melanoma, the duration of response is typically short-lived, with a median time to recurrence of 5 mo. The primary concern is its considerable regional toxicity, especially neurotoxicity, which limits its usage.

Doxorubicin (DOX) was also investigated in the ILP setting *(26,27)*, mostly for nonresectable STS, but was found ineffective when used alone or in combination with melphalan. No CRs were observed, the recurrence rate after delayed resection was high, and, most importantly, regional toxicity was unacceptable, with amputation rates reaching 40% in perfused patients.

3.3. Tumor Necrosis Factor

Tumor necrosis factor-α (TNF-α) was discovered in 1975, following the observation that intratumoral bacille Calmette-Guérin vaccine inoculations in metastatic melanoma nodules produced temporary tumor regression in immunocompetent animals and humans *(28)*. This regression has been correlated with a serum factor, later identified as TNF-α, produced by activated macrophages.

In 1985, the human TNF-α gene was cloned and expressed in *Escherichia coli*, and rTNF-α was made available for clinical usage *(29)*. TNF-α is able to produce very fast and effective necrosis of tumors *(3,30)*, as was demonstrated in a variety of tumor bearing mice and cultured cancer cells. However, attempts to clinically implement it in humans failed. Only anecdotal cases of partial response (PR) were described, from more than 800 cancer patients treated systemically with rTNF-α *(32–34)*. This failure was attributed to the inability to administer sufficient doses of TNF, because of life-threatening side effects *(31–35)*. The rTNF-α dose required to achieve the antitumor effect, based on data from murine tumor models, is 10–20× higher than the systemic maximal tolerated dose (MTD) in humans, (approx 200 μg/m²). Shortly after administration, higher doses result in a state mimicking the hemodynamics typically associated with septic shock: tachycardia, hypotension, decreased vascular resistance, increased cardiac index, as well as coagulopathy, thrombocytopenia, and metabolic impairment, such as increased bilirubin and liver enzymes, and decreased cholesterol levels, gradually leading to multiorgan failure *(35–37)*.

The novel idea of using rTNF-α in the ILP setting enables the dosage and systemic complications barrier to be overcome. The high dose of rTNF-α given via ILP (3–4 mg) was chosen by Lejeune *(38)* for two reasons. Historically, chemotherapeutic drug doses used in ILP have been approx 10× the MTD. Therefore, relative to the MTD dose of TNF (200 μg/m²), a 10-fold increase would result in a 4-mg dose. Furthermore, the limb isolation results in less than 10% systemic leakage, which itself is less than the MTD.

Higher TNF doses have not shown improved tumor response rates. A trial of TNF dose escalation demonstrated a dose-limiting regional toxicity at 6 mg, with response rates lower than those obtained with the 4-mg dose *(39)*. On the other hand, a much lower dose of rTNF-α (125–150 μg) was shown to induce a high CR rate of 100% *(40)*, but this was observed only in nine patients, and, for some unexplained reason, caused a high rate of regional toxicity, and thus a relatively low limb salvage rate. It should be noted, however, that lowering the TNF dose is no longer an objective, because the chief reason was to significantly improve systemic complications, and these have now been virtually prevented with improved isolation and monitoring. Nevertheless, defining the exact TNF dosage required for a maximal anticancer effect may be important in other settings, such as isolated hepatic or isolated lung perfusions.

Pharmacokinetic studies of rTNF-α in ILP demonstrate high plateaus of 1.5–2 μg/ml, with no decay attributable to degradation *(41)*. Thus, rTNF-α at a high concentration appears to be more stable, compared to the short half-life with systemic administration. The bypass in the liver during ILP may contribute to this stability.

TNF experts its antineoplastic effect through a variety of mechanisms. It has a direct cytolytic effect on several cancer cell lines *(30,42)*. The administration of TNF in vivo involves secondary mechanisms, because it induces the generation of many cytokines and mediators, such as interleukin (IL)-1, IL-6, IL-8, Interferon (IFN), oxgen free radicals, and arachidonic acid products, some of which have a definite anticancer effect *(36,43)*.

Observations in the sarcoma perfusion model in rats strongly suggest that neutrophils play a central role, because much of the TNF antitumor effect is lost in neutropenic rats *(44,45)*. Migration of leukocytes to the tumor may lead to adhesion to endothelium; to the release of oxygen free radicals, elastase, and other cytokines; and to an extensive local inflammatory reaction, and endothelial damage. This may result in tumor capillary bed destruction and hemorrhagic necrosis.

The most pronounced effect of TNF in vivo is attributed to its effect on the tumor's vasculature *(33,46,47)*. Using its procoagulant properties, TNF suppresses specific adhesion molecules, such as integrin-αVβ₃, on the surface of endothelial cells within the tumor and membranal receptors on macrophages and leukocytes *(48,49)*. Antagonists of αVβ₃ interfere with adhesion-dependent signals, causing apoptosis of angiogenic endothelial cells. This TNF-induced endothelial damage is exclusive to tumor vasculature, and normal vasculature is spared *(32,43,46)*. This is consistently demonstrated in angiograms performed in sarcoma patients before and after ILP–TNF (Fig. 2).

Nevertheless, the administration of TNF alone, as demonstrated in mouse tumor models and human tumor xenografts in nude mice, and in a pilot study in six patients,

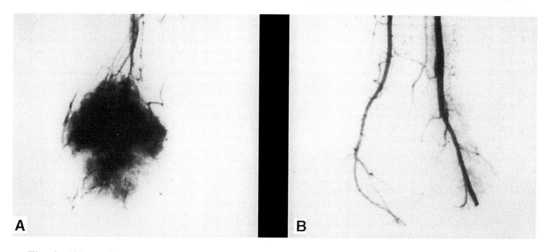

Fig. 2. (A) Angiogram performed before ILP in a patient with synovial sarcoma. Note the high vascularization of the tumor. **(B)** Ten d after ILP, the tumor vasculature has vanished, but normal vessels remained intact. *Cancer,* Vol. 79, 1997, pp. 1129–1137. Copyright © (1997) American Cancer Society. Reprinted with permission of Wiley-Liss, Inc., a subsidiary of John Wiley & Sons, Inc.

has only a transient antitumor effect, because there is regrowth of the tumor after its necrosis *(50)*. The addition of a cytotoxic drug is therefore mandatory for achieving a high and prolonged response rate. It has been speculated that, by damaging the tumor's vasculature, TNF increases microvascular permeability, thereby enhancing melphalan's penetration into the tumor *(51)*. This is, however, in contradiction to the observation that the increased diffusability through the tumor vasculature is unaffected by TNF, and that melphalan levels are comparable in tumor tissue with or without TNF *(52)*. What has been unequivocally demonstrated, in in vitro and in vivo studies, is a clear synergism between TNF and various cytotoxic drugs and hyperthermia *(53,54)*.

3.4. Other Cytokines

Interferon-γ (IFN-γ) has been shown to upregulate and increase the number of TNF-α receptors on malignant cells, which is an effect that has been shown in tumor cell cultures and human melanoma xenografts *(55)*. In addition, a synergistic antiproliferative activity of rTNF-α and IFN-γ and -α has been demonstrated in vitro and in vivo using human melanoma xenografts in nude mice *(56)*.

The highest tumor response rates have been achieved with the triple combination of TNF, melphalan, and IFN-γ, given both systemically and to the perfusate *(53)*. However, a comparative study with or without IFN-γ failed to demonstrate a significant improvement with IFN-γ *(10)*. Further studies are required to address the potential of IFN-γ.

IL-2 and lymphokine-activated killer cells administered via ILP and systemically postperfusion resulted in one short-lived (2 mo) CR and four PR (two short-lived) in six patients with extremity melanoma *(58)*. This study is too small to draw conclusions.

3.5. Hyperthermia

The fact that heat is effective against cancer and tumor growth has been known since the middle of the nineteenth century. A clinical trial demonstrated a good tumor response to isolation perfusion with a heated perfusate without cytotoxic drugs *(3)*. Based on this work, heat was added to the melphalan perfusion sytem, in the belief that hyperthermic melphalan perfusion is superior to normothermic ILP *(59)*. The

Table 2
Regional Toxicity: Weiberdink Classification

Wieberdink classification (grade)	Degree of Toxicity
I	No reaction.
II	Slight erythema/edema.
III	Considerable erythema/edema with some blistering. Slightly disturbed motility.
IV	Extensive epidermolysis and/or obvious damage to the deep tissues, causing definite functional disturbances; threatening or established compartmental syndrome.
V	Reaction that may necessitate amputation.

value of hyperthermia has been subjected to enormous experimental research that demonstrated a few possible mechanisms *(60–61)*. True hyperthermia (>41°C), decreases tissue pH and aerobic glycolysis, induces cycling of tumor cells, and changes the proportion of cells in the sensitive S and M phases. Cell membranes become more sensitive to active agents, rendering the tumor cells more vulnerable to cytotoxic drugs. There is an apparent decrease in DNA repair, possibly because of the development of oxygen-free radicals, which cause strand breaks in the DNA.

Hyperthermia appears to enhance both the antitumoral effect of TNF and melphalan *(62)*. However, true hyperthermia, exceeding 42°C, cannot be used in ILP, because of severe regional toxicity *(63)*. Mild hyperthermic conditions (39–40°C), commonly used, are still considered synergistic to melphalan and TNF, but without increasing the regional toxicity.

4. COMPLICATIONS OF ILP

Healing of the ILP wound is adversely affected by regional node dissection, when added to the procedure. The incidence of wound infection, seromas, and prolonged lymph drainage occur more frequently with lymph node dissection in conjunction with ILP. More importantly, long term lymphedema occurs more commonly *(63,64)*.

4.1. Regional Toxicity

The Wieberdink grading system of the regional toxic effect of ILP *(6)* is routinely used (Table 2). Mild edema, erythema, discomfort, and a warm limb (grade I) commonly develop within 2–3 d following ILP. Moderate to severe toxicity (grades III–IV) is not uncommon, and occurs in 15–30% of patients. Areas of the skin may develop blisters, particularly on the palms of the hand and soles of the feet. Only rarely is full-thickness loss encountered *(63,95)*. Pain and significant discomfort occur in 25–40% of patients, and are probably related to muscle swelling, compartmental syndrome, and direct neurotoxocity. Limb-threatening complications, with extensive tissue injury and severe edema, sometimes indicating compartmental syndrome, is uncommon, and occurs in less than 10% of patients. Limb loss is rare (0.5–1.5%), but is inevitably described in large series of ILP patients *(63,95)*.

Most of the complications following ILP resolve spontaneously within 2–3 wk. The redness may fade only partially and turn to brown, so that the limb may appear hyperpigmented. The blisters on the skin become dry. Inhibition of hair growth and temporary nail loss may occur.

In the vast majority experiencing grades II–III toxicity, the long-term functional sequelae of ILP are minimal. However, following moderate-to-severe toxicity (grades IV–V), the overall long-term limb dysfunction rate is 15–42% *(63,66)*. Lymphedema, often related to the addition of node dissection during ILP, is the most common (20–30%) complication, and is more often noted in the lower limb. Muscle atrophy, mobility restriction mostly caused by ankylosis of the ankle, is encountered in 15% of patients after grade IV–V toxicity. Chronic pain is also a long-term troublesome sequela in 2–4% of patients.

Some contributing factors correlate with regional toxicity, and can sometimes be manipulated for prevention. The toxicity is closely related to the melphalan peak concentration in the perfusate *(63,67,68)*, which only obviates the need to adjust the dosage according to limb volume, and to standardize circuit-priming volume, because it directly affects drug concentrations in the perfusate.

In the authors' experience, and in that of others, the addition of TNF-α to melphalan does not appear to increase regional toxicity *(4,69)*. Other groups *(70)* reported that the rapid onset, severity, and duration of limb toxicity are more prominent with TNF-α added to melphalan. Also, during a phase I study *(71)*, escalating the dose of TNF-α to 6 mg, combined with melphalan, induced severe muscle and nerve toxicity, but TNF alone elicited no regional toxicity. It is, therefore, possible that, combined with melphalan, TNF is more deleterious to the limb, compared to melphalan perfusion. This must be studied and confirmed prospectively.

With true hyperthermia (>42°C) the incidence of limb-threatening complications and loss was so high that, despite impressive tumor responses, it was abandoned *(63,65,68,72)*.

Reduced oxygenation and low pH during ILP augment local toxicity, and should be avoided. When the distal part of the limb is unaffected by tumor, it can be protected from degeneration, epidermolysis, and nail loss of the sole or palm, by wrapping the foot or hand with an Esmark band prior to injecting the drugs into the perfusate.

Compartmental syndrome and muscle damage is uncommon, but are probably underestimated because of subclinical forms *(63)*. Monitoring of compartmental pressure is rarely performed. The monitoring of serum creatine kinase, in addition to circumference measurements of the limb, clearly adds to the early diagnosis of severe toxicity *(73)*. Creatine kinase values exceeding 1000 U/L are highly indicative of severe toxicity. Prophylactic fasciotomy is rarely performed, and is indicated only after very complicated ILP, with vascular problems, prolonged ischemia, or impaired venous return.

Regional toxicity and long term complications are also more common and pronounced following double ILP (with an interval of a few weeks) or repeat ILP *(63,74)*.

Nerve toxicity, manifested by shooting pain or parathesias, occurs relatively late: 2–3 wk after ILP in 25–40% of patients. It usually resolves within a few months. Long-term neuropathy is considered more rare (1–4% in most series), but, with close follow-up and attention, it is recorded in as high as 48% of patients *(63,75)*. Such neuropathy may result from a direct neurotoxic effect of melphalan or cisplatin, or secondary to prolonged pressure induced by compartmental syndrome. However, neurological evaluation with the aid of electromyography usually attributes the neural damage to local pressure caused by an overtight tourniquet. Unfortunately, long-term or permanent nerve damage is more common in the upper limb. The brachial plexus is unprotected by heavy muscles and tissue, and therefore is prone to direct injury from the snugly applied Esmark rubber band. With more distal ILP, when an inflatable cuff is used, tourniquet pressure can be monitored, and neuropathy is far less common.

Vascular complications may also develop following ILP. Arterial complications are rare and unrelated to the drugs used in ILP. The incidence of thrombosis at the arteriotomy site is 2.5% *(63)*, necessitating reexploration, with minimal long-term morbidity. In patients with peripheral atherosclerosis, the manipulation and perfusion of arteries may lead to emboli and distal ischemia.

The incidence of DVT is significant (~10%), despite heparizination during ILP. The thrombogenic effect of the tumor, the cytotoxic drugs, and the surgical trauma, coupled with edema and increased compartmental pressure and decreased mobility, are all contributing factors. The clinical diagnosis may be difficult, given the expected limb edema seen following ILP. Preventive measures and Doppler flow studies, whenever DVT is suspected, are therefore indicated *(63,76)*.

Another important category of complications is associated with the rapid necrosis induced by TNF. This is a real threat in patients with ulcerated tumors, in whom existing bacterial colonization may turn into overt sepsis. This was the authors' experience with a 14-yr-old adolescent whose ulcerated sarcoma underwent liquification necrosis, abscess formation, and uncontrolled sepsis, necessitating urgent amputation. Staphylococcal sepsis was also encountered, which originated in the infected necrotic tumor of a 78-yr-old patient, and eventually led to his death *(69)*.

4.2. Systemic Side Effects

A direct leakage of drugs from the perfusate into the systemic circulation during ILP is responsible for most of the systemic side effects. However, even with complete isolation and a thorough washout of the perfusate on completion of the ILP, the drug may remain in the tissue of the perfused limb, or in its intravascular compartment, and redistribute systemically once normal circulation is reestablished. Systemic toxicity from melphalan perfusion is limited, if systemic leakage is less than 10% *(63,77)*. Because melphalan rapidly declines from the perfusate 10 min after administration, its systemic toxicity is chiefy related to early leakage *(15,63,78)*. This only obviates the need to monitor leakage, and to achieve a stable perfusion with no leakage prior to melphalan injection. With limited systemic leakage of melphalan, patients typically experience some nausea and vomiting immediately following ILP, and, at 10–14 d develop mild, short-lived neutropenia. When systemic leakage exceeds 20%, severe toxicity is encountered, manifested by a more severe bone marrow depression, hair loss, macropapular rash, pruritus, nausea, vomiting, and stomatitis.

The addition of TNF introduces the potential risk of immediate life-threatening complications. In contrast to melphalan, a stable and high TNF level in the perfusate and limb during the entire ILP occurs, so that a small but continuous leak may divert a systemically significant dose of TNF *(63,79)*. Furthermore, TNF-α induces the generation of secondary cytokines and mediators, which can, by themselves, elicit many side effects, some of which are similar to those observed following rTNF-α administration *(43)*.

The systemic side effects of TNF-α may be divided into three categories: cardiovascular, metabolic, and hematologic *(4,34,69)*. The immediate effect is to the cardiovascular system, manifested by a hyperdynamic state, with tachycardia, hypotension, increased cardiac index, and a marked decreased in systemic vascular resistance (SVR). Unlike many types of shock in which vasoconstriction dominates, TNF-like septic shock leads to a pathognomonic vasodilatation. There is good correlation (regression analysis = 0.8) between the severity of the decrease in SVR and the high systemic levels of TNF-α.

Also of importance is the cardiac effect of TNF-α. Despite the hyperdynamic state and increase in cardiac index, there is an overall cardio-depressant effect manifested by a decrease in left ventricular strike work index. The metabolic effects of TNF-α mostly relate to hepatic toxic effects, with hyperbilirubinemia, increased levels of liver enzymes, and a marked hypocholesterolemia. The hematologic systemic side effects are manifested by leukopenia, thrombocytopenia, and coagulopathy.

Finally, despite the ability of TNF-α to impair and slow wound healing by inhibiting neovascularization and decreasing collagen synthesis, no such effect has been observed. It is likely that when neovascularization in the surgical wound is required some 3–5 days following the perfusion, TNF-α has no further influence *(80)*.

With standardization of the ILP technique, and by meticulous isolation, systemic leakage is minimized. This virtually eliminates side effects and greatly simplifies the entire procedure. No special monitoring and intensive care are required, and patients are transferred to the surgical ward some 2–3 h following the procedure.

When leakage is prevented, the systemic toxicity is restricted to fever. After ILP–TNF, all patients experience fever that is probably attributable to pyrogens, such as IL-1 and IL-6, which are generated during and after perfusion *(4,63)*.

5. ILP FOR MALIGNANT MELANOMA

ILP has been establishing its role in the management of malignant melanoma for the past 40 yr. Its variability in staging, surgical technique, drugs administered, degree of hyperthermia, indications, and response evaluation, and the retrospective nature of most reported patient series, did not preclude its implementation by many surgical oncologists.

There are two clinical situations in which ILP is considered. The first is as an adjuvant treatment following complete removal of primary melanoma in a high-risk patient, and the second is as therapeutic ILP in the presence of recurrent or regionally metastatic melanoma.

The concept of adjuvant ILP in melanoma is a very appealing one; high-risk tumors (1.5 mm and deeper) have probably shed tumors cells into the surrounding skin and lymphatic channels. The standard care, wide excision (WE) of the lesion, with about 2-cm margins, does not address this risk. Perfusion of the entire limb with high doses of a chemotherapeutic drug can result in eradication of these tumor cells, but hard evidence that this concept is correct are lacking. Most studies report retrospective, single-institutional experience *(81–89)*. The controls are historical, and there is significant variability in dosage, technique, and the use of hyperthermia. Some of these studies show efficacy of adjuvant ILP, compared to historical controls in all *(81,83,84)* or subgroups of patients *(87)*, but others do not confirm this *(82,89)*. Martijn et al. *(85)*, in the Netherlands, compared the results of ILP with melphalan, following surgical excision of the tumor, with matched controls treated by surgical excision alone at the Sydney Melanoma Unit in Australia, and showed improved survival in women with limb melanoma deeper than 1.5 mm. However, a later study *(86)*, comparing the survival of 227 melanoma patients treated at one institution with 238 matched controls from five other hospitals in Europe, did not demonstrate any benefit.

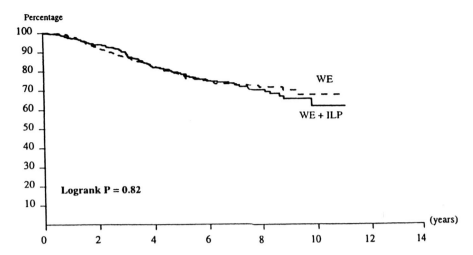

Fig. 3. EORTC/WHO/North American Perfusion Group prospective randomized adjuvant perfusion trial of patients with high-risk primary melanoma (Breslow thickness >1.5 mm). Survival by treatment group. (We = wide excision; ILP = isolated limb perfusion). Lienard D, et al., *Seminars in Surgical Pathology,* Vol. 14, 1998, pp. 202–209. Copyright © 1998. Reprinted by permission of Wiley-Liss, Inc., a division of John Wiley & Sons, Inc.

The question of adjuvant ILP in melanoma, and its impact on survival, has been addressed by three randomized trials *(16–18)*. The first two, done more than a decade ago, presented relatively small series from single institutions *(16,17)*. In a study conducted by Ghussen et al. *(16)*, the advantage of ILP was so significant that the investigators stopped randomization, considering that it was not ethical to continue the trial. This study was criticized on two issues: its small size (less than 20 patients per stage of melanoma in each arm); and the higher-than-expected survival in the perfusion group, 98% 5-yr survival, including 66% of patients with stages II and III melanoma. In the second prospective study, by Hafstrom et al. *(17)*, in which 69 patients were randomized, there was an improved local recurrence rate and disease-free survival in the perfusion group, but overall survival did not improve significantly.

The third study is a recently published, large, multcenter study, sponsored by the European Organization for Research and Treatment of Cancer, the World Health Organization, and the North American Perfusion Group *(18)*, and composed of 832 melanoma patients (>1.5 mm thickness) from 16 centers. Patients were randomized to undergo WE alone or WE and ILP with melphalan and mild hyperthermia. Lymph node dissection was optional, but the same policy was applied for patients with or without ILP. The treatment groups were matched for age, gender, anatomical location, Breslow thickness, presence of ulceration, and previous biopsy. Data analysis, performed at a median of 6.4 yr, demonstrated a transient effect of ILP in terms of regional recurrence; the rate for in-transit metastases was reduced from 6.6 to 3.3%, with an improved disease-free interval from 62 to 75% at 6 yr. However, these effects were nullified by the higher rate of distant metastases in the ILP group (12.9 vs 9.7%). The overall survival was practically identical in both groups and subgroup analysis also did not reveal any survival benefit (Fig. 3). This study indicates that adjuvant ILP is not justified.

The issue of adjuvant ILP, following a complete excision of local recurrence or in-transit metastases, is different, and has not been fully addressed. Ghussen et al. *(90)*

Table 3
Therapeutic ILP/Melphalan in Melanoma: Response Rates

Author	Yr	(ref.)	No. pts	ILP Melphalan leg/arm	Temp (C°)	Duration (min)	RR (%)	CR (%)	PR (%)
Stehlin	1969	(3)	12	NA	42	120	83	NA	
Hafstrom and Johnson	1980	(93)	10	0.9/0.45 mg/kg	38–40	120	80	10	70
Bulman and Jamieson	1980	(94)	70	1.5 mg/kg	37	60	48	NA	
Lejeune et al.	1983	(59)	23	1.5/0.75 mg/kg	39	60	88	65	23
Minor et al.	1985	(11)	22	1.5/0.75 mg/kg	39–40	60	100	82	18
Kroon et al.	1987	(95)	254	10/13 mg/L	37–38	60	86	39	47
Skene et al.	1990	(96)	67	2.0 mg/kg	39–40	60	78	NA	
Klaase et al.	1994	(97)	102	10/13 mg/L	37–38	60	NA	54	NA
Klaase et al.	1994	(97)	18	10/13 mg/L	41–42	60	NA	54	NA

NA, not available.

found increased survival in a small group of stage III patients treated by complete excision of all measurable disease and ILP, compared to those treated by surgical excision alone. However, Hafstrom et al. (17) could not confirm such an advantage in their series. Undoubtedly, a large-scale controlled study addressing this issue is required.

The biological rationale behind the performance of therapeutic ILP in patients with regional melanoma metastases relies on the fact that about 40–50% of melanomas occur in the extremities, and 10–20% of tumor recurrences or in-transit metastases are confined to the affected limb (19). Although the prognosis of these patients is poor, the disease remains regional, and, in some cases, allows long survival. The best evidence for this is contained in two studies in which major amputations were performed in patients with multiple in-transit metastases, resulting in 42 and 21% 5- and 10-yr survival, respectively (91,92).

The results of therapeutic ILP with melphalan for recurrent or in-transit melanoma metastases vary considerably (3,11,59,93–98). Typically, time period to maximal response was approx 7–8 wk. Response rates range from 48 to 100%, and CR rates from 10 to 82% (Table 3). A large series in therapeutic ILP, which also reflects the acceptable responses, is from a multicenter Netherlands study (97). The overall response was 79%, with 54% CR. Klaase et al. managed to improve the CR rate by applying a second normothermic ILP with melphalan 3–4 wk following the first. The response rate in the double perfusion group (n = 42) was 90%, compared to 68% in the retrospective, single-perfusion group (45 patients, well balanced with respect to their melonoma characteristics). The vast difference was in the CR rate, which was 76 vs 48% in favor of the double-perfusion group.

The variation in response rates probably reflects patient selection, perfusion technique and drug concentrations. Klasse et al. (97) performed a detailed analysis of prognostic factors associated with CR in a group of 120 patients: CR was achieved in 54%. The investigators concluded that the absence of lymph node metastases, leg (compared to foot or arm) location, and a double perfusion were associated with a higher CR rate.

Patients experiencing PR following ILP may still benefit from the procedure, because the disease is usually arrested for a period, and the time to progression may be several months. The duration among complete responders ranges from 8 to 20 mo: In the large Dutch study *(97)*, the median time was 9 mo. Double perfusion did not result in a long recurrence-free interval.

Limb recurrence following ILP (both local and in-transit) occurs in 29–50% *(17,99–100)*. Even in the double-perfusion setting, approximately half of the patients with CR developed recurrence in the perfused area. Major risk factors for limb recurrence were tumor left *in situ*, number of previous recurrences, and high tumor burden *(100)*.

Therapeutic ILP has an impact on survival, but exact rates vary, and are not fully documented. Oldhoff and Koops *(101)* reported 52 and 38% 3- and 5-yr survival in 100 stage II–III patients. They found a significant improvement in survival when they compared 82 patients who had hyperthermic perfusion with 18 who had normothermic ILP. These numbers are in accordance with the Tulane experience *(102)*, with 36% 5-yr survival in 468 stage III patients. The Dutch groups have shown better results for stage IIIA (71 patients, 45% 5-yr survival) and significantly worse for stage IIIB (78 patients, 25% 5-yr survival) *(100)*. It is generally accepted that long term survival (>10 yr) and cure is a reasonable goal in 25–30% of patients experiencing CR following ILP with melphalan.

A number of chemotherapeutic drugs other than melphalan were used via ILP. Cisplatin was evaluated because of its increased tumor concentration when delivered in hyperthermic conditions. Response rates were comparable to melphalan *(20)*, but the duration was shorter *(103)*.

DTIC is the most active single agent in melanoma. It was therefore tested in ILP, although a passage in the liver is necessary for its conversion to the active metabolite. Didolkar et al. *(104)* demonstrated a 76% response rate in a group of 32 patients, but others demonstrated only a 33% response rate *(105)*. Other drugs, such as nitrogen mustard *(102,106)*, thio-TEPA and actinomycin-D *(102)*, were used, but the results were inferior to those obtained with melphalan alone.

The initial report by Lienard and Lejeune *(4)*, of 100% response (90% CR), using the combination of TNF, melphalan, and IFN-γ caused great interest in this combination therapy, and many centers embarked on trials to study the effect and specific contribution of TNF. Besides the high CR (close to double that of melphalan alone), the pattern of response was different: Tumors become soft, and even necrotic, within hours to a few days. This pattern was obviously different than that caused by melphalan alone, and resembled the kinetics observed in preclinical studies using TNF *(28)*.

IFN-γ was added to the original protocol, following the observation that it upregulates TNF receptors on the membrane of both the tumor and endothelial dells *(55)*. However, a phase III study comparing the response to ILP with melphalan and TNF, with or without IFN-γ, showed no significant difference between the two regimens *(18)*. Based on this study, most centers omitted use of IFN-γ.

Since its introduction, ILP with TNF and melphalan is being performed in centers in Europe, the United States, and Israel *(38,107–109;* Table 4). In a multicenter European study *(38)* (groups from Lausanne, Groningen, Amsterdam, and Rotterdam), 53 patients (of whom 34 were stage IIIA [in-transit metastasis], 15 stage IIIAB [same, plus lymph node metastasis], and 4 stage IV) were treated by TNF and melphalan. Response rate was 100%, with 91% CR. The authors compared their results to a group of 103 matched historical controls treated at the same institutions by ILP with melphalan alone: The response rate was 77.6%, with 52% CR. Duration of response was similar in both groups.

The authors' experience within a phase II study in 43 melanoma patients, 28 of whom (65%) had bulky disease (tumor measuring >3 cm in diameter or >10 lesions),

Table 4
Therapeutic ILP/TNF + Melphalan in Melanoma Response Rates

Author	Yr	(ref.)	No. pts	RR (%)	CR (%)	PR (%)	Comments
Lienard et al.	1992	(4)	29	100	90	10	
Hill et al.	1993	(40)	4	100	100		(Low-dose TNF)
Lienard et al.	1994	(18)	53	100	90	10	(Multicentric)
Fraker et al.	1996	(107)	25	92	76	16	TNF-4 mg
			11	100	36	64	TNF-6 mg
Hoehenberger and Kettelhack	1997	(109)	20	83	65	18	
Gutman et al.	1998	(108)	43	86	60	26	

Response spans the RR, CR, PR columns.

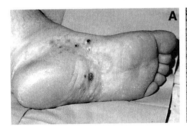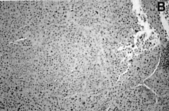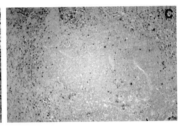

Fig. 4. (A) Eight wk post-ILP for metastatic melanoma with numerous lesions on the foot. The lesions have dried, but the black color has remained as a tattoo. Punch biopsies showed CR. (B) Prior to ILP, sheaths of atypical melanoma cells. (C) After treatment, CR of tumor cells is evident, surrounded by fibroblasts and hemosidene pigment.

shows an overall response of 86%, with 60% CR (Fig. 4), which was significantly lower in patients with high disease volume (108).

In order to establish whether ILP with TNF and melphalan is more advantageous than melphalan alone, a multicenter, prospective, randomized trial, including 11 cancer centers from Europe and Israel, was initiated in 1997. Its aim is to focus not only on response rates, but specifically on duration of response, local recurrence, and survival.

A phase III trial at the NCI in Bethesda, MD, compared perfusions using the TNF–melphalan–IFN-γ combination, to ILP using melphalan alone. The experimental arm had 80% CR, compared to 61% in the melphalan-alone arm. The duration of response was identical. Subgroup analysis disclosed that the advantage of TNF was more significant in patients with high tumor burden (110). In a second NCI trial, two groups of patients, who were not eligible for the aforementioned phase III study, received ILP with TNF and melphalan. One group consisted of 17 patients who had previously failed ILP with a melphalan. Reperfusion with TNF was associated with an 94% overall response rate and 65% CR (111).

The role of ILP in melanoma has recently been refined. Adjuvant melphalan perfusion is not justified routinely in primary melanoma. Its role following the excision of metastatic disease should be evaluated. Therapeutic ILP is the most effective therapy for local recurrence or in-transit metastasis. The addition of TNF caused a marked increase in response rates, but long-term effect of TNF is yet to be determined.

Table 5
ILP/Chemotherapy in Soft Tissue Sarcoma

Author	Yr	(ref.)	Drug	No. pts	RR (%)	CR (%)	PR (%)	Limb Salvage (%)
Krementz et al.	1977	(116)	Melphalan/Act-D/NH₂	17	35	0	35	NS
Krementz et al.	1977	(116)	Melphalan/Act-D/NH₂	39	31	10	21	NS
Pommier et al.	1988	(117)	Cisplatin	17	18	0	18	82
Klaase et al.	1989	(26)	Melphalan/doxorubicin	13	7	7	0	61
Rossi et al.	1994	(27)	Doxorubicin	22	74	0	74	61

NS, not stated.

6. ILP FOR EXTREMITY STS

As it became evident that amputation is not mandatory in STS, and that comparable survival rates can be achieved with adequate tumor resection (112), limb preservation became a major goal. However, limb-sparing surgery is not always possible, especially when the tumor is large, expanding into more than one compartment, adjacent to or invading a major blood vessel or nerve, or when there is a multifocal appearance, making amputation, disarticulation, or mutilating surgery almost inevitable. Several treatment modalities have been developed that facilitate limb-sparing, even in cases of advanced tumor. Neoadjuvant therapy is an option, which is principally preoperative radiation or a combined preoperative (intra-arterial and/or systemic) chemotherapy and RT (113,114). For example, in a few series, intra-arterial DOX resulted in a 50% response rate, whereas combining intra-arterial chemotherapy with systemic chemotherapy increased response rates, but at the cost of significant complications.

Brachytherapy, applied to the tumor bed when only marginal resections are possible, can also avoid amputation, and improve local control (115).

Although these multimodality therapies have led to a significant reduction in amputation rates (which were 50% prior to 1977), 8–15% of patients with extremity sarcoma still undergo amputation (113).

The use of ILP in sarcoma was suggested as a neoadjuvant treatment, with the major goal of reducing tumor size, thus facilitating subsequent resection. The drugs used in ILP for sarcoma included melphalan, actinomycin-D, nitrogen mustard, DOX, and cisplatin (Table 5). However, ILP with chemotherapeutic drugs was found unsatisfactory and disappointing. None of the regimens could be considered superior to surgery combined with RT. The clinical response was poor, with a negligible CR and a low rate of PR. Even ILP with DOX, which appears to be the most effective systemic chemotherapy, was proven ineffective in ILP, and resulted in considerable regional toxicity. Because ILP entails major surgery and delays in definite treatment, it was neglected by surgical oncologists for sarcomas, even in centers utilizing it effectively for melanoma. Interest rose again after Lienard and Lejeune (4) published promising results, following the introduction of high-dose TNF-α in ILP. Although most of their patients had in-transit melanoma metastases, four had recurrent STSs, and all experienced complete remission.

This initial report led to a phase II, multicenter study to determine the effect of ILP with TNF-α and melphalan ± IFN-γ in patients with nonresectable STS confined to the limb, utilizing it in most patients as a neoadjuvant treatment, followed several weeks later by resection of the tumor or its remnants.

The primary objective of ILP with high-dose TNF is to render a nonresectable extremity sarcoma resectable, by reducing its size. Candidates for such treatment are those 8–15% of patients with extremity sarcoma, considered either nonresectable or resectable only at the cost of major functional morbidity. Included in this category are large STSs, which are single tumors that are adjacent or fixated to the neurovascular bundle and/or bone. Even a small reduction in size distances the tumor margin from vital structures, and may facilitate efficient resection, and thus limb salvage. Patients with such characteristics, however, should not be immediately offered ILP, because the physician should first estimate the chances for limb salvage. At times, even the best scenario for CR will not result in limb sparing. This is particularly true for large tumors, occupying extensive parts or the circumference of the limb, when the delayed resection, even of the tumor bed after complete necrosis, mandates amputation. An ILP for such tumors is indicated only as a palliative measure in the presence of metastases, in order to avoid amputation.

Multifocal primary or recurrent sarcomas are another group usually benefiting from this modality. Amputation is almost always unavoidable in this group, because resection is impossible. Despite their dismal prognosis, this subset of patients often require local control, because the lesions multiply, penetrate, and ulcerate. ILP may therefore be their only option for limb salvage and palliation, and may be performed as a sole treatment, without delayed resection.

ILP–TNF is also indicated as a palliative measure in selected patients who have a reasonable life expectancy, even in the presence of distant STS metastasis, with avoidance of amputation being the chief goal.

What are the typical tumor changes following ILP–TNF *(10,57,69)*?

1. In large, bulky tumors, marked softening of the tumor can be noticed in the first days post-ILP, but this is not an accurate measure for response, because it may sometimes be secondary to edema following perfusion.
2. Reduction in tumor mass, which can evolve into its complete disappearance clinically, and on imaging studies (Fig. 5). At times, the mass reduction is only limited, but, in cases in which the tumor is adherent to a major nerve (e.g., sciatic nerve) or blood vessel (e.g., popliteal vessels), even a small change in size (2–3 cm) can enable safe margin resection, with preservation of these structures. However, even when the size of the mass is not reduced after ILP, this does not necessarily indicate treatment failure, because in a considerable number of these masses, only necrosis and fibrosis are found with no viable tumor cells.
3. In ulcerated tumors, penetrating the skin, hemorrhagic necrosis can be seen even a few hours after the perfusion (Fig. 6). This is noticeable, not only in clear-cell and epitheloid sarcomas, which may not represent typical STS, since they resemble some of the characteristics of melanoma, but also in synovial and other subtypes of sarcoma (Fig. 7).

However, despite these clinical responses, an accurate assessment of response in STS following ILP–TNF is difficult. The disappearance of the vascular bed, as demonstrated by postoperative angiograms, is usually a good indicator of massive necrosis (Fig. 2). Newer techniques, such as magnetic resonance spectroscopy and positron-emission tomography scanning *(118,119)*, can be useful in assessing the extent of necrosis vs tumor viability, and ease the accuracy of response.

Histopathology is obviously the most accurate method for response assessment. Typical histologic changes 6–8 wk after TNF perfusion include huge cystic hemorrhagic necrosis in the central area of the remaining tumor. Although spontaneous necrosis is

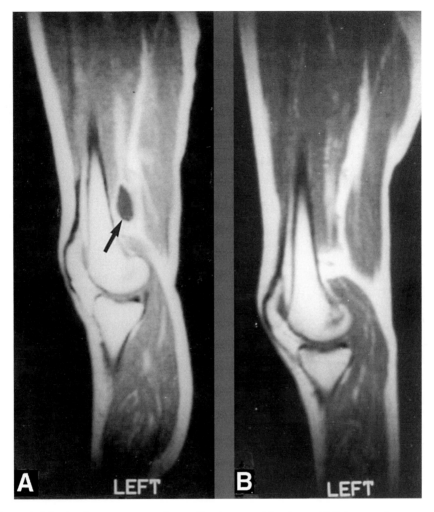

Fig. 5. An MRI of a liposarcoma at the popliteal area: **(A)** prior to ILP (arrow demonstrates the tumor mass); **(B)** at 8 wk post-ILP, the tumor has vanished completely.

encountered in STS, the magnitude and extent of necrosis following ILP–TNF is unique. Usually, if any viable tumor cells exist, they are observed in the periphery of these cysts, but, even then, the malignant potential of these remaining cells is not fully determined. Other histological changes include extensive interstitial and pericystic fibrosis, which can also be seen following neoadjuvant chemotherapy. No correlation has been found between tumor size, histological subtype, and the pattern of response.

There is a notable discrepancy between the clinical response assessment and the pathological one. Histological examination upgrades the overall response rate because masses that remain unchanged, or only partially regress, may be converted into a CR (no viable tumor cells) following pathological examination. Therefore, because studies performed on sarcoma patients undergoing ILP with cytostatic drugs in the pre-TNF era were based on clinical and radiological assessment only, the reported response rates may have been underestimated relative to pathologically based TNF studies. Nevertheless, clinically based TNF response rates are still significantly superior *(10)*.

A review of worldwide experience with ILP, using rTNF-α and melphalan ± IFN-γ (Table 6), discloses an overall response rate of 82–100%, with a CR of 29–67% and

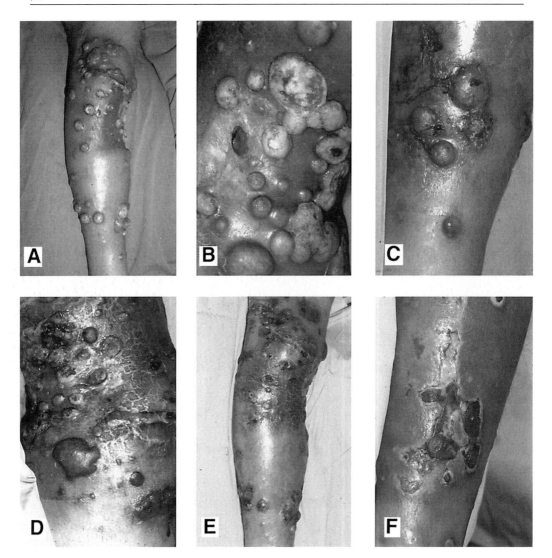

Fig. 6. The lower limb of a patient with clear-cell sarcoma, manifested by dozens of nodules occupying the entire limb. The patient had failed with systemic chemotherapy and radiation, and was a candidate for hemipelvectomy. (**A**) At the knee area, multiple lesions are shown eroding the skin. (**B**) Close-up photo of the lesions. (**C**) Three h after isolated limb perfusion (ILP) with TNF and melphalan via external iliac approach. Bluish discoloration was noted. (**D**) Twelve h after ILP. (**E**) At 48 h, softening and necrosis of the lesions was evident. (**F**) At 6 d, only dry crust remained, and all lesions disappeared from the entire limb. *Cancer,* Vol. 79, 1997, pp. 1129–1137. Copyright © (1997) American Cancer Society. Reprinted with permission of Wiley-Liss, Inc., a subsidiary of John Wiley & Sons, Inc.

PR of 22–56%, and only up to 18% of no response or progression of disease. In 20% of PRs, a near-total response, with >95% necrosis, was found, and only the finding of several tumor cells precluded categorizing them as CRs.

These results were obtained in a selected group of patients with extensive disease, who were all candidates for amputation or mutilating surgery. The average tumor size was 16 cm, most tumors were of high grade (85%), and 43% were recurrent. There was also a relatively high rate of multifocal disease (23%) *(10).*

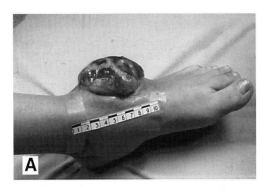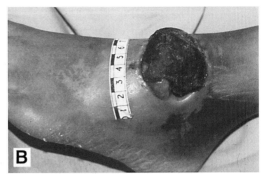

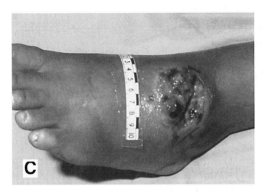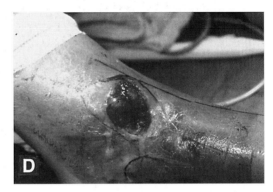

Fig. 7. Synovial sarcoma occupying the entire foot of a young woman. The patient was a candidate for below-knee amputation: **(A)** before isolated limb perfusion (ILP) with high-dose TNF and melphalan; **(B)** six h after ILP; **(C)** three wk later; **(D)** at 2 mo, no residual tumor remained. The patient was ready for tumor-bed excision and grafting. At histopathologic examination, no viable tumor cells were found. *Cancer,* Vol. 79, 1997, pp. 1129–1137. Copyright © (1997) American Cancer Society. Reprinted with permission of Wiley-Liss, Inc., a subsidiary of John Wiley & Sons, Inc.

Table 6
ILP/TNF + Melphalan in Soft Tissue Sarcoma

Author	Yr	(ref.)	Drug	No. pts	RR (%)	CR (%)	PR (%)	Limb Salvage (%)
Schraffordt-Koops et al.	1993	*(120)*	TNF + melphalan + IFN-γ	23	100	44	56	87
Vagilini et al.	1994	*(121)*	TNF + melphalan	9	89	67	22	89
Gutman et al.	1996	*(69)*	TNF + melphalan	35	94	37	57	85
Eggermont et al.	1996	*(57)*	TNF + melphalan + IFN-γ	55	87	36	51	84
Eggermont et al.	1996	*(10)*	TNF + melphalan ± IFN-γ	186	82	29	53	82
Hill et al.	1993	*(40)*	TNF low-dose + melphalan	9	100	100	0	63.5

Limb salvage has been achieved in 85% of these patients. This high rate is the most valuable and proven benefit of ILP–TNF in advanced sarcoma patients. Achieving CR *per se* is not crucial. Whether the tumor responds completely or partially is irrelevant, so long as it becomes amenable to resection without loss of limb function. In patients in whom the tumor completely disappeared, resection of the tumor bed was mandatory, but without risking the limb.

At times, a definite PR with significant tumor shrinkage is still insufficient to render it resectable without endangering limb function. A second perfusion with TNF may be considered, to achieve further tumor shrinkage. The authors' experience with nine PR patients with sizable tumors, who underwent two TNF perfusions scheduled 6–10 wk apart, resulted in the conversion of six to CR and two to further tumor shrinkage, enabling limb salvage in 8 of 9 patients. One patient did not benefit from the second ILP–TNF.

The benefit of limb salvage is particularly noticeable in patients with multiple lesions. The authors' experience is that 85% of such patients achieved limb sparing and palliation with improvement in their life quality *(122)*.

Tumor control and avoidance of amputation are also possible in patients in the presence of distant metastases. Eggermont et al. *(10)* described a 92% limb salvage rate in 23 such patients, in whom a single ILP with TNF and melphalan provided rapid and life-long (up to 2 yr) local control and limb salvage.

The response to ILP–TNF is remarkable, but is it long standing? Recurrent local disease, in patients whose limbs are considered salvaged after ILP–TNF, ranges from 10 to 15% after 3–24 mo, during a median follow up of 22 mo *(10,69)*. This local recurrence rate is relatively low, considering the large median tumor size and the percentage of recurrent sarcomas treated. Local recurrence rates could probably be further improved by the administration of postresection RT in a higher percentage of patients.

Given the unique selection of patients in this group of ILP–TNF, it is difficult to compare these results with other sarcoma studies. Comparison of response rates and limb salvage in this selected group of locally advanced sarcoma patients appears superior to other neoadjuvant modalities, but this should be addressed in a prospective study.

REFERENCES

1. Creech O, Krementz ET, Ryan RF, et al. Chemotherapy of cancer: regional perfusion utilizing an extracorporeal circuit, *Ann. Surg.,* **148** (1958) 616–631.
2. Cavaliere R, Ciocatto EC, Giovanella BC, et al. Selective heat sensitivity of cancer cells: biochemical and clinical studies, *Cancer,* **20** (1967) 1351–1381.
3. Stehlin JS. Hyperthermic perfusion with chemotherapy for cancers of the extremities, *Surg. Gyncol. Obstet.,* **129** (1969) 305–308.
4. Lienard D, Ewalenko P, Delmotti JJ, et al. High dose recombinant tumor necrosis factor alpha in combination with interferon gamma and melphalan in isolation perfusion of the limbs for melanoma and sarcoma, *J. Clin. Oncol.,* **10** (1992) 52–60.
5. Muchmore JH, Krementz ET, and Kerstein MD. Noninvasive evaluation of peripheral vasculature following regional hyperthermic chemotherapeutic perfusion (RHCP), *Am. Surg.,* **53** (1987) 94–96.
6. Wieberdink J, Benckhuysen C, Braat RP, et al. Dosimetry in isolation perfusion of the limbs by assessment of perfused tissue volume and grading of toxic tissue reactions, *Eur. Cancer Clin. Oncol.,* **18** (1982) 905–910.
7. Sorkin P, Abu-Abid S, Lev D, et al. Systemic leakage and side effects of tumor necrosis factor administered via isolated limb perfusion can be manipualted by flow rate adjustment, *Arch. Surg.,* **130** (1995) 1079–1084.
8. Barker WC, Andrich MP, Alexander HR, et al. Continuous intraoperative external monitoring of perfusate leak using I-131 human serum albumin during isolated perfusion of the liver and limbs, *Eur. J. Nucl. Med.,* **22** (1995) 1242–1248.
9. Thom AK, Alexander HR, Andrich MP, et al. Cytokine levels and systemic toxicity in patients undergoing isolated limb perfusion (ILP) with high-dose TNF, interferon-gamma and melphalan, *J. Clin. Oncol.,* **13** (1995) 264–273.
10. Eggermont AMM, Schraffordt-Koops H, Klausner JM, et al. Isolated limb perfusion with tumor necrosis factor and melphalan for limb salvage in 186 patients with locally advanced soft tissue

extremity sarcomas: the cumulative multicenter European experience, *Ann. Surg.,* **224** (1996) 756–765.

11. Minor DR, Allen RE, Alberts D, et al. Clinical and pharmacokinetic study of isolated limb perfusion with heat and melphalan for melanoma, *Cancer,* **55** (1985) 2638–2644.

12. Stehlin JS. Hyperthermic perfusion for melanoma of the extremeties: experience with 165 patients 1976 to 1979, *Ann. NY Acad. Sci.,* **335** (1980) 352–355.

13. Benckhuijsen C, Kroon BBR, Van Geel AN, et al. Regional perfusion treatment with melphalan for melanoma in a limb. An evaluation of drug kinetics, *Eur. J. Surg. Oncol.,* **14** (1988) 157–163.

14. Scott RN, Kerr KJ, Blackie R, et al. Pharmacokinetic advantages of isolated limb perfusion with melphalan for malignant melanoma, *Br. J. Cancer,* **68** (1992) 159–166.

15. Briele HA, Dyuric M, Jung DT, et al. Pharmacokinetics of melphalan in clinical isolation perfusion of the extremities, *Cancer Res.,* **45** (1985) 1885–1889.

16. Ghussen F, Kruger I, Groth W, et al. Role of hyperthermic cytostatic perfusion in the treatment of extremity melanoma, *Cancer,* **61** (1988) 654–659.

17. Hafstrom L, Rudenstam CM, Blomquist E, et al. Regional hyperthermic perfusion with melphalan after surgery for recurrent melanoma of the extremities, *J. Clin. Oncol.,* **9** (1991) 2091–2094.

18. Lienard D, Eggermont AM, Kroon BBR, et al. Isolated limb perfusion in primary and recurrent melanoma: indications and results, *Semin. Surg. Oncol.,* **14** (1998) 202–209.

19. Balch CM, Soong SJ, Shin HM, et al. Changing trends in the clinical and pathologic features of melanoma, In Balch CM, et al. (eds), *Cutaneous Melanoma.* Lippincott, Philadelphia, (1992) pp. 40–45.

20. Klein ES and Ben-Ari GY. Isolation perfusion with cisplatin for malignant melanoma of the limbs, *Cancer,* **59** (1987) 1068–1071.

21. Guchelaar JH, Hoekstra HJ, de Vries EG, et al. Cisplatin and platinum pharmacokinetics during hyperthermic isolated limb perfusion for human tumors of the extremities, *Br. J. Cancer,* **65** (1992) 898–902.

22. Fletcher WS, Pommier R, and Small K. Results of cisplatin hyperthermic isolation perfusion for stage IIIA and IIIAB extremity melanoma, *Melanoma Res.,* **4** (1994) 17–19.

23. Roseman JM. Effective management of extremity cancers using cisplatin and etoposide in isolated limb perfusions, *J. Surg. Oncol.,* **35** (1987) 170–172.

24. Martijn H, Oldhoff J, and Koops HS. Hyperthermic regional perfusion with melphalan and a combination of melphalan and actinomycin D in the treatment of locally metastasized malignant melanomas of the extremities, *J. Surg. Oncol.,* **20** (1982) 9–13.

25. Didolkar MS, Fitzpatrick JL, Jackson AJ, et al. Toxicity and complications of vascular isolation and hyperthermic perfusion with imidazole carboxamide (DITC) in melanoma, *Cancer,* **57** (1986) 1961–1966.

26. Klaase JM, Kroon BBR, Benckhuysen C, et al. Results of regional isolation perfusion with cytostatics in patients with soft tissue tumors of the extremities, *Cancer,* **64** (1989) 616–621.

27. Rossi CR, Vecchiato A, Foletto M, et al. Phase II study on neoadjuvant hyperthermic-antiblastic perfusion with doxorubicin in patients with intermediate or high grade limb sarcomas, *Cancer,* **73** (1994) 2140–2146.

28. Carswell EA, Old LJ, Kassel RL, et al. Endotoxin-induced serum factor that causes necrosis of tumors, *Proc. Natl. Acad. Sci. USA,* **72** (1975) 3666–3670.

29. Aggarwal BB, Kohr WJ, Hass PE, et al. Human tumor necrosis factor: production, purification and characterization, *J. Biol. Chem.,* **260** (1985) 2345–2354.

30. Haranaka K, Satomi N, and Sukari A. Antitumor activity of murine tumor necrosis factor against transplanted murine tumors and heterotransplanted human tumors in nude mice, *Int. J. Cancer,* **34** (1984) 263–267.

31. Asher AL, Mule JY, Reichert CM, Shiloni E, and Rosenberg SA. Studies of the antitumor efficacy of systemically administered recombinant tumor necrosis factor against several murine tumors in vivo, *J. Immunol.,* **138** (1987) 963–974.

32. Spriggs DR, Sherman ML, Michie H, et al. Recombinant human tumor necrosis factor administered as a 24-hour intravenous infusion. A phase I and pharmacologic study, *J. Natl. Cancer Inst.,* (1988) 1039–1044.

33. Chapman PB, Lester TJ, Casper ES, et al. Clinical pharmacoogy of recombinant human tumor necrosis factor in patients with advanced cancer, *J. Clin. Oncol.,* **5** (1987) 1942–1951.

34. Feinberg B, Kurzrock R, Talpaz M, et al. Phase I trial of intravenously administered recombinant tumor necrosis factor alpha in cancer patients, *J. Clin. Oncol.,* **6** (1988) 1328–1334.

35. Tracey KJ, Beutler B, Lowry SF, et al. Shock and tissue injury induced by recombinant human cachectin, *Science,* **234** (1986) 470–473.

36. Beutler B and Cerami A. Tumor necrosis, cachexia shock and inflammation; a common mediator, *Ann. Rev. Biochem.,* **57** (1988) 505–518.

37. Bevilcqua MP, Pober JS, Majeau GR, et al. Recombinant tumor necrosis factor induces coagulant activity in cultured human vasculature endothelium; characterization and comparison with actions of interleukin-1, *Proc. Natl. Acad. Sci. USA,* **83** (1986) 4533–5437.

38. Lejeune FJ. High-dose recombinant tumour necrosis factor (rTNFα) administered by isolation perfusion for advanced tumours of the limbs: a model for biochemotherapy of cancer, *Eur. J. Cancer,* **B1A** (1995) 1009–1016.

39. Alexander HR, Fraker DL, and Bartlett DL. Isolated limb perfusion for malignant melanoma, *Semin. Surg. Oncol.,* **12** (1996) 416–426.

40. Hill S, Fawcett WJ, Sheldon J, et al. Low-dose tumour necrosis factor alpha and melphalan in hyperthermic isolated limb perfusion, *Br. J. Surg.,* **80** (1993) 995–997.

41. Spriggs DR, Sherman ML, Frei E III, et al. Clinical studies with tumor necrosis factor, In Old LJ (ed), *Ciba Foundation Symposium 131, Tumor Necrosis Factor and Related Cytotoxins.* Wiley, New York, (1987) 206–227.

42. Sugarman BJ, Aggarwal BB, Hass PF, et al. Recombinant tumor necrosis factor-α: effects of proliferation of normal and transformed cells in vitro, *Science,* **230** (1985) 943–945.

43. Quinn TD, Polk HC Jr, and Edwards J. Hyperthermic isolated limb perfusion increases circulating levels of inflammatory cytokines, *Cancer Immunol. Immunother.,* **40** (1995) 272–275.

44. Renard N, Lienard D, Gaspanard L, et al. Early endothelian activation and polymorphonuclear cell invasion precede specific necrosis of human melanoma and sarcoma treated by intravascular high-dose tumor necrosis factor alpha (TNF-α), *Int. J. Cancer,* **57** (1994) 656–663.

45. Manusoma ER, Stavast J, Marquet RC, et al. Total body irradiaiton (TBI) attenuates antitumor effects of TNFα in isolated limb perfusion (ILP) in the rat, *Eur. J. Surg. Res.,* **27** (1995) 110(Abstract).

46. Watanabe N, Niitsu Y, Umeno H, et al. Toxic effect of TNF on tumor vasculature in mice, *Cancer Res.,* **49** (1988) 2179–2183.

47. Nawroth PP and Stern DM. Modulation of endothelial cell hemostatic properties by tumor necrosis factor, *J. Exp. Med.,* **163** (1986) 740–745.

48. Cheresh DA. Death to a blood vessel, death to a tumor, *Nature Med.,* **4** (1998) 395–396.

49. Ruegg C. Evidence for the involvement of endothelial cell integrin αVβ3 in the disruption of the tumor vasculature induced by TNF and IFN-γ, *Nature Med.,* **4** (1998) 408–414.

50. Regeness A, Muller M, Curschellas E, et al. Antitumor effects of tumor necrosis factor in combination with chemotherapeutic agents, *Int. J. Cancer,* **39** (1987) 266–273.

51. Folli S, Pelegrin A, Chalandon Y, et al. Tumor necrosis factor can enhance radio-antibody uptake in human colon carcinoma xenografts by increasing vascular permeability, *Int. J. Cancer,* **53** (1993) 829–836.

52. Brown CK, Bartlett SK, Libuth E, et al. Augmental capillary leak during isolated hepatic perfusion (IHP) occurs via ILP independent mechanisms (abstract). 51st Annual Cancer Symposium, SSO, San Diego, 26–29 March 1998, **24,** 12.

53. Krosnick JA, Mule JJ, McIntosj JK, et al. Augmentation of antitumor efficacy by the combination of recombinant tumor necrosis factor and chemotherapeutic agents in vivo, *Cancer Res.,* **49** (1989) 3729–3733.

54. Watanabe N, Niitso Y, Umeno N, et al. Synergistic cytotoxic and antitumor effects of recombinant human tumor necrosis factor and hyperthermia, *Cancer Res.,* **48** (1988) 650–653.

55. Aggarwell BB, Eessalu TE, and Hass PE. Characterization of receptors for tumor necrosis factor and their regulation by gamma-interferon, *Nature,* **318** (1985) 665–667.

56. Balkwill FR, Lee A, Aldam G, et al. Human tumor xenografts treated with recombinant human necrosis factor alone or in combination with interferons, *Cancer Res.,* **46** (1986) 3990–3993.

57. Eggermont AMM, Schraffordt Koops H, Lienard D, et al. Isolated limb perfusion with high-dose tumor necrosis factor-α in combination with interferon-γ and melphalan for non-resectable extremity soft tissue sarcoma: a multicenter trial, *J. Clin. Oncol.,* **14** (1996) 2653–2665.

58. Belli F, Arienti F, Rivoltini L, et al. Treatment of recurrent in-transit metastases from cutaneous melanoma by isolation perfusion in extracorporeal circulation with interleukin-2 and lymphokine activated killer cells. A pilot study. *Melanoma Res.,* **2** (1992) 263–271.

59. Lejeune FJ, Deloof T, Ewalenko P, et al. Objective regression of unexcised melanoma in-transit metastases after hyperthermic isolation perfusion of the limbs with melphalan. Recent results, *Cancer Res.,* **86** (1983) 268–276.

60. Dickson JA and Calderwood SK. Temperature range and selective sensitivity of tumors to hyperthermia. A critical review, *Ann. NY Acad. Sci.,* **335** (1980) 180–201.

61. Dietzel F. Basic principles in hyperthermic tumor therapy. Recent results, *Cancer Res.,* **86** (1983) 177–190.

62. Robbins HI, d'Oleire F, Kutz M, et al. Cytotoxic interactions of tumor necrosis factor, melphalan and 41.8°C hyperthermia, *Cancer Lett.,* **89** (1995) 55–62.

63. Vrouenraets BC, Klaase JM, Nieweg OE, et al. Toxicity and morbidity of isolated limb perfusion, *Semin. Surg. Oncol.,* **14** (1998) 224–231.

64. Baas PC, Schraffordt Koops H, Hoekstra HJ, et al. Groin dissection in the treatment of lower-extremity melanoma: short- and long-term morbidity, *Arch. Surg.,* **127** (1992) 281–286.

65. Klaase JM, Kroon BB, van Geel AN, et al. Patient and treatment related factors associated with acute regional toxicity after isolated perfusion for melanoma of the extremities, *Am. J. Surg.,* **167** (1994) 618–620.

66. Vrouenraets BC, Klaase JM, Kroon BB, et al. Long-term morbidity after regional isolated perfusion with melphalan for melanoma of the limbs. The influence of acute regional toxic reactions, *Arch. Surg.,* **130** (1995) 43–47.

67. Klaase JM, Kroon BB, van Slooten GW, et al. Relation between calculated melphalan peak concentrations and toxicity in regional isolated perfusion for melanoma, *Reg. Cancer Treat.,* **4** (1992) 309–312.

68. Thompson JF, Eksborg S, Kam PC, et al. Determinants of acute regional toxicity following isolated limb perfusion for melanoma, *Melanoma Res.,* **6** (1996) 267–271.

69. Gutman M, Inbar M, Shlush-Lev D, et al. High-dose tumor necrosis factor alpha and melphalan administered via isolated limb perfusion for advanced soft tissue sarcoma results in a >90% response rate and limb preservation, *Cancer,* **79** (1997) 1129–1137.

70. Fraker DL and Alexander HR. Isolated limb perfusion with high-dose tumor necrosis factor for extremity melanoma and sarcoma, *Important Adv. Oncol.,* **1994** (1994) 179–192.

71. Yang JC, Fraker DL, Thom AK, et al. Isolation perfusion with tumor necrosis factor-α, interferon-γ, and hyperthermia in the treatment of localized and metastatic cancer, *Recent Res. Cancer Res.,* **138** (1995) 161–166.

72. Kroon BB, Klaase JM, van Geel BN, et al. Application of hyperthermia in regional isolated perfusion for melanoma of the limbs, *Reg. Cancer Treat.,* **4** (1992) 223–226.

73. Lai DT, Ingvar C, and Thompson JF. Value of monitoring serum creatine phosphokinase following hyperthermic isolated limb perfusion for melanoma, *Reg. Cancer Treat.,* **1** (1993) 36–39.

74. Klaase JM, Kroon BB, van Geel AN, et al. Retrospective comparative study evaluating the results of a single-perfusion versus double-perfusion schedule with melphalan in patients with recurrent melanoma of the lower limb, *Cancer,* **71** (1993) 2990–2994.

75. Vrouenraets BC, Eggermont AM, Klaase JM, et al. Long-term neuropathy after regional isolated perfusion with melphalan for melanoma of the limbs, *Eur. J. Surg. Oncol.,* **20** (1994) 681–685.

76. Rosin DR. Isolated limb perfusion: past experience and present studies using a minimal-access approach, *Melanoma Res.,* **4(suppl 1)** (1994) 51–55.

77. Hoekstra HJ, Naujocks T, Schraffordt Koops H, et al. Continuous leakage monitoring during hyperthermic isolated regional perfusion of the lower limb: techniques and results, *Reg. Cancer Treat.,* **4** (1992) 301–304.

78. Thompson JF, Kam PC, Razan D, et al. Clinical pharmacokinetics of melphalan in isolated limb perfusion; compartmental modelling and moment analysis, *Reg. Cancer Treat.,* **8** (1994) 83–87.

79. Gerain J, Lienard D, Ewalenko P, et al. High serum levels of TNFα after its administration for isolation perfusion of the limbs, *Cytokine,* **4** (1992) 585–591.

80. Salomon GD, Kasid A, Cromack DT, et al. Local effects of cachectin/tumor necrosis factor in wound healing, *Ann. Surg.,* **214** (1991) 175–180.

81. McBride CM, Sugarbaker EV, and Hickey RC. Prophylactic isolation-perfusion as the primary therapy for invasive malignant melanoma of the limbs, *Ann. Surg.,* **192** (1975) 316–324.

82. Golomb FM, Bromberg J, and Dubin N. Controlled study of the survival experience with primary malignant melanoma of the distal extremities treated with adjuvant isolated perfusion, In Jones SE and Solomon SE (eds), *Adjuvant Therapy of Cancer II.* Grune & Stratton, New York, 1979, pp. 519–526.

83. Rege VB, Leone LA, Soderberg CH, et al. Hyperthermic adjuvant perfusion chemotherapy for stage I malignant melanoma of the extremity with literature review, *Cancer,* **52** (1983) 2033–2039.

84. Fletcher JR, White CR, and Fletch WS. Improved survival rates of patients with acral lentiginous melanoma treated with hyperthermic isolation perfusion, wide excision and regional lymphadenopathy, *Am. J. Surg.,* **151** (1986) 593–598.

85. Martijn H, Koops HS, Milton GW, et al. Comparison of two methods of treating primary melanomas Clark IV and V, thickness 1.5mm and greater localized on the extremities—wide surgical excision with and without adjuvant regional perfusion, *Cancer*, **57** (1986) 1923–1930.

86. Franklin H, Koops HS, Oldhoff J, et al. To perfuse or not to perfuse? A retrospective comparative study to evaluate the effect of adjuvant isolated regional perfusion in patients with stage I extremity melanoma with a thickness of 1.5mm or greater, *J. Clin. Oncol.*, **6** (1988) 701–708.

87. Edwards MJ, Soong SJ, Boddie AW, et al. Isolated limb perfusion for localized melanoma of the extremity, *Arch. Surg.*, **125** (1990) 317–321.

88. Vrouenraets BC, Kroon BBR, Klaase JM, et al. Adjuvant regional isolated perfusion with melphalan for patients with Clark C melanoma of the extremities, *J. Surg. Oncol.*, **52** (1993) 249–254.

89. Schraffordt-Koops H, Kroon BBR, Oldhoff J, et al. Controversies concerning adjuvant isolated perfusion for stage I melanoma of the extremities, *World J. Surg.*, **16** (1992) 241–245.

90. Ghussen F, Kruger I, Smalley RV, et al. Hyperthermic perfusion with chemotherapy for melanoma of the extremities, *World J. Surg.* **13** (1989) 598–602.

91. Turnbull A, Shah J, and Fortner J. Recurrent melanoma of an extremity treated by major amputation, *Arch. Surg.*, **106** (1973) 496–498.

92. Jaques DP, Coit DG, and Brenman MF. Major amputation for advanced malignant melanoma, *Surg. Gynecol. Obstet.*, **169** (1989) 1–6.

93. Hafstrom L and Jonsson PE. Hyperthermic perfusion of recurrent malignant melanoma of the extremities, *Acta. Chir. Scand.*, **146** (1980) 313–318.

94. Bulman AS and Jamieson CW. Isolated limb perfusion with melphalan in the treatment of melanoma, *Br. J. Surg.*, **67** (1980) 660–662.

95. Kroon BB, van Geel AN, Benckhuijsen C, et al. Normothermic isolation perfusion with melphalan for advanced melanoma of the limbs, *Anticancer Res.*, **7** (1987) 441–442.

96. Skene AI, Bulman AS, Williams TR, et al. Hyperthermic isolated perfusion with melphalan in the treatment of advanced malignant melanoma of the lower limb, *Br. J. Surg.*, **77** (1990) 765–767.

97. Klaase JM, Kroon BB, van Geel AN, et al. Prognostic factors for tumor response and limb recurrence-free interval in patients with advanced melanoma of the limbs treated with regional isolated perfusion using melphalan, *Surgery* **115** (1994) 39–45.

98. Bryant PJ, Balderson GA, Mead P, et al. Hyperthermic isolated limb perfusion for malignant melanoma: response and survival, *World J. Surg.*, **19** (1995) 363–368.

99. Lejeune FJ, Lienard D, el Douaihy M, et al. Results of 206 isolated limb perfusions for malignant melanoma, *Eur. J. Surg. Oncol.*, **15** (1989) 510–519.

100. Klaase JM, Kroon BB, van Geel AN, et al. Limb recurrence-free interval and survival in patients with recurrent melanoma of the extremities treated with normothermic isolated perfusion, *J. Am. Coll. Surg.*, **178** (1994) 564–572.

101. Oldhoff HM and Koops HS. Regional perfusion in the treatment of patients with locally metastasized, malignant melanoma of the limbs, *Eur. J. Cancer*, **17** (1981) 471–476.

102. Krementz ET, Sutherland CM, and Muchmore JH. Isolated hyperthermia chemotherapy perfusion for limb melanoma, *Surg. Clin. N. Am.*, **76** (1996) 1313–1331.

103. Hoekstra HJ, Koops HS, de Vries LG, et al. Toxicity of hyperthermic isolated limb perfusion with cisplatin for recurrent melanoma of the lower extremity after previous perfusion, *Cancer*, **72** (1993) 1224–1229.

104. Didolkar MS, Viens ML, Suter CM, et al. Phase II study of isolation perfusion with DITC in stage IIIa-IIIab melanoma of the extremity, *Proc. Am. Soc. Clin. Oncol.*, **9** (1990) 276.

105. Cavaliere R, Cavaliere F, Deeraco M, et al. Hyperthermic antiblastic perfusion in the treatment of stage IIIA-IIIB melanoma patients. Comparison of two experiences, *Melanoma Res.*, **4** (1994) 5–11.

106. Shiu MH, Knapper WH, Fortner JG, et al. Regional isolated limb perfusion of melanoma in-transit metastases using mechlorethamine (nitrogen mustard), *J. Clin. Oncol.*, **4** (1986) 1819–1826.

107. Fraker DL, Alexander HR, Andrich MP, et al. Treatment of patients with melanoma of the extremity using hyperthermic isolated limb perfusion with melphalan, tumor necrosis factor, and interferon-gamma: results of a tumor necrosis factor dose-escalation study, *J. Clin. Oncol.*, **14** (1996) 479–489.

108. Gutman M, Lev-Chelouche D, Abu-Abeid S, Inbar M, and Klausner JM. Isolated limb perfusion with tumor necrosis factor and melphalan for locally advanced malignant melanoma. Ninth Congress of the European Society of Surgical Oncology, Lausanne, Switzerland, 3–6 June 1998.

109. Hohenberger P and Kettelhack C. Clinical management and current research in isolated limb perfusion for sarcoma and melanoma, *Oncology*, **55** (1998) 89–102.

110. Fraker DL, Alexander HR, Bartlett DL, et al. Prospective randomized trial of therapeutic isolated limb perfusion (ILP) comparing melphalan (M) versus melphalan, tumor necrosis factor (TNF) and interferon-gamma (IFN): an initial report, *Soc. Surg. Oncol.,* **49** (1996) 6 (Abstract).

111. Barlett DL, Ma G, Alexander HR, et al. Isolated limb reperfusion with tumor necrosis factor and melphalan in patients with extremity melanoma after failure of isolated limb perfusion with chemotherapeutics, *Cancer,* **80** (1997) 2084–2090.

112. Gaynor JJ, Tan CC, Casper ES, et al. Refinement of clinicopathologic staging for localized soft tissue sarcoma of the extremity: a study of 423 adults, *J. Clin. Oncol.,* **10** (1992) 1317–1327.

113. Lawrence W, Donegan WL, Natrajan N, et al. Adult soft tissue sarcomas: a pattern of care survey of the American College of Surgeons, *Ann. Surg.,* **205** (1987) 349–359.

114. Eilber FR, Eckhardt JF, Rosn G, et al. Neoadjuvant chemotherapy and radiotherapy in the multidisciplinary management of soft tissue sarcomas of the extremity, *Surg. Oncol. Clin. North. Am.,* **2** (1993) 611–620.

115. Hoekstra HJ, Mehta DN, Wigffels RT, et al. Local tumor control by intraoperative radiotherapy (IORT): a pilot experience, *Eur. J. Surg. Oncol.,* **17** (1996) 364–369.

116. Krementz ET, Carter RD, Sutherland CM, et al. Chemotherapy of sarcomas of the limbs by regional perfusion, *Ann. Surg.,* **185** (1977) 555–564.

117. Pommier RF, Moseley HS, Cohen J, et al. Pharmacokinetics, toxicity and short-term results of cisplatin hyperthermic isolated limb perfusion for soft tissue sarcoma and melanoma of the extremities, *Am. J. Surg.,* **155** (1988) 667–671.

118. Sijens PE, Eggermont AMM, van Dijk P, et al. 31P magnetic resonance spectroscopy as predictor for clinical response in human extremity sarcoma treated by single dose TNF-alpha and melphalan isolated limb perfusion, *NMR Biomed.,* **8** (1995) 215–221.

119. Nieweg OF, Pruim J, Hoekstra HY, et al. Positron emission tomography with fluorine-18-fluorodeoxyglucose for the evaluation of therapeutic isolated regional limb perfusion in a patient with soft tissue sarcoma, *J. Nucl. Med.,* **35** (1994) 90–92.

120. Schraffordt-Koops H, Lienard N, Eggermont AMM, et al. Isolated limb perfusion with high-dose ENF-alpha, gamma-IFN, and melphalan in patients with irresectable soft tissue sarcomas; a highly effective limb saving surgery. 46th Annual Cancer Symposium, Society of Surgical Oncology, Los Angeles, 18–21 March 1998, **4** 1 (Abstract).

121. Vaglini M, Belli F, Ammatuna M, et al. Treatment of primary or relapsing limb cancer by isolation perfusion with high-dose alpha-tumor necrosis factor gamma interferon and melphalan, *Cancer,* **73** (1994) 483–492.

122. Lev D, Abu-Abid S, Issakov J, et al. Isolated limb perfusion (ILP) with tumor necrosis factor (TNF) and melphalan for multifocal soft tissue sarcoma (STS): Limb salvage in fatal disease. 51st Annual Cancer Symposium WFSOS (World Federation of Societies of Surgical Oncology), San Diego, 26–29 March 1998, W47, p. 42 (Abstract).

6 Lung Perfusion for Treatment of Metastatic Sarcoma to the Lungs

David Liu, Michael Burt, and Robert J. Ginsberg

CONTENTS

1. INTRODUCTION

The lung is among the most common sites involved in metastatic disease *(1)*. Approximately 30% of patients with cancer will develop pulmonary metastases at some point in the course of their disease *(2)*, and, more importantly, 20% of these patients will have metastatic disease limited to the lungs only *(3)*. Soft tissue sarcomas (STSs) of an extremity metastasize almost exclusively to this organ *(4)*. It is in this group of patients that pulmonary resection of metastases is most commonly performed, yielding 5-yr survival rates of 25–30% *(5)*. However, a significant portion of these patients are unresectable, and systemic chemotherapy remains the only available option, which, in most patients, has not proven to be effective in prolonging survival or producing a durable response *(6)*. This is may, in part, result from inadequate delivery of the drug to the lungs, when the chemotherapeutic agent is given by the intravenous (iv) route, because of dose-limiting toxicities. In an attempt to increase the therapeutic index of antineoplastic agents in this setting, lung perfusion was developed as an alternate method of delivering chemotherapy to minimize the drug's systemic effects, and to allow larger doses to be delivered to the tumor.

2. HISTORICAL PERSPECTIVE

2.1. Isolated Lung Perfusion

The first recorded case of lung perfusion was performed by Creech et al. *(7)* in 1958, for a patient with unresectable carcinoma. Complete isolation and simultaneous

From: *Current Clinical Oncology: Regional Chemotherapy: Clinical Research and Practice*
Edited by: M. Markman © Humana Press Inc., Totowa, NJ

perfusion of both lungs was accomplished using two extracorporeal circuits: a systemic circuit and a pulmonary circuit. The following year, a method for performing unilateral isolated lung perfusion in dogs was developed by Pierpont and Blades *(8)*. Using radioactive chromium-tagged red blood cells, they demonstrated that there were no leaks into the systemic circulation. Isolated lung perfusions were performed with escalating doses of nitrogen mustard, and the maximum tolerated dose (MTD) was determined to be 0.4 mg/kg, or 175–200× that which could be given intravenously. Jacobs et al. *(9)*, in 1960, improved the technique of Pierpont and Blades by utilizing gravity drainage of the effluent, as opposed to closed suction, allowing for drainage of additional blood from the bronchial circulation, thus reducing pulmonary vascular pressure and injury. This enabled them to use concentrations of nitrogen mustard up to 1.6 mg/kg without adverse effects.

2.2. Regional Lung Perfusion with Inflow Pulmonary Artery Occlusion

A less invasive method of unilateral lung perfusion was reported by Smyth and Blades *(10)* in 1960, first in dogs and then in humans. Using a balloon-tipped cardiac catheter, inserted percutaneously and positioned radiographically, the right or left pulmonary artery was occluded, and nitrogen mustard was infused distal to the balloon. Occlusion times up to 15 min were well tolerated. Four perfusions were performed in three patients, two with inoperable primary lung cancer and one with metastatic osteosarcoma. The patient with bilateral metastases had the left lung perfused first, and the right a month later. The advantages of this technique, compared to isolated lung perfusion, are that access to the pulmonary artery supplying the tumor can be accomplished less invasively, and selective lobe and multiple perfusions are possible without the need for a thoracotomy. Karakousis et al. *(11)*, in 1981, demonstrated this by performing a total of 56 injections with doxorubicin (DOX), using a Swan-Ganz catheter, through individual lobar arteries in seven patients with STSs metastatic to the lungs. Most of the perfusions were performed at 2-wk intervals. Although this was not an isolated system, and, therefore, any remaining drug not absorbed by the tumor and the lung parenchyma was released into the systemic circulation following deflation of the balloon, high tissue concentrations of the drug were still obtained. In canine experiments, Karakousis et al. found a 29-fold increase in lung tissue drug levels when DOX was infused through the Swan-Ganz catheter, with inflow occlusion of the pulmonary artery, compared to an equivalent dose delivered via the iv route. In a similar study performed on a rat model, we demonstrated that regional lung perfusion through the pulmonary artery with 0.5 mg/kg DOX (at one-tenth the iv dose) resulted in a five-fold increase in lung tissue concentrations, compared with iv delivery *(12)*.

2.3. Bronchial Artery Infusion

Many studies have demonstrated that the blood supply to primary lung cancers come from the bronchial arterial circulation *(13)*. Some have also suggested that the bronchial arteries supply metastatic neoplasms, as well *(14)*. Therefore, infusion of various anticancer agents through the bronchial artery has been proposed as an alternate method of lung perfusion for the treatment of both primary and metastatic tumors. The technique of bronchial artery infusion was first described by Cliffton and Mahajan *(15)* in 1963, using a double-balloon catheter to isolate and infuse nitrogen mustard into the segment of the aorta from which the bronchial arteries arose. The advantages are similar to that for inflow occlusion of the pulmonary artery, in addition to utilization of the blood supply to primary bronchogenic tumors and the ability to treat both lungs simultaneously.

Lung perfusions via the bronchial artery for metastatic tumors to the lung have also been performed. In 1965, Ohno *(16)* performed prophylactic bronchial artery infusions with three anticancer agents (mitomycin C, nitrogen mustard, and 5-flourouracil), using the Mahajan-Cliffton catheter, described previously *(15)*, for patients with pulmonary metastases from osteosarcoma of the extremities. Thirty-five patients, all without radiographic evidence of pulmonary metastases, first underwent prophylactic isolated lung perfusion, using the technique of Creech et al. *(7)*, 2 wk prior to radical operation of the extremity. Following the operation, they then received 1–4 postoperative bronchial artery infusions at 6–8 wk intervals. Aortic occlusion times of 20 min were well tolerated. The results appeared promising. The estimated 5-yr survival for the 35 patients who received isolated lung perfusion, radical operation of their extremity, and bronchial artery infusions, was 37%, compared with 30% for patients who underwent isolated lung perfusion and surgery only (*n* = 21), and 17% for patients who had surgery only (*n* = 41).

For bronchogenic carcinomas involving one lung or a portion of a lung, selective bronchial artery catheterization may be more appropriate. Tate et al. *(17)* performed the first selective bronchial artery infusion with nitrogen mustard in 1964, followed by 13 other infusions in patients with unresectable bronchogenic carcinoma, using either nitrogen mustard or cyclophosphamide. Two patients received two perfusions each. Only one patient showed an objective improvement.

Since then, others have performed selective bronchial artery infusions in patients with primary lung cancers, using a variety of other agents including 5-fluorouracil, thio-TEPA, methotrexate, mitomycin-C, and cisplatin *(18–22)*. In one study, 6 of 7 patients with far-advanced bronchogenic carcinomas were treated with continuous infusions of methotrexate, maintained by a pump. Three patients had catheters in place for 9–15 d *(18)*.

These bronchial artery infusions were used as treatment for symptoms in unresectable tumors, as primary treatment for lung cancer, or as induction therapy prior to surgical resection. Many patients had either partial responses or marked regression of their tumor as a result of treatment, and, in some cases, converted an inoperable tumor into an operable one. In a few patients who underwent induction therapy prior to surgical resection, no cancer cells could be found in the resected specimens. Therefore, bronchial artery infusions may be of therapeutic value in patients with inoperable lung cancer, for the purpose of relieving symptoms or causing such significant regression of the tumor as to make them resectable.

3. PRECLINICAL ANIMAL STUDIES

3.1. Animal Models

Numerous studies have been performed in dogs and pigs for evaluating the physiologic responses to lung perfusion and the pharmacokinetics of drug delivery via isolated lung perfusion. However, no tumor model existed with these two animal species for evaluating the efficacy of treatment. Consequently, our laboratory developed a tumor-bearing rat model that was convenient and economical for evaluating the efficacy of isolated lung perfusion in treating cancers metastatic to the lungs *(23)*. Metastases were established in the lungs by injecting tumor cells via the jugular vein. Once the animal was anesthetized and intubated, isolated lung perfusion was performed. The technique of isolated lung perfusion consisted of performing a left thoracotomy, isolating the pulmonary vessels, clamping the pulmonary artery and vein, cannulating the pulmonary artery, and performing a pulmonary venotomy, with the effluent collected by a suction catheter placed nearby.

3.2. Toxicity Studies

Doxorubicin is considered to be one of the most active single agents against sarcomas *(24)*. In canine studies, Johnston et al. *(25)* demonstrated the technique of isolated lung perfusion to be safe, with no apparent systemic or local toxicity at doxorubicin doses of 0.5 µg/mL in the plasma perfusate. Minchin et al. *(26)* carried out further pharmacokinetic and toxicity studies in dogs, and showed a dose-related complication following isolated lung perfusion with DOX. Using lactate dehydrogenase (LDH) activity as a marker of tissue injury, LDH activity, from both the perfusate and circulating plasma, increased with increasing DOX concentrations used, and remained elevated over the week following lung perfusion. Similarly, serum angiotensin-converting enzyme, another indicator of cellular injury, increased with higher doses of DOX and continued to increase in the group of animals that eventually died following contralateral pneumonectomy 2 wk later. The increase in serum ACE activity was reversible in the groups of animals perfused with the lower doses of DOX, and generally indicated survival following pneumonectomy, possibly reflecting reversible cellular injury. It was determined that substantial damage to the lungs occurred with perfusate concentrations of DOX above 11.6 µg/mL. Baciewicz et al. *(27)* performed similar perfusion studies, and found that significant histologic injury occurred at perfusate concentrations of DOX above 7.61 µg/mL. The finding of pulmonary toxicity at lower doses may be related to the fact their perfusions were done under relative hyperthermic (39°C) conditions, in contrast to Minchin's studies, which were at normothermic (37°C) temperatures.

Our laboratory found DOX delivery by isolated lung perfusion to be superior to iv injection in a rodent model *(28)*. We were able to achieve lung levels of DOX that were 20× higher, and heart concentrations that were 7× lower, with isolated lung perfusion than that of iv injection. The animals that underwent perfusion gained weight normally; the animals that received iv injections failed to thrive. From long-term (>2 mo) toxicity studies in Fisher F344 rats, we determined the median lethal dose of DOX delivered by isolated lung perfusion to be 10 µg/mL *(29)*.

Cisplatin is another drug that has demonstrated antitumor activity in STSs, with objective responses of approx 20% *(30,31)*. Ratto et al. *(32)* examined various methods of lung perfusion with cisplatin in pigs. Four groups of animals underwent cisplatin (2.5 mg/kg) infusion through the pulmonary artery, using inflow occlusion with or without outflow occlusion, isolated lung perfusion with 2.5 mg/kg cisplatin, or isolated lung perfusion with 5 mg/kg cisplatin. The animals that received cisplatin inflow occlusion only (group 2) had the worst profile (high systemic plasma and low lung tissue platinum levels) of all the groups. There were no significant differences in regional and systemic platinum concentrations between the animals that underwent cisplatin infusion through the pulmonary artery and those that underwent inflow/outflow occlusion (group 1) and ILP (groups 3 and 4). However, isolated lung perfusion produced higher mediastinal node and lower bone marrow platinum values than infusions through the pulmonary artery with either the inflow alone or inflow/outflow occlusion techniques. Lung damage was assessed by measuring gas-exchange parameters, and by light and electron microscopy, 1 hr after restoration of the pulmonary circulation. Acute morphologic and functional changes were found to be independent of the methods used, and appeared to return to normal during the 1-h recovery period.

Tumor necrosis factor (TNF) has been shown, in murine studies, to have significant antitumor effects against a variety of subcutaneous tumors (33). However, results from phase I human trials of iv recombinant TNF have been disappointing, with low response rates and a high frequency of systemic toxicities, such as fevers, chills, hypotension, and leukopenia (34). The method of isolated lung perfusion, with its inherent advantage of allowing one to deliver higher concentrations of a toxic substance without the systemic side effects, seemed suited for the delivery of TNF in the treatment of lung cancers. Pogrebniak et al. (35) used a swine model to evaluate the toxicity of isolated lung perfusion with TNF alone, or in conjunction with hyperthermia. They first determined the MTD iv of TNF to be 40 µg/kg. The left lung was then perfused with TNF at doses of 40 µg/kg, with ($n = 2$) or without hyperthermia ($n = 3$), or 80 µg/kg at normothermic conditions ($n = 3$). All the animals perfused with 40 µg/kg, with or without hyperthermia, survived. In the animals perfused with 80 µg/kg of TNF, 2 of 3 animals had life-threatening complications as a result of systemic leaks, or high local TNF levels that resolved with removal of the lung. There were no long-term changes seen on histologic analysis of the lungs 6–9 mo later.

3.3. Efficacy Studies

Our efficacy studies were performed in the rodent model. DOX was the first chemo-therapeutic agent studied with this model (36). Methylcholanthrene (MCA)-induced rat sarcoma cells were injected via the jugular vein to develop pulmonary metastases. One wk after injection, the rats were subjected to isolated lung perfusion at various doses of DOX, ranging from 10 to 320 µg/mL for 10 min at 500 µL/min, followed by a washout period of 5 min with buffered Hespan. One wk later, the rats were sacrificed and the lungs examined. At 320 µg/mL DOX, all evidence of sarcoma cells in the perfused lung was completely eradicated, either by gross examination or histologic evaluation (Fig. 1).

However, isolated lung perfusion with DOX, at a dose of 320 µg/mL resulted in long-term pulmonary toxicity (29). Buthionine sulfoximine (BSO), a potent inhibitor of glutathione synthesis, was examined as a possible adjunct for enhancing the effects of isolated lung perfusion with DOX, thus reducing the dose of DOX needed to achieve similar benefits. The efficacy of isolated lung perfusion with 10 µg/mL of DOX, with ($n = 12$) or without BSO pretreatment ($n = 12$), against lung metastases from MCA sarcomas, was evaluated (37). Overall, there was a 13-fold reduction in the number of tumor nodules in the rats that had undergone pretreatment with BSO intraperitoneally (2 mmol/kg × 3 doses), followed by isolated lung perfusion, compared with the perfusion only group. Furthermore, there were five complete responses in the perfusion + BSO group, and no complete responses in the perfusion only group. Pretreatment with BSO reduced the dose of DOX required for eradication of lung metastases, and presumably this would translate into a reduction of local pulmonary toxicity from isolated lung perfusion with DOX.

In addition to DOX, we have evaluated other agents delivered by isolated lung perfusion against various tumors. Rats perfused with human TNF, at doses of 420 µg, had a significant reduction in the number of MCA sarcoma nodules in the perfused lung, compared with the unperfused right lung (38). Similar doses of TNF delivered intravenously were ineffective, resulting in massive replacement of both lungs by tumor. Isolated lung perfusion with floxuridine was demonstrated to be safe and effective in significantly reducing the number of pulmonary nodules from Sp-5 colorectal adenocar-cinoma cells in BDIX rats (39). Isolated lung perfusion with melphalan, at a dose of

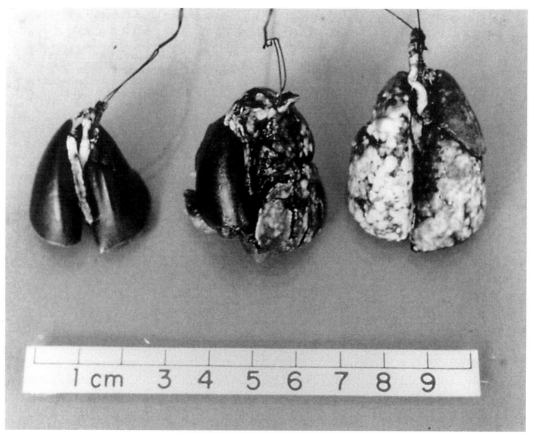

Fig. 1. Posterior view of the lungs of three rats. **Left,** Normal untreated lungs; **middle,** lungs after left isolated lung perfusion with DOX; **right,** lungs after left lung perfusion with saline solution. Normal lung tissue stains black, and tumors are white.

2 mg, resulted in significant reduction of MCA sarcoma nodules in Fisher F344 rats, compared with the unperfused right lung *(40)*. Rats that received an equivalent dose of melphalan intravenously died within 5 d, and rats that received 1 mg melphalan intravenously had no effect on the pulmonary nodules.

4. CLINICAL TRIALS OF ISOLATED LUNG PERFUSION

4.1. Doxorubicin

Following preclinical studies in dogs *(25)*, Minchin et al. *(41)*, in 1984, reported on the pharmacokinetics of isolated lung perfusion with DOX in patients who had unresectable metastatic pulmonary sarcoma nodules. Three patients underwent 50 min of isolated lung perfusions, which were performed at 25°C, with DOX concentrations ranging from 1 to 2 nmol/mL (0.58–1.16 μg/mL). Systemic DOX levels were not detected at any time during or after the perfusions. Tissue DOX levels increased steadily with time of perfusion, but DOX levels in the tumor nodules (range 0 to 0.4 nmol/g) were always lower than the immediate surrounding pulmonary tissue (range 0 to 1.2 nmol/g).

A pilot trial of isolated lung perfusion in humans was reported by Johnston et al. *(42)* in 1994. Four patients with metastatic sarcoma to the lungs and four patients with diffuse bronchiolo-alveolar carcinoma were the subjects of this study. Three patients underwent single-lung perfusion and five patients underwent perfusion of both lungs simultaneously (total lung perfusion) with either cisplatin (range 14 to 20 µg/mL) or DOX (range 1 to 10 µg/mL). Single-lung perfusion was accomplished by cannulation of the pulmonary artery and left atrial appendage. Total lung perfusion required a systemic circuit and a pulmonary circuit. For the systemic circuit, standard cardiopulmonary bypass was used, with arterial cannulation of the ascending aorta and a venous cannula placed in the right atrial appendage. The pulmonary circuit consists of a pulmonary artery cannula and a venous cannula in the left atrial appendage. Patients were perfused with either cisplatin or DOX, at times ranging from 40 to 60 min, followed by a washout with 200 mL systemic blood in single-lung perfusions or 500–1000 mL low-mol wt dextran in total lung perfusions.

Drug levels were measured in systemic blood, pulmonary perfusate, lung, tumor, and, occasionally, lymph node samples. In the three patients who underwent single-lung perfusion, there were no detectable levels of the drug in the systemic circulation, either during the perfusion or following restoration of the pulmonary circulation. There was minimal leak of the drug into the systemic circulation in the patients who underwent total lung perfusion, with an average of 7% of the peak pulmonary perfusate drug level being detected systemically. Significant tumor drug levels were detected in all patients. In the four patients who had sampling of their mediastinal nodes, three patients had detectable drug levels in their lymph nodes. Contrary to popular belief that the blood supply of most primary lung cancers arises from the bronchial circulation, these findings suggest that both primary and metastatic cancers in the lung are at least partially perfused by the pulmonary circulation. Demonstrable tumor response was not found, either by radiographic studies or survival. However, because dose-limiting toxicity was never reached, it was not possible to speculate whether perfusion at higher doses would have resulted in any clinical response.

Our phase I study consisted of single isolated lung perfusion with DOX in patients with unresectable metastatic sarcoma to the lungs. The objectives were to determine the MTD of DOX by isolated lung perfusion in humans, describe the toxicity of such therapy in humans, study the pharmacokinetics of DOX in this setting, and look for evidence of a therapeutic effect. Eight patients were enrolled. The primary histologies included leiomyosarcomas (two), synovial cell sarcoma (one), spindle cell sarcoma (one), extraosseous chondrosarcoma (one), alveolar soft part sarcoma (one), malignant fibrous histiocytoma (one), and osteogenic sarcoma (one). Our technique of single isolated lung perfusion consisted of cannulating the pulmonary artery and pulmonary vein, instead of the left atrial appendage. The bronchial arteries were temporarily clipped (Fig. 2). All perfusions were completed, with no perioperative deaths.

Preliminary results show that the MTD of DOX by single isolated lung perfusion is 40 mg/m^2 with peak perfusate concentrations ranging from 6 to 15 µg/mL. One patient who was perfused with 80 mg/m^2 of DOX, corresponding to a peak perfusate level of 50 µg/mL, had significant pulmonary toxicity, with evidence of consolidation and injury upon gross examination 2 wk postperfusion, and absence of ipsilateral ventilation or perfusion on lung scan 8 wk later. In the seven patients who had arterial blood samples available for analysis, the systemic levels of DOX were undetectable in five patients and minimal in two patients. None of the patients developed any evidence of systemic toxicity. Although this was a phase I trial designed to evaluate the MTD of isolated lung perfusion with DOX, we assessed the responses and survival in the treated patients. For example, a patient who underwent left isolated lung perfusion for unresectable pulmonary metastases from a high-grade, clear-cell paraspinal sarcoma

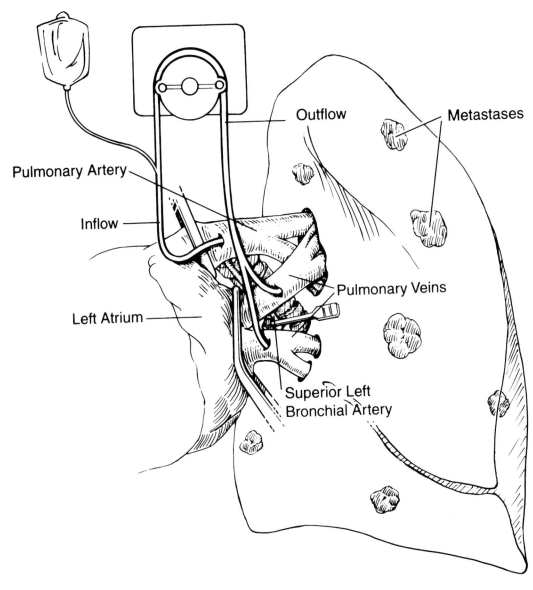

Fig. 2. The technique of isolated lung perfusion.

showed stabilization of the perfused lung; the unperfused right lung had rapid progression of her lesions at 2 and 4 mo after perfusion (Fig. 3).

4.2. Tumor Necrosis Factor

In 1996, Pass et al. *(43)* published the results of a phase I trial of hyperthermic isolated lung perfusion with TNF-α in conjunction with subcutaneous interferon-α, for pulmonary metastases from a variety of cancers, including STSs (five), melanomas (five), Ewing's sarcoma (two), adenoid cystic carcinoma (one), renal cell carcinoma (one), and colon cancer (one). Fifteen patients underwent 16 lung perfusions, most at moderate hyperthermia (38°C), for 90 min, with one patient receiving bilateral, staged perfusions. A dose-escalation scheme was performed, starting at 0.3 mg and ending at

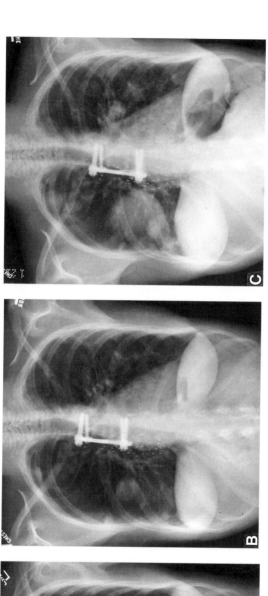

Fig. 3. Patient with unresectable pulmonary metastases from paraspinal sarcoma. **Left,** preoperative chest X-ray; **middle,** 2 mo after left isolated lung perfusion; **right,** 4 mo after left isolated lung perfusion. Note the progression of the lesions in the unperfused right lung.

6.0 mg of TNF. There were no significant changes in the hemodynamic parameters (e.g., heart rate, systemic and pulmonary artery blood pressures, right atrial pressures, wedge pressures, cardiac output, venous oxygen saturation) among the groups receiving different doses of TNF. The majority of patients had no evidence of leaks into the systemic circulation, either by use of radiolabeled albumin or enzyme-linked immunoassays for TNF. Only one person, perfused at the lowest TNF dose of 0.3 mg, had a significant leak rate of 10%, resulting in sequelae of TNF toxicity that included hypotension requiring pressors, transient rise in creatinine, and pulmonary insufficiency requiring intubation. This may have been complicated by excessive hyperthermia to the lung (peak of 45.3°C). There was a late complication seen in one patient, in whom necrosis developed in one of his large melanoma metastases, resulting in a lung abcess that required antibiotics and percutaneous drainage.

In the patients who underwent follow-up pulmonary function testing, the forced vital capacity (FVC), forced expiratory volume in 1 s (FEV_1), and diffusing capacity to carbon monoxide (DLCO) returned to 85% of preoperative values. Eight wk after their procedure, ventilation and perfusion of the TNF-exposed lung returned to 80 and 90% of preoperative values, respectively. There were three partial responses seen in the patients with melanoma, adenoid cystic carcinoma of the breast, and renal cell cancer. These responses were short-lived, with progression of their disease occurring within 9 mo after their operations.

4.3. Cisplatin

Following their experiments in pigs, Ratto et al. (44) evaluated the feasibility of isolated lung perfusion with cisplatin in humans. Six patients with metastatic sarcoma to the lungs were the subjects of their study. Perfusions were performed for 60 min at normothermic conditions, with a 200 mg/m² cisplatin dose, similar to the highest dose used in their animal experiments (5 mg/kg). At the end of perfusion, the volume in perfusion circuit was increased by 50% (700 mL), as a result of bronchial flow into the pulmonary circulation, because the bronchial arteries were not occluded. There were two postoperative complications as a result of contusion syndrome, resulting in interstitial and alveolar edema, which resolved after standard therapy. There were no systemic toxicities, such as myelosuppression, nausea and vomiting, and electrolyte abnormalities. Pulmonary function testing, at either 10 or 30 d postperfusion, revealed significant decreases in the FVC, FEV_1, and DLCO. Although no ventilation/perfusion mismatches were seen on lung scanning, there were scattered areas of defects in both ventilation and perfusion. Total platinum concentrations were minimally detected, and ultrafilterable platinum was never detected in the systemic circulation, indicating that the leak rate was very small. At the end of the perfusion, similar concentrations of platinum between normal lung and tumor suggested that the neoplastic tissue takes up the drug at a rate similar to normal lung.

5. FUTURE DIRECTIONS

Patients who are rendered disease-free after pulmonary resection of their sarcoma metastases are at high risk for recurrences. These recurrences occur almost exclusively in the lungs (4). Presumably, this is because of microscopic disease still present in the lungs following resection. To address this issue, we are currently considering a phase II trial of isolated lung perfusion with DOX as an adjuvant therapy to be performed concurrently with pulmonary resection. This adjuvant trial may translate into improved disease-free intervals for these patients with resectable disease.

Although the tumor responses to isolated lung perfusion with various agents have been short-lived, most of these patients received only one perfusion. Multiple perfusions may be required, but, because isolated lung perfusion is an invasive procedure that requires a thoracotomy, multiple perfusions are not particularly feasible or convenient for the patient. Regional perfusion with inflow blood occlusion of the pulmonary artery, using a balloon-tipped catheter, is a less-invasive technique that allows for multiple perfusions without an operation. We plan to evaluate this technique in a phase I study of regional perfusion with cisplatin, for patients with unresectable metastatic sarcoma to the lungs.

In the laboratory, we continue to investigate the use of isolated lung perfusion to deliver chemotherapeutic agents, including cisplatin, in conjunction with hyperthermia. Other treatment strategies being evaluated include gene therapy (e.g., suicide genes, cytokines) and modulators of drug resistance (e.g., cyclosporine, verapamil).

6. CONCLUSION

The outlook for patients with metastatic STS to the lung is dismal. Because current systemic chemotherapeutic agents have been unable to have a significant impact on the overall survival of these patients, novel methods of delivering antineoplastic agents, including lung perfusion, have been investigated. Regional lung perfusion has been demonstrated to be feasible in humans, and advantageous in providing a higher therapeutic index, compared to the standard iv route. Encouraging results have been reported, with a demonstration of a partial response in some patients with unresectable disease. This technique for delivery of antineoplastic agents to the lungs may hold promise in the adjuvant treatment of patients with resectable pulmonary metastases.

REFERENCES

1. Gilbert HA and Hagan AR. Metastases: incidence, detection, and evaluation without histologic confirmation, In Weiss L (ed), *Fundamental Aspects of Metastasis,* North-Holland, Amsterdam, 1976, pp. 385–405.
2. Van Dongen J and Van Slooten E. Surgical treatment of pulmonary metastases, *Cancer Treat. Rev.,* **5** (1978) 29–44.
3. Viadana E, Bross IDJ, and Pickern JW. Cascade spread of blood-borne metastases in solid and nonsolid cancers in humans, In Weiss L, Gilbert HA (eds), *Pulmonary Metastases,* GK Hall, Boston, 1978, pp. 142–167.
4. Potter DA, Glenn J, and Kinsella T. Patterns of recurrence in patients with high grade soft-tissue sarcomas, *J. Clin. Oncol.,* **3** (1985) 353–366.
5. Casson AG, Putnam JB, Natarajan G, et al. Five-year survival after pulmonary metastasectomy for adult soft tissue sarcoma, *Cancer,* **69** (1992) 662–668.
6. O'Bryan RM, Luce JK, Talley RW, et al. Phase II evaluation of Adriamycin in human neoplasia, *Cancer,* **32** (1973) 1–8.
7. Creech O, Krementz ET, Ryan RF, and Winblad JN. Chemotherapy of cancer: regional perfusion utilizing an extracorporeal circuit, *Ann. Surg.,* **148** (1958) 616–632.
8. Pierpont H and Blades B. Lung perfusion with chemotherapeutic agents, *J. Thorac. Cardiov. Surg.,* **39** (1960) 159–165.
9. Jacobs JK, Flexner JM, and Scott HW. Selective isolated perfusion of the right or left lung, *J. Thorac. Cardiov. Surg.,* **42** (1961) 546–552.

10. Smyth NP and Blades B. Selective chemotherapy of the lung during unilateral pulmonary arterial occlusion with a balloon-tipped catheter, *J. Thorac. Cardiovasc. Surg.,* **40** (1960) 653–666.

11. Karakousis CP, Park HC, Sharma SD, and Kanter P. Regional chemotherapy via the pulmonary artery for pulmonary metastases, *J. Surg. Oncol.,* **18** (1981) 249–255.

12. Wang HY, Ng B, Blumberg D, et al. Pulmonary artery perfusion of doxorubicin with blood flow occlusion: pharmacokinetics and treatment in a metastatic sarcoma model, *Ann. Thorac. Surg.,* **60** (1995) 1390–1394.

13. Cudkowicz L, Armstrong JB. Blood supply of malignant pulmonary neoplasms, *Thorax,* **8** (1953) 152–156.

14. Liebow AA. Pulmonary carcinoma: pathogenesis, diagnosis, and treatment, In Mayer E, Maier HC (eds), *Pathologic Aspects,* New York University Press, New York, 1956, pp. 62–149.

15. Cliffton EE and Mahajan DR. Technique for visualization and perfusion of bronchial arteries: suggested clinical and diagnostic applications, *Cancer,* **16** (1963) 444–452.

16. Ohno T. Bronchial artery infusion with anticancer agents in the treatment of osteosarcoma: prevention of pulmonary metastasis and improvement of prognosis, *Cancer,* **27** (1971) 549–557.

17. Tate CF, Viamonte M, and Agnew JR. Bronchial arterial perfusion with cytotoxic agents for bronchogenic carcinoma, *Am. Rev. Res. Dis.,* **97** (1968) 685–693.

18. Kahn PC, Paul RE, and Rheinlander HF. Selective bronchial arteriography and intra-arterial chemotherapy in carcinoma of the lung, *J. Thorac. Cardiovasc. Surg.,* **50** (1965) 640–647.

19. Haller JD, Bron KM, Wholey MJ, Poller S, and Enerson DM. Selective bronchial artery catheterization for diagnostic and physiologic studies and chemotherapy for bronchogenic carcinoma, *J. Thorac. Cardiov. Surg.,* **51** (1966) 143–152.

20. Heelekant C, Boijsen E, and Svanberg L. Preoperative infusion of mitomycin-C in the bronchial artery in squamous cell carcinoma of the lung, *Acta. Radiol. Diagn.,* **19** (1978) 1045–1056.

21. Uchiyama N, Kobayashi H, Nakajo M, and Shinohara S. Treatment of lung cancer with bronchial artery infusion of cisplatin and intravenous sodium thiosulfate rescue, *Acta. Oncol.,* **27** (1988) 57–61.

22. Ekholm SE, Dahlback O, and Tylen U. Preoperative treatment of squamous cell carcinoma of the lung with mitomycin-C in the bronchial artery, *Eur. J. Radiol.,* **6** (1986) 9–11.

23. Weksler B, Schneider A, Ng B, and Burt M. Isolated single lung perfusion in the rat: an experimental model, *J. Appl. Physiol.,* **74** (1993) 2736–2739.

24. O'Bryan RM, Luce JK, Talley RW, et al. Phase II evaluation of Adriamycin in human neoplasia, *Cancer,* **32** (1973) 1–8.

25. Johnston MR, Minchin R, Shull JH, et al. Isolated lung perfusion with Adriamycin: a preclinical study, *Cancer,* **52** (1983) 404–409.

26. Minchin RF, Johnston MR, Schuller HM, et al. Pulmonary toxicity of doxorubicin administered by *in situ* isolated lung perfusion in dogs, *Cancer,* **61** (1988) 1320–1325.

27. Baciewicz FA, Arredondo M, Chaudhuri B, et al. Pharmacokinetics and toxicity of isolated perfusion of lung with doxorubicin, *J. Surg. Res.,* **50** (1991) 124–128.

28. Weksler B, Ng B, Lenert JT, and Burt ME. Isolated single lung perfusion with doxorubicin is pharmacokinetically superior to intravenous injection, *Ann. Thorac. Surg.,* **56** (1993) 209–214.

29. Liu D, Kaneda Y, Burt M, and Ginsberg R. Long-term pulmonary toxicity of doxorubicin in isolated lung perfusion, unpublished data.

30. Dirix LH and Oosterom AT. Diagnosis and treatment of soft tissue sarcomas in adults, *Curr. Opin. Oncol.,* **6** (1994) 372–383.

31. Budd GT, Metch B, Weiss SA, et al. Phase II trial of ifosfamide and cisplatin in the treatment of metastatic sarcomas: a SWOG study, *Cancer Chemother. Pharmacol.,* **31** (1993) S213–216.

32. Ratto GB, Esposito M, Leprini A, et al. *In situ* lung perfusion with cisplatin, *Cancer,* **71** (1993) 2962–2970.

33. Asher AL, Mulé JJ, Reichert CM, Shiloni E, and Rosenberg SA. Studies on the antitumor efficacy of systemically administered recombinant tumor necrosis factor against several murine tumors *in vivo,* *J. Immunol.,* **138** (1987) 963–974.

34. Schiller JH, Witt PL, Storer B, et al. Clinical and biologic effects of combination therapy with gamma-interferon and tumor necrosis factor, *Cancer,* **69** (1992) 562–571.

35. Pogrebniak HW, Witt CJ, Terrill R, et al. Isolated lung perfusion with tumor necrosis factor: a swine model in preparation of human trials, *Ann. Thorac. Surg.,* **57** (1994) 1477–1483.

36. Weksler B, Lenert J, Ng B, and Burt M. Isolated single lung perfusion with doxorubicin is effective in eradicating soft tissue sarcoma lung metastases in a rat model, *J. Thorac. Cardiovasc. Surg.,* **107** (1994) 50–54.

37. Port JL, Hochwald SN, Wang HY, and Burt ME. Buthionine sulfoximine pretreatment potentiates the effect of isolated lung perfusion with doxorubicin, *Ann. Thorac. Surg.,* **60** (1995) 239–244.
38. Weksler B, Blumberg D, Lenert J, Ng B, Fong Y, and Burt M. Isolated single-lung perfusion with TNF-α in a rat sarcoma lung metastases model, *Ann. Thorac. Surg.,* **58** (1994) 328–332.
39. Port JL, Ng B, Ellis JL, et al. Isolated lung perfusion with FUDR in the rat: pharmacokinetics and survival, *Ann. Thorac. Surg.,* **62** (1996) 848–852.
40. Nawata S, Abecasis N, Ross HM, et al. Isolated lung perfusion with melphalan for the treatment of metastatic pulmonary sarcoma, *J. Thorac. Cardiovasc. Surg.,* **112** (1996) 1542–1548.
41. Minchin RF, Johnston MR, Aiken MA, and Boyd MR. Pharmacokinetics of doxorubicinin isolated lung of dogs and humans perfused *in vivo, J. Pharmacol. Expt. Ther.,* **229** (1984) 193–198.
42. Johnston MR, Minchen RF, and Dawson DA. Lung perfusion with chemotherapy in patients with unresectable metastatic sarcoma to the lung or diffuse bronchioloalveolar carcinoma, *J. Thorac. Cardiovasc. Surg.,* **110** (1994) 368–373.
43. Pass HI, Mew DJY, Kranda KC, Temeck BK, Donington JS, and Rosenberg SA. Isolated lung perfusion with tumor necrosis factor for pulmonary metastases, *Ann. Thorac. Surg.,* **61** (1996) 1609–1617.
44. Ratto GB, Toma S, Passerone GC, et al. Isolated lung perfusion with platinum in the treatment of pulmonary metastases from soft tissue sarcomas, *J. Thorac. Cardiov. Surg.,* **112** (1996) 614–622.

7 Regional Chemotherapy of Cancer of the Pancreas

James H. Muchmore and Jyoti Arya

CONTENTS

1. INTRODUCTION

Pancreatic cancer (PC) is the fifth most common cause of cancer death among males and females in the United States. In 1999, the American Cancer Society estimated that there would be 29,000 new cases of PC (14,100 men and 14,900 women). Even though 20% of patients elsewhere in the United States may live up to 2 yr, in Louisiana, essentially every patient will die within 2 yr. The longest survival time from the Charity Hospital of Louisiana in New Orleans is only 21 mo *(1–3)*.

The incidence of PC has continued to be virtually flat over the past 20 yr; previously, incidence, from the 1920s through 1973, had noticeably increased, according to the Charity Hospital Tumor Registry *(4,5)*. A similar trend in the incidence of PC is seen in England, as reported from data of the West Midlands Region Cancer Registry *(6)*. PC in Louisiana currently remains more prevalent in the African-American population, compared to the Caucasian population *(7)*. It is also essentially a disease of an older population, with the incidence increasing after the age of 40 yr; the majority of cases occur after 60 yr of age *(2,8)*.

From: *Current Clinical Oncology: Regional Chemotherapy: Clinical Research and Practice*
Edited by: M. Markman © Humana Press Inc., Totowa, NJ

Table 1
Extent of Disease at Diagnosis

	(%)
Local regional	80
Regional lymph nodes	86
Liver metastases	23–40
Peritoneal surfaces	25–35
Positive peritoneal cytology	30–75

The relative improvement in survival of patients with PC during the past two decades is derived primarily from a decrease in perioperative mortality. However, scarcely 0.4–4% of patients survive 5 yr or more, except in selected series (2,8–10). Median survival for patients with resectable PC, from several large series during the past decade, remains only around 6–23 mo, with an average of 14.6 mo (11,12). The dismal prognosis of this disease relates to the fact that 85–90% of patients come to diagnosis with an advanced, inoperable tumor and/or metastatic disease.

The last review of patients (60) with pancreatic ductal adenocarcinoma (ACA), from 1987 to 1991, recorded in the Charity Hospital Tumor Registry, showed that the majority (65%) had stage IV distal metastases at diagnosis. Only a small percentage (10.5%) had stage I/II resectable localized disease. Six patients had undergone a curative resection, but the longest-lasting survivor died of recurrent disease at 21 mo. Incredibly, the median survival for the entire group of patients was just 1 mo (3). During the years 1992 and 1993, there were 27 new patients with PC cancer for whom there was no improvement in survival. However, a slight improvement in the resectability rate (18.5%) was achieved. Thus, the prognosis for this disease in Louisiana remains poor and zero.

Regional chemotherapy for the treatment of PC addresses two of the major problems of this disease: local-regional failure, as well as that of the liver metastases; and the impressive resistance to systemic chemotherapy.

2. PATTERNS OF FAILURE

The patterns of failure in PC are no more than a reflection of the extent of disease at diagnosis, because 80% of patients come to diagnosis with advanced, local-regional disease (Table 1). Local-regional aggressiveness is a hallmark of this disease, in that small tumors (0.4–24%) are seldom found in most series, and only a small percent are well differentiated (2–8%) (2,13–15). Normally, in patients with pancreatic ductal ACA, 80% are diagnosed with a T4 lesion, that is, with local-regional invasion of the retroperitoneum (16,17).

The majority of patients, also, will come to diagnosis with tumors greater than 2 cm in size. Thus, they usually (86%) will have early involvement of multiple, lymph nodal sites, including regional nodes outside of the peripancreatic lymph nodes (18,19). Even small tumors produce regional, distal lymph nodal spread (20,21).

Liver metastases are commonly found in 23–40% of patients at diagnosis, and a significant proportion, approx 25–35%, will have peritoneal metastases (PMs) (11,22).

Table 2
Patterns of Failure in Resectable PC

	Postoperative adjuvant therapy (%)	Preoperative neoadjuvant therapy (%)
Local-regional	50–73	11–30
Regional lymph nodes	63	19
Liver metastases	50–62	54–100
Peritoneal surfaces	42	11–50
Positive peritoneal cytology	30–67	27
Extra-abdominal metastases	27	12.5–33

Laparoscopic staging of patients, now part of the preoperative (pre-op) workup, demonstrates that 30% of patients with resectable tumors will have positive peritoneal cytologies *(23)*. However, other studies of peritoneal cytology suggest that the incidence of positive cytologies in cases of resectable pancreatic disease may be only 7–8% *(24,25)*.

2.1. A Three-Compartment Problem

Pancreatic malignancies typically involve three different compartments within the abdominal cavity: the pancreatic, tumor-bearing region, including the peripancreatic lymph notes; the liver; and the peritoneal surfaces. Failure to effectively treat each of these different compartments, in patients with advanced disease, will result in the ultimate demise of the patient within 6–14 mo.

The primary site of initial failure of PC is local-regional in 19–33% of cases, following a curative resection *(26,27)*. Hepatic metastases are the second most common sole site of failure (15–24%), followed by peritoneal disease in 4–10% of cases. Only rarely (3%) are distal sites, outside the abdominal cavity, the initial or sole sites of failure. Commonly published is the incidence for combined, multiple sites of failure (Table 2): local-regional, 72–73%; hepatic, 62%; peritoneal, 42%; and distal, 27% *(26,27)*.

Local-regional failure is the most frequent site of recurrence, because a relatively high frequency of positive surgical margins (29–73%) are encountered following a curative resection. This is indicative of both the local-regional aggressiveness and advanced state of this malignancy at diagnosis *(15,28,29)*. Unfortunately, the local-regional failure rate is not significantly affected by adjuvant chemotherapy or radiotherapy (RT), except in cases of a margin, tumor-free resection *(29–31)*. Also, the majority of local treatment failures result in recurrences just outside the radiation field of the pancreatic bed, independent of the use of either intraoperative or external beam RT *(32,33)*.

Preoperative RT vs surgery alone improves the resectability rate and 1-yr survival rate, but downstaging of the local disease status does not translate into any long-term survival advantage *(34)*. Preoperative RT accomplishes a significant reduction of the tumor size, but there is no local-regional effect on the incidence of nodal metastases, nor a decrease in the development of perineural invasion. Also, very troublesome is the increased incidence of liver metastases in those patients treated with pre-op RT *(34)*.

Liver metastases are encountered at diagnosis in 23–40% of patients with PC *(11,22)*, and 27–75% of patients with operable disease will have liver metastases not detectable on pre-op staging *(35,36)*. In addition, liver metastases represent a primary site of failure in over 50% of patients, following a curative resection *(8,26)*. Adjuvant RT reduces local recurrences, but seems to induce an increased incidence of liver and PMs *(37,38)*. Preoperative RT improves local control, but then patients were found to principally fail with liver metastases *(14,34)*. Patients undergoing neoadjuvant chemoradiotherapy develop liver metastases, in 25% of cases, during restaging prior to laparotomy *(38)*. Hoffman et al. *(39)*, in a series of 63 patients, also noted a significant failure (73%), with hepatic metastases, following both pre-op chemotherapy and RT *(39)*.

Peritoneal cytologies are positive in 7–30% of cases deemed resectable by standard pre-op criteria *(23–25)*. Moreover, peritoneal seeding will be a component of failure in 42% of patients undergoing resection *(23,26)*. Also, patients with unresectable disease on initial exploration, had positive cytologies in 17.6% of the cases. This percentage increased to 67% when these patients were reexplored for treatment with interstitial RT *(40,41)*. Another study of patients with locally unresectable disease, treated with pre-op chemoradiotherapy found that 50% of the patients failed, with progression of the peritoneal surfaces *(42)*.

3. SURGICAL IMPROVEMENTS:
NOT ENOUGH TO CHANGE SURVIVAL

The sole contribution of the major cancer centers in treating patients with PC during the past decade has been to better select patients for surgical exploration and possible curative resection. The perioperative mortality for most major cancer centers is less than 2% *(15,43,44)*, but even the smaller institutions have recently shown that pancreaticoduodenectomy can be performed with a mortality of less than 5% and a 15% 5-yr survival rate *(45)*. The resectability rate for patients with PC has gone from approx 10% to, in some cases, over 25% *(14)*. The Memorial Sloan-Kettering Cancer Center (MSKCC) data shows that 18% of their patients, after their pre-op evaluation, had resectable disease, and, of those patients explored, 25% were resectable for cure *(11,46,47)*. Also, the Johns Hopkins Hospital data shows that the average size of the resected lesion is only 3 cm; the incidence of positive margins is decreased, as was the incidence of positive nodes in these selected patients *(15)*. Subsequently, the larger series show the survival for patients with PC to be 15–25% at 5 yr. However, even when the patients with the best prognostic variables are selected out, their survival, at best, remains only around 20% at 5 yr *(11,15,29)*, Unfortunately, in larger and nonselected series, the overall survival for all patients with resectable PC has not been appreciatively affected, and long-term survival remains less than 10% at 5 yr *(2,6,14)*.

Most patients undergoing a standard pancreaticoduodenectomy, or even the more limited pylorus-sparing procedure, eventually will fail, with local or distant disease. Thus, it must be assumed that the curative resection for PC is a misnomer, except for a minority of patients. Demonstration of this concept comes from the MSKCC series of 684 patients with PC: 118 had a curative resection, and only 12 patients survived 5 yr. However, 50% of the surviving patients later developed recurrent disease *(47)*.

Total pancreatectomy and the radical pancreaticoduodenectomy add little or no survival benefit to that of the two lesser procedures *(11,14,46)*. The essence of the Fortner radical operation proved that even an extensive *en bloc* resection lymph node dissection had no effect on survival *(48,49)*. The surgical rationale was to include the nodal basins containing a high incidence of metastatic disease, in 86% of the cases studied *(18,49,50)*.

The Japanese data *(51,52)* also demonstrates that there is no improvement in survival from a radical pancreatic resection, which leads to a much higher local-regional failure rate (87%), and the development of hepatic metastases, in 53% of the cases *(53)*. Thus, the surgical extent of treating local-regional disease, irrespective of tumor size or stage, does not change local-regional failure. Furthermore, local-regional disease is not the sole determining survival factor, because most patients also fail with liver or PMs.

4. LIMITATIONS OF CURRENT ADJUVANT THERAPIES

Postoperative chemotherapy and RT bring about limited survival benefit, mostly for only those patients with negative resection margins and negative nodal involvement *(30)*. Unfortunately, local-regional failure is not significantly altered by adjuvant chemotherapy or RT, in patients with involved surgical margins or with positive nodal disease *(29,30)*. Also, after postsurgical treatment of the pancreatic bed with intraoperative or external beam RT, most patients will fail, with recurrences just outside the radiation field *(35,37)*. Even though pancreatic bed failure is significantly reduced by local adjuvant therapies, the liver and peritoneal surfaces still remain the principal sites of failure *(38,39)*. Preoperative RT alone improves resectability and local control of the primary PC. However, the improvement in resectability does not translate into improved patient survival *(34)*. Detrimentally, the patients treated with pre-op RT experience an increase in the incidence of liver metastases *(34)*. All current strategies are aimed at improving the control and failure of only the local-regional disease. Not a single surgical and adjuvant treatment regimen yet improves the control of the two other principal sites of failure: the liver and the peritoneal surfaces.

5. RATIONALE FOR REGIONAL CHEMOTHERAPY

In 1950, the first reports of intra-arterial chemotherapy using nitrogen mustard were published simultaneously by Klopp et al. *(54)* and Beirman et al. *(55)*. Intra-arterial chemotherapy was found to enhance the local-regional tumor response rates, compared to that of systemic chemotherapy. The theoretical basis of regional chemotherapy remains essentially unchanged since the 1950s. The dose of a chemotherapeutic agent delivered intra-arterially to a tumor-bearing region can be effectively increased, compared to that of systemic chemotherapy. Simultaneously, the local-regional tumor response will be improved, while limiting systemic toxicity.

Data from in vitro tissue culture assays show that gastrointestinal (GI) tract malignancies are usually resistant to the systemic dosages of most chemotherapeutic agents *(56)*. Also, selection of those tumors with minimal sensitivity to systemic chemotherapy might benefit from an incremental increase in a locally delivered drug dose, particularly because most chemotherapeutic agents have a very steep dose–response curve.

With regional intra-arterial chemotherapy, the maximum regional drug escalation is only 1.5–2-fold that of systemic chemotherapy, but, for most solid tumors, there has not been the predicted improvement in response and survival. However, at Tulane University, School of Medicine, in the 1950s, the isolated regional perfusion technique was developed. This system employed complete vascular isolation of the tumor-bearing region, i.e., limb or liver, which was connected to a heart–lung perfusion pump *(57)*. With this regional chemotherapy system, regional drug delivery can be escalated 6–10× that of a systemic dose. Regional perfusion effectively controls local-regional metastatic malignant melanoma, normally exquisitely resistant to the entire spectrum of systemic chemotherapeutic agents *(57,58)*. Thus, theoretically, from this system, it was learned that the local-regional drug dose needs to be escalated approx 5–10× that of the systemic dose, in order to induce a complete (CR) or significant partial response (PR). A curative surgical resection of the tumor and tumor-bearing tissues should then follow regional chemotherapy to improve the long-term survival of patients with an advanced cancer. This rationale appears also to apply to the treatment of PC.

5.1. Limitations of Drug Delivery

Effective drug delivery of chemotherapeutic or biological agents remains a major obstacle in the treatment of PC. Normally, the microvascular environment of a primary pancreatic malignancy is a dense, poorly vascularized fibrotic envelope resulting from the chronic pancreatitis surrounding the tumor. The tumor itself can be composed of several regions with varying blood flow, because tumors, as they grow, compress their central blood supply. The peripheral region, with active neovascularization, can be hypervascular; the central portion is usually necrotic, or even avascular *(59,60)*. The blood flow within a PC has been measured to be about 45 cc/min/100 g; the blood flow of the normal pancreatic parenchyma is on the order of 87 cc/min/100 g *(61)*. The intratumor pressure is significantly elevated, because neoplasms do not develop a neolymphatic system to drain the extravascular fluid from within the tumor nodule *(59,60,62)*. Intratumor vascular shunts (tissue hypertension causing hypoxia within the tumor) are additional factors leading to ineffective drug delivery *(63)*. The major portion of a systemic drug dose is therefore shunted around and away from the primary tumor; thus, the pancreatic tumor is almost impenetrable by any systemic therapeutic modality.

5.2. Multidrug Resistance

A primary reason for the treatment failure of PC is the remarkable inefficacy of systemic, neoadjuvant, or adjuvant chemotherapy. 5-fluorouracil (5-FU), or 5-FU in combination with other chemotherapeutic agents, at best produces response rates only in the range of 7–28% *(64–66)*. Mitomycin C (MMC), likewise, in a large clinical trial, produced a response rate of only 21%, but the response was only of short duration *(67)*. Ductal PC is exquisitely resistant to the entire spectrum of chemotherapeutic agents. The response rate of PC to all chemotherapeutic agents is unexplainably ineffective, or essentially zero, in 50% of the majority of single agents studied (Table 3; *11,12,68*). Because the response rate average is so poor, less than 20%, Taylor *(89)* has suggested that the use of chemotherapy for PC should be entirely abandoned. Even gemcitabine (2′, 2′-difluorodeoxycytidine), touted currently as the most effective agent for advanced PC, produces only a 11% PR, with a median duration of 13 mo *(76)*. Another phase II trial with gemcitabine found a response rate of only 6.25%, and the median duration of survival was only 6.3 mo *(77)*. Also, in both clinical trials, there was not a single patient with a CR to gemcitabine.

One fundamental reason that ductal carcinoma is exquisitely resistant to chemotherapy is that this malignancy usually expresses moderate-to-high levels of a 170-kDa plasma membrane glycoprotein. P-glycoprotein, the multidrug resistance gene (MDR1) product, functions as an energy-dependent efflux enzyme system that rapidly clears toxins and natural-product chemotherapeutic agents from the tumor cell *(11,90)*. Consequently, a pancreatic malignancy can easily avoid the tumor cytotoxic effects of most systemically delivered chemotherapeutic agents.

Second, the majority of pancreatic ACAs (80–95%) contain gene mutations involving K-*ras* at codon 12 *(91–93)*. Malignancies with K-*ras* gene mutations maintain an

Table 3
Investigational Studies
of Chemotherapeutic and Biological Agents for Pancreatic Cancer

Agent (ref.)	Responses/Patients (response rate %)	Median survival (mo)
Aclacinomycin (69)	0/16 (0)	3
Amonafide (70)	0/36 (0)	2.5
Azinidinylbenzoquinone (71)	0/21 (0)	2
Brequinar sodium (72)	0/17 (0)	
Dihydroxyanthracenedione (69)	0/23 (0)	2.5
Docetaxel (73)	5/29 (17)	NA
Edatrexate (74)	2/40 (5)	3.5
Fludarabine (75)	0/20 (0)	3
Gemcitabine (76)	5/44 (11.4)	5.6
Gemcitabine (77)	2/34 (5.8)	6.3
Goserelin (78)	0/18 (0)	5
Iproplatin (79)	3/32 (9.4)	NA
Irinotecan (80)	3/32 (9.4)	5.2
Merbarone (81)	2/29 (6.9)	NA
Mitoguazone (71)	2/32 (6.3)	7.6
Octreotide (82)	0/22 (0)	5
Paclitaxel (83)	3/39 (8)	5
Piroxantrone (84)	0/35 (0)	3
Pirarubicin (85)	0/17 (0)	NA
Spirogermanium (69)	0/20 (0)	3
Topotecan (86)	3/30 (10)	4.5
Tomudex (87)	2/42 (5)	NA
Tumor necrosis factor (88)	0/22 (0)	2.9
Median	(5)	4

NA = not available.

active upregulated state of membrane-associated tyrosine kinases, and increased signal transduction, with resultant cellular proliferation. Also, a host of other membrane functions are activated by the ras protein product through raf (94–96). Other data shows that p53 tumor suppressor gene mutations are commonly found in over 50% of PC (97). The importance of both the K-ras oncogene mutation and p53 tumor suppressor gene loss is that these activate the expression of the MDR1 gene promoter (98). Consequently, the MDR1 gene will be upregulated in the majority of patients with PC.

Recently, other non-P-glycoprotein mechanisms of multidrug resistance have been delineated in pancreatic tumors: the multidrug resistance-associated protein, a 190-kDa, adenosine triphosphate-dependent efflux protein similar to P-glycoprotein; and the lung cancer resistance-associated protein (99,100). Furthermore, the amplification or upregulation of thymidylate synthase expression, the target enzyme of 5-FU, is responsible for the reduced chemosensitivity to 5-FU in gastric and colorectal malignancies, and quite possibly also in PC (101–103). Thus, it becomes clear why the majority of the chemotherapeutic agents delivered systemically have had little or no cytotoxic effect on pancreatic ductal ACA, and little impact on the survival of these patients with this malignancy.

6. REGIONAL CHEMOTHERAPY AND PHARMACOKINETICS

Inherent in the strategy of effective regional chemotherapy should be the means of overcoming the drug delivery difficulties within the microvascular environment of a pancreatic tumor, and, second, the multidrug resistance. The theory supporting the use of regional chemotherapy is based on two assumptions: First, intra-arterially delivered chemotherapeutic agents generate a higher drug concentration within the tumor-bearing area, and thus should improve the overall response, compared to systemic chemotherapy; second, if the infused target region clears the agent-limiting systemic toxicity, the drug dose can be significantly escalated.

Eckman et al. *(104)*, in 1974, developed a mathematical model detailing the potential drug concentration advantage derived from an intra-arterial infusion vs iv administration. This model describes an advantage from intra-arterial drug delivery vs systemic therapy as an integral equation of concentration multiplied by time (C × T). The regional advantage, most aptly described in terms of the area under the drug concentration–time curve (AUC), is also dependent on the rate of drug delivery, the regional blood flow, and the rate of total body clearance.

Further drug-delivery models evaluating the potential drug exposure to a tumor-bearing region were described by Chen and Gross *(105)* and Collins and Dedrick *(106)*. The model of Chen and Gross is based on the liver as the primary target organ for regional chemotherapy *(83)*. The regional drug advantage is determined by three factors: regional drug extraction or metabolism, regional blood flow, and the total body clearance of the drug. The efficacy of regional drug extraction, metabolism, and clearance in this model, then, defines the advantage of regional drug delivery. There is relatively no regional advantage, if the infused drug is cleared more rapidly systemically than regionally. This lack of advantage is particularly true in the cases of an extrahepatic intra-arterial infusion.

Collins *(107)* characterizes the therapeutic index as

the ratio of drug concentration in the tumor (AUC_T) . . . to drug concentration in the systemic circulation (AUC_S). . . . The therapeutic advantage for drug delivery, R_d, can be expressed as the ratio of the therapeutic index for intra-arterial (IA) versus the therapeutic index for intravenous (IV) administration:

$$R_d = (AUC_T/AUC_S) \text{ IA}/(AUC_T/AUC_S) \text{ IV}$$

For that region or organ that metabolizes and clears the infused drug, i.e., the liver, the therapeutic advantage is increased in proportion to the regional drug clearance. The R_d also depends on the fraction of drug, E, removed during a single pass through the target tissue:

$$R_d = Cl_{TB}/Q \; (1 - E) + 1$$

For that region not metabolizing or clearing the infused agent, the R_d is a function of the regional blood flow (Q_i) and total body clearance (Cl_{TB}).

$$R_d = Cl_{TB}/Q_i + 1$$

Chemotherapeutic agents rapidly cleared systemically, such as 5-FU, may allow some regional benefit when the drug is delivered as a continuous regional infusion.

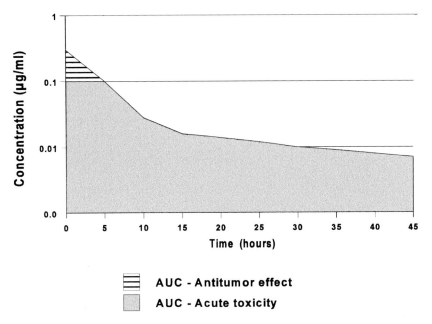

Fig. 1. Drug pharmacologic profile (AUC) for an intra-arterial bolus dose of DOX 30 mg/m². Only that part of the drug dose (AUC) above 0.1 μg/mL contributes to the tumorcidal effect of DOX. All of the drug dose (AUC) below 0.1 μg/mL contributes primarily to the systemic toxicity. Adapted with permission from ref. *110.*

6.1. Regional Drug Scheduling, Dose, and Drugs

Most chemotherapeutic agents have essentially the same antineoplastic activity, irrespective of whether it is administered as a single bolus dose once a month, as a weekly dose, or as a prolonged infusion. However, it is important to remember that their antineoplastic activity and acute toxicity (i.e., primarily myelosuppression) correspond to the integral equation of $C \times T$, or the area under the drug concentration–time curve (AUC), rather than the peak plasma concentration, C_{max}, achieved following bolus administration *(110,111).* Both the antitumor effect and toxicity are directly proportional to AUC. However, the antitumor effect is determined more by the C_{max}, and the time this concentration is maintained above a certain tumor cytotoxic threshold (Fig. 1). Also, increasing the delivered drug dose does not significantly produce an increase in the C_{max}, but usually increases only the half-life of the terminal phase *(112).* It is the AUC of the terminal phase that contributes most to the toxicity of a particular chemotherapeutic agent.

The alkylating agents, nitrogen mustard, melphalan, and nitrosoureas, plus the antitumor antibiotics, MMC, dacarbazine, and cisplatin, have commonly been used in most regional chemotherapy systems *(57,58).* These drugs, which interact rapidly with the DNA, tend to be noncell-cycle-dependent and are primarily concentration-dependent for their cytotoxic effect. On the other hand, antimetabolites (floxuridine [FUDR], 5-FU, and methotrexate) are time-dependent, and require a prolonged exposure time for their antitumor effect (Table 4). Thus, theoretically, tumor cytotoxicity can be better facilitated by significantly increasing the regional drug peak concentration, rather than increasing the time exposure of a tumor-bearing region to a chemotherapeutic agent *(113).* The anthracyclines and anthracenes are primarily concentration-dependent cytocidal drugs having some time dependence *(113).*

Table 4
Concentration Vs Time Dependency
of Chemotherapeutic Agents Used in Treating PC

| Drug | IC_{50} ($\mu g/mL$) | | SDR |
	1-h exposure	24-h exposure	
5-fluorouracil	220	0.23	957
Methotrexate	97	0.32	303
Etoposide	3.3	0.032	103
Cisplatin	19	0.30	63
Melphalan	1.3	0.13	10
Mitomycin C	0.48	0.06	8.0
Doxorubicin	0.13	0.022	5.9

IC = inhibitory concentration; SDR = schedule dependency ratio: <24 implies concentration dependency; >24 implies time dependency.
Adapted with permission from ref. *112*.

Therefore, the appropriate scheduling of agents used for regional chemotherapy would be alkylating agents or antitumor antibiotics of a high-dose bolus, or a high-dose, short-term infusion of approx 1–2 h. This type of scheduling generates a maximal plasma level, or C_{max}, of drug capable of producing the appropriate intratumor drug levels.

Most clinical data on regional chemotherapy is derived from clinical trials using hepatic artery infusions with antimetabolites to treat metastatic colorectal cancer of the liver. Ensminger and Gyves' data *(114,115)* shows that only FUDR and 5-FU have a regional therapeutic advantage when infused through the hepatic artery. The regional clearance of FUDR delivered by the hepatic artery is better than 90% on the first pass through the liver. 5-FU has a 50% hepatic extraction rate on the first pass through the liver. Because FUDR and 5-FU are effectively cleared by the target organ, the drug dose can be increased proportionally to their regional drug clearance *(90)*. The rest of the chemotherapeutic agents (MMC, doxorubicin [*DOX*], nitrosoureas, and cisplatin) have little or no regional advantage, because they undergo modest-to-minimal hepatic extraction *(114,115)*.

For PC, the drugs that have been commonly used for regional treatment are 5-FU, DOX, MMC, cisplatin, and mitoxanthrone (MTZ). The lack of any efficient regional drug clearance presents a real problem in using standard intra-arterial chemotherapy techniques in treating PC. However, by using extracorporeal devices, the total body clearance of chemotherapeutic agents can be artificially increased, and the regional advantage of regional chemotherapy significantly improved (*see* subheading 9).

7. LIMITATIONS OF INTRA-ARTERIAL CHEMOTHERAPY

Because total body clearance, Cl_{TB}, is inversely proportional to AUC, and principally the toxicity of a chemotherapeutic agent, the rapidity of the clearance determines the usefulness of regional drug infusion.

$$Cl_{TB} = \text{drug dose}/AUC$$

The antimetabolite, FUDR, used in treating hepatic metastases from colon cancer, is the only chemotherapeutic agent that has a truly worthwhile regional advantage. This agent has a hepatic extraction ratio of approx 92%, and therefore the hepatic tumor

Table 5
Relative Advantage (R_d) Regional Infusion for Antineoplastic Agents

Drug	Cl_{tb}	Q = 10 (mL/min)	Q = 100 (mL/min)	Q = 1000 (mL/min)
Floxuridine	25,000	2500	251	26
5-fluorouracil	4000	400	41	5
BCNU	1000	100	11	2
Doxorubicin	900	90	10	1.9
Cisplatin	400	40	5	1.4

BCNU, 1, 3-*bis*(2-chloroethyl)-1-nitrosourea.
Adapted with permission from ref. *116*.

drug exposure can be increased 100–400-fold *(115)*. However, 5-FU, DOX, MMC, nitrosoureas, and cisplatin are not as effectively cleared by the liver. In addition, because of the high regional blood flow (~1450 cc/min) within the liver, the tumor uptake of these agents is modest, and their effectiveness on tumor response is minimal (Table 5; *116*). The regional pharmacokinetics of MMC, DOX, and 5-FU show that, during a hepatic artery infusion, the extraction ratios were only 23–50%. At best, the hepatic exposure is increased only 5–10-fold *(114,115,117,118)*. Thus, most chemotherapeutic agents do not have a realistic regional therapeutic advantage, even in treating hepatic colorectal metastases or, for that matter, PC.

Another problem is evident after analyzing the pharmacokinetics of intra-arterial DOX. Studies with intra-arterial DOX show that the hepatic clearance, or detoxifying mechanism, becomes saturated at higher drug levels *(105)*. Similarly, with increasing higher DOX doses, the hepatic extraction fraction decreased from 0.33 to 0.22 in a rat isolation–perfusion model *(119)*. Also, in patients with liver metastases, there can be a tremendous variation in hepatic DOX clearance, and, in one study, the hepatic extraction ratio ranged from a low of 0.05 to 0.5, a more normal extraction fraction *(117)*.

The therapeutic advantage for regional drug delivery for extrahepatic sites is not well defined. Thus, for the pancreas, the major portion of the infused drug dose will be cleared systemically. Systemic toxicity, then, remains the principal dose-limiting factor. However, the venous effluent following a pancreatic, celiac infusion passes mostly through the portal system of the liver. The total body clearance of the drugs used (5-FU, MMC, cisplatin, DOX, and MTZ) will be only partly dependent on the first pass, hepatic extraction, and metabolism, but the hepatic extraction will never be enough to create a regional therapeutic advantage.

The question of the actual concentration of drug delivered to a target area presents another notable problem for regional chemotherapy. The regional drug dose is increased by intra-arterial delivery by only 1–1.5× that of systemic drug delivery. The initial experience in treating PC with regional chemotherapy produced no difference in survival, compared to systemic chemotherapy *(120,121)*. Even though tumor response to the small increment in delivered dose is significantly better, the survival advantage for patients with pancreatic or GI tract malignancies remains minimal *(120–122)*. In fact, tissue culture data shows that significant improvement in response for most GI malignancies comes only after increasing the drug dose 5–10× above the systemic C_{max} of the drug *(123,124)*.

With current techniques, regional chemotherapy, at most, increases the regional drug dose by 2–3× that of the systemic dose *(118,125)*. Thus, the regional advantage and drug delivery are not increased enough to overcome the tumor cell resistance stemming from the P-170 drug efflux enzyme system. 5-FU should be escalated more than 10× the normal systemic C_{max} to be effective. MMC, DOX, MTZ, and cisplatin only produce increased response rates of GI tract malignancies in vitro when the plasma dose is increased from 1 to 10 μg/mL (123,126). Likewise, gemcitabine demonstrates only a modest in vitro activity against sensitive, human tumor cell lines, after increasing the dosage from 1 to 10 μg/mL, but resistant cell lines require that drug dose be escalated up to 100 μg/mL (127).

8. REGIONAL INTRA-ARTERIAL CHEMOTHERAPY

8.1. Regional Chemotherapy for Inoperable PC

Only a few studies are published on using regional chemotherapy for the treatment of advanced PC. The first study, by Theodors et al. (120) in 1982, using an infusion, over 4 d, of 5-FU, DOX, MMC, and streptozotocin, produced a response rate of 47%. Unfortunately, the 19 treated patients had a rather short median survival of only 5 mo. Bengmark and Andren-Sandberg (121) reported a mean survival of more than 12 mo for 19 patients treated with regional infusion of 5-FU of 10 mg/kg/d for 1 mo. However, these patients were also treated with oral 50 mg/kg 5-FU and 50 mg testolactone tid. Because of significant complications with regional infusions, and because the survival was no better than that of systemic therapy, the use of intra-arterial chemotherapy for PC was discontinued for more than 15 yr.

Using a celiac artery infusion, Aigner et al. (122) treated 26 patients with unresectable PC. A response rate of 77% was obtained in these patients, with a median survival of 9–13.8 mo, using a combination of 5-FU, MMC, and cisplatin. A Japanese study (128) of 15 patients with unresectable PC, using a splenic and gastroduodenal arterial infusion, produced a median survival of 14 mo. The treatment protocol in this study used a combination of 5-FU with leucovorin, methotrexate + angiotensin. Notably, 13% of these patients developed liver metastases. A larger Italian study (129) of 38 unresectable patients with stage III and IV PC evaluated the combination of intra-arterial 5-FU, leucovorin, epirubicin, and cisplatin. The median survival for the entire group of patients was only 6.2 mo: 13.4 mo for those with stage III disease and 3.6 months for stage IV. The only randomized study comparing regional to systemic chemotherapy is another small Japanese study of 16 patients (130). The reported survival of those receiving intra-arterial chemotherapy was 10.6 vs 1.6 mo for those treated with systemic therapy.

Two studies have looked at the combination of regional chemotherapy and RT for unresectable PC. McCracken et al. (131) studied a small group of 18 patients using a celiac infusion of 5-FU and MMC followed by radiation. A reported 44% response was elucidated in 8 of 18 patients.

Another study (132) of combined regional chemotherapy and radiotherapy also looked at primary irradiation of the pancreas (60 Gy) and hepatic artery 5-FU + low-dose irradiation (20 Gy) to the liver. The median survival was 50 wk, and the incidence of hepatic metastatic disease was only 6%.

The average survival in these studies is only 9–14 mo, even though there is a significant improvement in the overall response rates. However, like the studies using systemic neoadjuvant chemoradiation, the average survival is about the same, because most of these patients will still fail from uncontrolled PMs.

8.2. Preoperative Regional Chemotherapy

Regional intra-arterial chemotherapy should be able to improve local-regional control by improving resectability, and facilitate a margin free of tumor curative resection. Using a celiac artery infusion, Aigner et al. *(122)* treated a group of 26 patients with advanced stage III and IV disease, achieving a response rate of 77%. The average survival of these patients was only 9–13.8 mo. In 1993, Aigner et al. *(123)* updated the data on 164 patients from four different studies with unresectable stage II and IV disease. This combined data showed that at least 30% of these patients could be converted to candidates for a curative resection, but the average survival for the entire group of patients remained 9.8–12 mo.

One other case study *(130)* investigated the disease control of the resection margin using pre-op intra-arterial chemotherapy for an unresectable tumor of the head of the pancreas. A short course of intra-arterial 5-FU, methotrexate + angiotensin II produced a significant reduction in tumor size. Also, the authors noted that, following resection, the margins were clear of tumor, and there was no evidence of extrapancreatic perineural invasion.

8.3. Adjuvant Regional Chemotherapy

Regional chemotherapy for resectable PC has only been considered recently. Using a postoperative celiac infusion, Link et al. *(134)* treated 20 patients whose median survival was 21 mo, and the hepatic disease progression appeared to be decreased. Ishikawa et al. *(135)* demonstrated an effective reduction in incidence of liver metastases (8%) following pancreaticoduodenectomy, using an hepatic artery and portal vein infusion of 5-FU. The most impressive aspect of this study was the reported, 5-yr survival rate of 54%. The only randomized trial, involving 80 patients following pancreatectomy, showed a significant difference in median survival of 30 vs 16.8 mo for those treated with regional chemoimmunotherapy *(136)*. Similar to the Japanese studies, the patients treated with regional therapy had a significant reduction in the development of hepatic metastases.

9. REGIONAL CHEMOTHERAPY PLUS EXTRACORPOREAL RECAPTURE

Regional intra-arterial chemotherapy, plus extracorporeal hemoperfusion or hemofiltration, was first employed by Oldfield and Dedrick et al. *(137,138)* to increase the drug exposure to primary brain tumors. Hemoperfusion employs a charcoal capsule or an absorbent resin capsule to recapture drug from within an extracorporeal circuit; hemofiltration utilizes a semipermeable, hollow tube filter to remove molecules of less than 10,000 mol wt within the extracorporeal circuit.

Hemoperfusion or hemofiltration, through rapid extracorporeal recapture of a chemotherapeutic agent, acts to detoxify the venous effluent from a tumor-bearing region. Significant reduction of systemic drug exposure and toxicity allows the regional drug dose to be markedly escalated.

9.1. Regional Chemotherapy plus Hemofiltration

Hemofiltration is a technique of extracorporeal drug clearance, related in part to both hemodialysis and hemoperfusion. Thus, extracorporeal hemofiltration acts to artificially

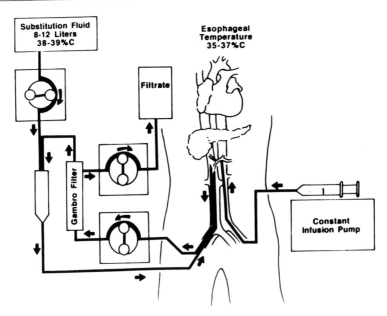

Fig. 2. Schema for regional intra-arterial chemotherapy with extracorporeal hemofiltration. A balanced hemofiltration is established with a flow rate of 400 mL/min and an ultrafiltration rate of 150 mL/min, and is continued for 60–70 min. The regional chemotherapy is delivered by means of a celiac artery catheter over the first 30–40 min.

increase the total body clearance, through a filtration process (Fig. 2). This method, used in conjunction with regional chemotherapy, permits the escalation of the total regional drug dose. Hemofiltration is most effective in recapturing the C_{max}s of an antineoplastic agent, when a steep drug gradient exists across the semipermeable membrane of the filter. Thus, hemofiltration rapidly clears through filtration the peak dose, but it then becomes inefficient as the dose on both sides of the filter equilibrates. Because filtration clears only the peak dose, this technique only effectively recaptures 20–25% of the total drug dose *(139)*.

In the case of hemofiltration, the regional advantage, R_d, is then related to the fraction of drug eliminated, E_r, on the first pass through the tumor-bearing region; second, the fraction cleared by the liver, E_l, plus, primarily, the fraction of drug cleared through the hemofiltration system E_{hf} *(139)*:

$$R_d = Cl_{TB}/Q \ [1 - (E_r + E_l + E_{hf})] + 1$$

A modified Gambro® hemofiltration system (Stockholm, Sweden) was used in the Tulane University trials for rapid extracorporeal clearance of the chemotherapeutic agents. This system then allowed the regional drug dose to be escalated only 3–5× that of a systemically delivered drug dose. However, the total drug dose infused is only twofold greater than the total systemic dose normally used.

A strategy and procedure similar to that of Dedrick et al. *(137)* was collaboratively modified by Aigner et al. *(140)* and Muchmore et al. *(141,142)* for the treatment of patients with liver metastases and advanced intra-abdominal malignancies. Current treatments with regional chemotherapy plus hemofiltration allow an estimated drug dosage of 3–4× that of the systemic dose to be infused into the tumor-bearing region.

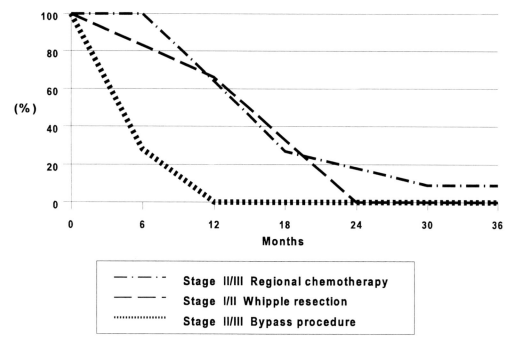

Fig. 3. Survival of patients with stage II/III inoperable cancer treated with regional chemotherapy, compared with other stages treated by surgery alone, at Charity Hospital. Stage I/II patients were treated by a curative resection. Stage II/III treated by hepatic and gastric bypass procedures.

Response rates of advanced PC to regional chemotherapy plus hemofiltration are reported from 45.5 to 77%. These are approx 2–3× the average response rates of 20–28% achieved through the use of systemic chemotherapy *(11,122,142)*.

Aigner and Gailhofer *(143)* reported on using celiac axis infusion of MMC and MTZ with starch microspheres, combined with hemofiltration. Using this method, a 27% CR rate was obtained in 15 patients with unresectable PC.

At Tulane University School of Medicine, 45.5% of patients (5 of 11) with unresectable PC achieved a PR using intra-arterial chemotherapy plus hemofiltration. The resectability rate after regional chemotherapy in this series was 25%, and the entire group had a median survival of 14 mo *(3)*. The longest-lasting survivor of this group with unresectable PC was one of three patients from the Charity Hospital. On initial exploration, she was found to have tumor involving the portal vein. After regional treatment and reoperative pancreaticoduodenectomy, she died of pulmonary metastases at 38 mo, without any evidence of intra-abdominal disease. Overall, patients with inoperable disease have an average survival of only 10–14 mo (Fig. 3).

The best responses to regional chemotherapy were found with the first two cycles of treatment. By the third cycle, there was generally no further response. This is not so surprising, because the abrupt increase in tumor cell resistance may be caused by the upregulation of *MDR1*, and by the other inducible, non-P-glycoprotein mechanisms of resistance normally found in pancreatic tumors *(11,90,99,103)*. All the studies of patients with advanced PC demonstrated that the small group of patients with survival past 24 mo were only those with a CR or PR tumor response followed by a curative surgical resection.

9.2. Regional Chemotherapy plus Hemoperfusion

Systemic chemotherapy using an extracorporeal, activated-charcoal hemoperfusion capsule, was initially investigated by Winchester et al. *(144,145)*, to study the enhancement of total body elimination of DOX. Extracorporeal drug recapture in conjunction with regional chemotherapy was then proposed by Dedrick and Oldfield as a means for increasing the local-regional drug dose *(125,137,138)*. The hemoperfusion system effectively and rapidly expedites the total body clearance of most chemotherapeutic agents, permitting the regional escalation of the total drug dose on the scale of 2–8-fold *(138)*. Thus, the regional advantage, R_d, depends on the fraction of drug eliminated within the tumor-bearing region, E_r, the fraction cleared by the liver, E_l, plus, primarily, the fraction of drug cleared by the hemoperfusion capsule, E_{hp}:

$$R_d = Cl_{TB}/Q \, [1 - (E_r + E_l + E_{hp})] + 1$$

The regional chemotherapy plus hemoperfusion can be more effective than using an extracorporeal hemofiltration system. Using multiple hemoperfusion capsules allows a greater percentage of the total drug dose to be rapidly and effectively recaptured. Thus, the regionally infused drug dose can be increased up to $6-10 \times$ that of systemic chemotherapy *(146,147)*.

Regional therapy plus hemoperfusion has not been fully tested for the treatment of patients with advanced PC. The proficiency of a single charcoal capsule has been the limiting factor, because it rapidly fills with the recaptured drug, but the use of multiple capsules in parallel has solved this problem *(147,148)*. Also, the reported injury to platelets initially caused doubt about the utility of this technique for pancreatic malignancies. However, Japanese studies *(147)* have demonstrated a greater efficacy of this technique, compared to intra-arterial chemotherapy plus hemofiltration, for hepatic malignancies. Also, studies in the United States have demonstrated the capability of safely tripling the infused, regional drug dose using a hemoperfusion system *(149)*. A single Japanese study *(150)* in animals shows that it is possible to achieve a 90% reduction in the systemic drug exposure, permitting escalation of the drug dose during a regional infusion of the pancreas.

10. THEORETICAL MODELING OF REGIONAL DRUG DELIVERY

Antineoplastic efficacy is chiefly a function of tumor cell drug exposure over time $(C \times T)$, but only when an effective cytotoxic concentration threshold is reached *(125)*. In vitro, most GI tumors demonstrate chemosensitivity in 79–100% of the cases, only when the dosages of 5-FU, MMC, DOX, MTZ, and cisplatin are increased to 10-fold, from 1 to 10 µg/mL *(123,126)*. Also, gemcitabine shows a similar requirement of at least a 10-fold drug dose escalation in vitro, to improve its efficacy against human pancreatic cell lines *(127)*. However, relatively little data exists comparing in vitro chemosensitivity and in vivo tissue levels. Only at an in vitro dose of 10 µg/mL does DOX effectively kill most tumors of GI tract origin. Unfortunately, the tumor tissue levels of DOX derived from patients showed that the tissue drug levels were never near the concentration needed to achieve a cytotoxic level of drug *(110)*.

Dedrick *(125)* and Dedrick et al. *(137)* have shown that the rate and time of infusion into a limited region is a means by which local concentration can be increased at least 10-fold or more, and systemic exposure can be limited. The best means of describing the pharmacokinetic efficiency of each antitumor agent is in terms of AUC. Thus, AUC is defined as the area under the drug concentration–time curve. AUC also defines the effective cytotoxicity as well as the resultant systemic toxicity. Both the plasma and intracellular AUC, and not just the C_{max}, are the determining factors in antineoplastic efficacy of a drug *(113,151)*. If drug dose exposure is shortened to 1 h, and the C_{max} is significantly elevated, then the cytotoxicity can be increased. Drewinko et al. *(152)* showed, with a 1-h exposure of a colon cancer cell line to DOX, that cytotoxicity could be maximized. Likewise, dihydroxyanthracenedione is more effective against pancreatic tumors in vitro as a short-term exposure of 1 h, as opposed to a 5-d exposure *(153)*.

By manipulating the AUC, i.e., shortening the time of infusion to 2 h, the peak concentration can be increased above the tumorcidal threshold, then using extracoporeal rapid reduction of the total drug dose will limit the systemic exposure and toxicity. Using this system, one Japanese case report *(146)* and one small study *(147)* have shown that the regional hepatic dose of DOX can be increased up to 140–150 mg/m² without significant systemic exposure. The drug was infused over 10–30 min, and then rapidly cleared through extracoporeal hemoperfusion. The pharmacokinetic data in the case study matches the Dedrick *(125)* model data for increasing local drug exposure and limiting systemic toxicity. The importance of this model is that the antineoplastic efficacy of most chemotherapeutic agents, except antimetabolites, is chiefly a function of tumor cell exposure (C × T) to the drug, but only once an effective concentration threshold is reached.

The isolated regional perfusion system remains the basic model for using regional chemotherapy *(57,58)*. With this system, it is possible to deliver a high drug dose to the tumor-bearing region. Because there is complete vascular isolation of the tumor, the rest of the patient is protected from systemic toxicity. In an animal model using a totally isolated liver perfusion system, the hepatic plasma level of DOX can be increased 5–10 × over that of the peak systemic plasma achievable by iv bolus delivery, and can be maintained for up to 3 h *(154)*, with relatively little hepatic toxicity. There is only one report of an isolated perfusion of the pancreas-duodenum within the recent literature, using MMC *(155,156)*. The dose of MMC used for the 45-min perfusion was 0.25 mg/kg, but the C_{max} within the system remained above only 2 µg/mL for about 5 min, not at all close to the 5–10 µg/mL tumorcidal threshold for PC. Also, the technical difficulty of procedure and the operating room time of 4–5 h limits the use of this procedure.

Regional intra-arterial chemotherapy, in conjunction with extracorporeal drug recapture, can deliver the same drug dosage to a tumor-bearing region that is accomplished by isolated regional perfusion. The pharmacokinetics of the drugs used in these systems can be tailored to that achievable with regional perfusion. However, regional chemotherapy plus hemoperfusion remains more cost effective, because it can be used in the outpatient setting.

11. PATTERNS OF FAILURE OF REGIONAL THERAPY

Regional chemotherapy for PC only moderately improves the response rates for unresectable PC, with very little improvement in survival *(3,128,133)*. However, in a few adjuvant trials, using regional chemotherapy that targets local recurrence and primarily hepatic failure, is there some improvement in long-term survival *(134–136)*.

Survival improvement is dependent on the control of primary disease failure within the three principal sites of failure: the local-regional, tumor-bearing area; the liver; and the peritoneal surfaces. The current techniques of celiac artery or hepatic artery/portal

Table 6
Patterns of Failure After Regional
Chemotherapy

	(%)
Local regional	7–27
Liver metastases	9–13
Peritoneal surfaces	82
Extra-abdominal metastases	9

vein infusions limit the disease failure within the first two compartments, but have very little impact on disease failure of the peritoneal surfaces (Table 6). The principal area of improved distal failure is a significant reduction in liver metastases produced by either neoadjuvant or adjuvant regional chemotherapy. Treatment failure secondary to hepatic metastases is only 8–13% *(128,135,136)*. In the Japanese series of patients with operable PC, Ishikawa et al. *(135)* produced a significant improvement in survival (54%) at 5 yr with adjuvant hepatic regional chemotherapy. This improvement in survival was primarily the result of reduction in hepatic metastases from 34 to 8%. In the Tulane series *(3)* of inoperable PC, the incidence of hepatic metastases was reduced to only 9%, but the failure rate secondary to PMs increased to 82%. Thus, the survival impact, when the peritoneal disease is not controlled, would be minimal: only about 8–14 mo at best.

Until concurrent therapies include the peritoneal surfaces as one of the principal site of treatment failure, there can be little improvement in long-term survival of patients with advanced PC. Peritoneal chemotherapy may be beneficial, but only a single study *(157)*, in an animal model using MMC and cisplatin, shows complete inhibition of PMs from PC. Regional intraperitoneal chemotherapy has been postulated for the treatment of PMs, but there is no patient data on its use. Finally, for completeness, gene therapy for disseminated PC, targeting peritoneal disease, is still in the early stages *(158)*.

12. CONCLUSION

Regional chemotherapy decreases the incidence of treatment failures within the tumor-bearing region and the liver. The most dramatic improvement from regional chemotherapy is in the adjuvant setting, with the decrease in incidence of hepatic metastases. Thus, at present, pre-op or postoperative regional chemotherapy seems more likely than any other treatment modality currently in use to improve long-term survival for PC. The thinking used in tackling the complexities of PC could also determine further treatment strategies for PC.

ACKNOWLEDGMENTS

The authors wish to thank Maria Alicia Jones, R.N., M.S. for her assistance in preparing and editing this manuscript.

REFERENCES

1. Landis SH, Murray T, Bolden S, and Wingo PA. Cancer statistics, 1998, *CA Cancer J. Clin.,* **48** (1998) 6–29.
2. Janes RH Jr, Niederhuber JE, Chmiel JS, et al. National patterns of care for pancreatic cancer, *Ann. Surg.,* **223** (1996) 261–272.

3. Muchmore JH, Preslan JE, and George WJ. Regional chemotherapy for inoperable pancreatic carcinoma, *Cancer,* **78** (1996) 664–673.
4. Krementz ET and Becker ML. Malignant diseases of the pancreas, *Adv. Surg.,* **6** (1972) 205–236.
5. Fontham ETH and Correa P. Epidemiology of pancreatic cancer, *Surg. Clin. N. Am.,* **69** (1989) 551–567.
6. Bramhall SR, Allum WH, Jones AG, Allwood A, Cummins C, and Neoptolemos JP. Treatment and survival in 13,560 patients with pancreatic cancer, and incidence of the disease, in the West Midlands: an epidemiological study, *Br. J. Surg.,* **82** (1995) 111–115.
7. Chen VW, Xiao-Cheng W, Andrews PA, Correa CN, and Lucas HF. Highlights of cancer incidence in Louisiana, 1988–1992, *J. LA. State Med. Soc.,* **149** (1997) 119–124.
8. Levin DL and Connelly RR. Cancer of the pancreas. Available epidemiologic information and its implications, *Cancer,* **31** (1973) 1231–1236.
9. Gudjonsson B. Cancer of the pancreas: 50 years of surgery, *Cancer,* **60** (1987) 2284–2303.
10. Menck HR, Garfinkel L, and Dodd GD. Preliminary report of the National Cancer Data Base, *CA.,* **41** (1991) 7–18.
11. Brennan MF, Kinsella TJ, and Casper ES. Cancer of the pancreas, In DeVita VT Jr, Hellman S, Rosenberg SA, (eds), *Cancer: Principles and Practice of Oncology,* 4th ed, Lippincott, Philadelphia, 1993, pp. 849–882.
12. Evans DB, Abbruzzese JL, and Rich TA. Cancer of the pancreas, In DeVita VT Jr, Hellman S, Rosenberg SA (eds), *Cancer: Principles and Practice of Oncology,* 5th ed. Lippincott, Philadelphia, 1997, pp. 1054–1087.
13. Bottger TC, Storkel S, Wellek S, Stockle M, and Junginger T. Factors influencing survival after resection of pancreatic cancer, *Cancer,* **73** (1994) 63–73.
14. Nitecki SS, Sarr MG, Colby TV, and van Heerden JA. Long-term survival after resection for ductal adenocarcinoma of the pancreas, *Ann. Surg.,* **221** (1995) 59–66.
15. Yeo CJ, Cameron JL, Sohn TA, et al. Six hundred fifty consecutive pancreaticoduodenectomies in the 1990s. Pathology, complications, and outcomes, *Cancer,* **226** (1997) 248–260.
16. Gall FP and Kockerling F. Problem of radical surgery in pancreatic cancer and its implications for a combined-treatment approach, *Rec. Res. Cancer,* **110** (1988) 79–86.
17. Kobari M, Sunamura M, Ohashi O, Saitoh Y, Yusa T, and Matsuno S. Usefulness of Japanese staging in the prognosis of patients treated operatively for adenocarcinoma of the head of the pancreas, *J. Am. Coll. Surg.,* **182** (1996) 24–32.
18. Cubilla AL, Fortner J, and Fitzgerald PJ. Lymph node involvement in carcinoma of the head of the pancreas, *Cancer,* **41** (1978) 880–887.
19. Nagakawa T, Kobayashi H, Ueno K, Ohta T, Kayahara M, and Miyazaki I. Clinical study of the lymphatic flow to paraaortic lymph nodes in carcinoma of the head of the pancreas, *Cancer,* **73** (1994) 1155–1162.
20. Nagai H, Kuroda A, and Morioka Y. Lymphatic and local spread of T1 and T2 pancreatic cancer: a study of autopsy material, *Ann. Surg.,* **204** (1986) 65–71.
21. Tsuchiya R, Oribe T, and Noda T. Size of the tumor and other factors influencing prognosis of carcinoma of the head of the pancreas, *Am. J. Gastroenterol.,* **80** (1985) 459–462.
22. Nix GAJJ, Dubbelman C, Wilson HP, Schutte HE, Jeekel J, and Postema RR. Prognostic implications of tumor diameter in carcinoma of the head of the pancreas, *Cancer,* **67** (1991) 529–535.
23. Warshaw AL. Implications of peritoneal cytology for staging of early pancreatic cancer, *Am. J. Surg.,* **161** (1991) 26–30.
24. Lei S, Kini J, Kim K, and Howard JM. Pancreatic cancer: cytologic study of peritoneal washings, *Arch. Surg.,* **129** (1994) 639–642.
25. Leach SD, Rose JA, Lowy AM, et al. Significance of peritoneal cytology in patients with potentially resectable adenocarcinoma of the pancreatic head, *Surgery,* **118** (1995) 472–478.
26. Sperti C, Pasquali C, Piccoli A, and Pedrazzoli S. Recurrence after resection for ductal adenocarcinoma of the pancreas, *World J. Surg.,* **21** (1997) 195–200.
27. Griffin JF, Smalley SR, Jewell W, et al. Patterns of failure after curative resection of pancreatic carcinoma, *Cancer,* **66** (1990) 56–61.
28. Allema JH, Reinders ME, van Gulik TM, et al. Prognostic factors for survival after pancreaticoduodenectomy for patients with carcinoma of the pancreatic head region, *Cancer,* **75** (1995) 2069–2076.
29. Willett CG, Lewandrowski K, Warshaw AL, Efird J, and Compton CC. Resection margins in carcinoma of the head of the pancreas, *Ann. Surg.,* **217** (1993) 144–148.
30. Kalser MH and Ellenberg SS. Pancreatic cancer: adjuvant combined radiation and chemotherapy following a curative resection, *Arch. Surg.,* **120** (1985) 899–903.

31. Gastrointestinal Tumor Study Group. Further evidence of effective adjuvant combined radiation and chemotherapy following a curative resection of pancreatic cancer, *Cancer,* **59** (1987) 2006–2010.

32. Hiraoka T, Watanabe E, Mochinaga M, et al. Intraoperative radiation therapy for patients with pancreatic carcinoma, *World J. Surg.,* **8** (1984) 766–771.

33. Shipley WU, Tepper JC, Warshaw AL, and Orlow EL. Intraoperative radiation therapy for patients with pancreatic carcinoma, *World J. Surg.,* **8** (1984) 929–934.

34. Ishikawa O, Hiroaki O, Imaoka S, et al. Is the long-term survival rate improved by preoperative irradiation prior to Whipple's procedure for adenocarcinoma of the pancreatic head?, *Arch. Surg.,* **129** (1994) 1075–1080.

35. Warshaw AL and Swanson RS. Pancreatic cancer in 1988. Possibilities and probabilities, *Ann. Surg.,* **208** (1988) 541–553.

36. Warshaw AL, Gu ZY, Wittenberg J, and Waltman AC. Preoperative staging and assessment of resectability of pancreatic cancer, *Arch. Surg.,* **140** (1990) 230–233.

37. Foo ML, Gunderson LL, Nagorney DM, et al. Patterns of failure in grossly resected pancreatic ductal adenocarcinoma treated with adjuvant irradiation ±5 fluorouracil, *Int. J. Radiat. Oncol. Biol. Phys.,* **26** (1993) 483–489.

38. Staley CA, Lee JE, Cleary KR, et al. Preoperative chemoradiation, pancreaticoduodenectomy, and intraoperative radiation therapy for adenocarcinoma of the pancreatic head, *Am. J. Surg.,* **171** (1996) 118–125.

39. Hoffman JP, Weese JL, Solin LJ, et al. Single institutional experience with preoperative chemoradiotherapy for Stage I–II pancreatic adenocarcinoma, *Am. Surg.,* **59** (1993) 772–781.

40. Van Heerden JA, McJhath DC, Jlsrup DM, and Weiland LH. Total pancreatectomy for ductal adenocarcinoma of the pancreas: an update, *World J. Surg.,* **12** (1988) 658–662.

41. Martin JK Jr and Goellner JR. Abdominal fluid cytology in patients with gastrointestinal malignant lesions, *Mayo Clin. Proc.,* **61** (1986) 467–471.

42. Jessup JM, Steele G Jr, Mayer RJ, et al. Neoadjuvant therapy for unresectable pancreatic adenocarcinoma, *Arch. Surg.,* **128** (1993) 559–564.

43. Trede M, Schwall G, and Salger H. Survival after pancreatoduodenectomy. 118 consecutive resections without an operative mortality, *Ann. Surg.,* **221** (1990) 447–458.

44. Fernandez-del Castillo C, Rattner DW, and Warshaw AL. Standards for pancreatic resection in 1990s, *Arch. Surg.,* **130** (1995) 295–300.

45. Ross Hm, Kurtzman SH, Maculy WP, Allen LW, Foster JH, and Deckers PJ. Resection for cure of adenocarcinoma of the head of the pancreas: the greater Hartford experience, *Conn. Med.,* **61** (1997) 3–7.

46. Geer RJ and Brennan MF. Prognostic indicators for survival after resection of pancreatic adenocarcinoma, *Am. J. Surg.,* **165** (1993) 68–73.

47. Conlon KC, Klimstra DS, and Brennan MF. Long-term survival after curative resection for pancreatic ductal adenocarcinoma: clinicopathologic analysis of 5-year survivors, *Ann. Surg.,* **223** (1996) 273–279.

48. Satake K, Nishiwaki H, Yokomatsu H, Kawazoe Y, Kim K, and Haku A. Surgical curability and prognosis for standard versus extended resection for T1 carcinoma of the pancreas, *Surg. Gynecol. Obstet.,* **175** (1992) 259–265.

49. Fortner JG. Surgical principles for pancreatic cancer: regional total and subtotal pancreatectomy, *Cancer,* **47(Suppl 6)** (1981) 1712–1718.

50. Nagakawa T, Kobayashi H, Ueno K, Ohta T, Kayahara M, and Miyazaki I. Clinical study of the lymphatic flow to paraaortic lymph nodes in carcinoma of the head of the pancreas, *Cancer,* **73** (1994) 1155–1162.

51. Hirata K, Sato T, Mukaiya M, et al. Results of 1001 pancreatic resections for invasive ductal adenocarcinoma of the pancreas, *Arch. Surg.,* **132** (1997) 771–776.

52. Mukaiya M, Hirata K, Satoh T, et al. Lack of survival benefit of extended lymph node dissection for ductal adenocarcinoma of the head of the pancreas: retrospective multi-institutional analysis in Japan, *World J. Surg.,* **22** (1998) 248–253.

53. Kayahara M, Nagakawa T, Ueno K, Ohta T, Takeda T, and Miyazaki I. Evaluation of radical resection for pancreatic cancer based on the mode of recurrence as determined by autopsy and diagnostic imaging, *Cancer,* **72** (1993) 2118–2123.

54. Beirman HR, Shimkin MB, Byron RL Jr, et al. Effects of intra-arterial administration of nitrogen mustard, *Fifth International Cancer Congress, Paris,* 1950, p. 186.

55. Klopp CT, Alford TC, Bateman J, Berry GN, and Winship T. Fractionated intra-arterial cancer chemotherapy with bis-amine hydrochloride: a preliminary report, *Ann. Surg.,* **132** (1950) 811–832.

56. Schroy PC III, Cohen A, Winawer SJ, and Friedman EA. New chemotherapeutic drug sensitivity assay for colon carcinomas in monolayer culture, *Cancer Res.,* **48** (1988) 3236–3244.

57. Krementz ET. Regional perfusion. Current sophistication, what next?, *Cancer,* **57** (1986) 416–432.

58. Muchmore JH, Carter RD, and Krementz ET. Regional perfusion for malignant melanoma and soft tissue sarcoma: a review, *Cancer Invest.,* **3** (1985) 129–143.

59. Folkman J. Clinical applications of research on angiogenesis, *N. Engl. J. Med.,* **333** (1995) 1757–1763.

60. Jain RK. Vascular and interstitial barriers to delivery of therapeutic agents in tumors, *Cancer Met. Rev.,* **9** (1990) 253–266.

61. Ishida H, Makino T, Kobayashi M, and Tsuneoka K. Laparoscopic measurement of pancreatic blood flow, *Endoscopy,* **15** (1983) 107–110.

62. Baxter LT and Jain RK. Transport of fluid and macromolecules in tumors. II. Role of heterogeneous perfusion and lymphatics, *Microvasc. Res.,* **40** (1990) 246–263.

63. Vaupal P. Hypoxia in neoplastic tissue, *Microvasc. Res.,* **13** (1977) 399–408.

64. Carter SK. Integration of chemotherapy into a combined modality approach for cancer treatment. VI. Pancreatic adenocarcinoma, *Cancer Treat. Rev.,* **3** (1975) 193–214.

65. Cullinan S, Moertel CG, Wieand HS, et al. Phase III trial on the therapy of advanced pancreatic carcinoma, *Cancer,* **65** (1990) 2207–2212.

66. DeCaprio JA, Mayer RJ, Gonin R, and Arbuck SG. Fluorouracil and high-dose leucovorin in previously untreated patients with advanced adenocarcinoma of the pancreas: results of phase II trial, *J. Clin. Oncol.,* **9** (1991) 2128–2133.

67. Crooke ST and Bradner WT. Mitomycin C: a review, *Cancer Treat. Rep.,* **3** (1976) 121–139.

68. Rothenberg ML, Abbruzzese JL, Moore M, Portenoy RK, Robertson JM, and Wanebo HJ. Rationale for expanding the endpoints for clinical trials in advanced pancreatic carcinoma, *Cancer,* **78** (1996) 627–632.

69. Asbury RF, Cnaan A, Johnson L, Harris J, Zaentz SD, and Haller DG. An Eastern Cooperative Oncology Group phase II study of single agent DHAD, VP-16, aclacinomycin, or spirogermanium in metastatic pancreatic cancer, *Am. J. Clin. Oncol.,* **17** (1994) 166–169.

70. Leichman CG, Tangen C, MacDonald JS, Leimert T, and Fleming TR. Phase II trial of amonafide in advanced pancreas cancer: a Southwest Oncology Group trial, *Invest. New Drugs,* **11** (1993) 219–221.

71. Bukowski RM, Fleming TR, Macdonald JS, Oishi N, Taylor SA, and Baker LH. Evaluation of combination chemotherapy and phase II agents in pancreatic adenocarcinoma: a Southwest Oncology Group study, *Cancer,* **71** (1993) 322–325.

72. Moore M, Maroun J, Robert F, et al. Multicenter phase II study of brequinar sodium in patients with advanced gastrointestinal cancer, *Invest. New Drugs,* **11** (1993) 61–65.

73. Rougier P, De Forni M, Adenis A, et al. Phase II study of Taxotere (RP56976, docetaxel) in pancreatic adenocarcinoma, *Proc. Am. Soc. Clin. Oncol.,* **14** (1995) 221 (Abstract).

74. Moore DF Jr, Pazdur R, Abbruzzese JL, et al. Phase II trial of edatrexate in patients with advanced pancreatic adenocarcinoma, *Ann. Oncol.,* **5** (1994) 286–287.

75. Kilton LJ, Benson AB, Greenberg A, et al. Phase II trial of fludarabine phosphate for adenocarcinoma of the pancreas: an Illinois Cancer Center study, *Invest. New Drugs,* **10** (1992) 201–204.

76. Casper ES, Green MR, Kelson DP, et al. Phase II trial of gemcitabine (2, 2'-difluorodeoxycytidine) in patients with adenocarcinoma of the pancreas, *Invest. New Drugs,* **12** (1994) 29–34.

77. Carmichael J, Fink U, Russell RC, et al. Phase II study of gemcitabine in patients with advanced pancreatic cancer, *Br. J. Cancer,* **73** (1996) 101–105.

78. Philip PA, Carmichael J, Tonkin K, et al. Hormonal treatment of pancreatic carcinoma: a phase II study of LHRH agonist goserelin plus hydrocortisone, *Br. J. Cancer,* **67** (1993) 379–382.

79. Hubbard KP, Pazdur R, Ajani JA, et al. Phase II evaluation of iproplatin in patients with advanced gastric and pancreatic cancer, *Am. J. Clin. Oncol.,* **15** (1992) 524–527.

80. Wagener DJ, Verdonk HE, Dirix LY, et al. Phase II trial of CPT-11 in patients with advanced pancreatic cancer, an EORTC early clinical trials group study, *Ann. Oncol.,* **6** (1995) 129–132.

81. Kraut EH, Fleming T, MacDonald JS, Spiridonidis CH, Bradof JE, and Baker LH. Phase II trial of merbarone in pancreatic carcinoma: a Southwest Oncology Group study, *Am. J. Clin. Oncol.,* **16** (1993) 327–328.

82. Friess H, Buchler M, Beglinger C, et al. Low-dose octreotide treatment is not effective in patients with advanced pancreatic cancer, *Pancreas,* **8** (1993) 540–545.

83. Whitehead RP, Jacobson J, Brown TD, Taylor SA, Weiss GR, and MacDonald JS. Phase II trial of paclitaxel and granulocyte colony-stimulating factor in patients with pancreatic carcinoma: a Southwest Oncology Group study, *J. Clin. Oncol.,* **15** (1997) 2414–2419.

84. Jenkins TR, Tangen C, MacDonald JS, Weiss GR, Chapman R, and Hertel A. Phase II trial of piroxantrone in adenocarcinoma of the pancreas: a Southwest Oncology Group study, *Invest. New Drugs,* **11** (1993) 329–331.

85. Mahjoubi M, Rougier P, Oliviera J, Herait P, Tigaud JM, and Droz JP. Phase II trial of pirarubicin in the treatment of advanced pancreatic cancer, *Cancer Invest.,* **12** (1994) 403–405.

86. Scher RM, Kosierowski R, Lusch C, et al. Phase II trial of topotecan in advanced or metastatic adenocarcinoma of the pancreas, *Invest. New Drugs,* **13** (1996) 347–354.

87. Pazdur R, Meropol NJ, Casper ES, et al. Phase II trial of ZD1694 (Tomudex) in patients with advanced pancreatic cancer, *Invest. New Drugs,* **13** (1996) 355–358.

88. Brown TD, Goodman P, Fleming T, MacDonald JS, Hersh EM, and Braun TJ. Phase II trial of recombinant tumor necrosis factor in patients with adenocarcinoma of the pancreas: a Southwest Oncology Group study, *J. Immunother.,* **10** (1991) 376–378.

89. Taylor I. Should further studies of chemotherapy be carried out in pancreatic cancer?, *Eur. J. Cancer,* **29A(Suppl 8)** (1993) 1076–1078.

90. Goldstein LJ, Galski H, Fojo A, et al. Expression of multidrug resistance gene in human cancers, *J. Nat. Cancer Inst.,* **81** (1989) 116–124.

91. Almoquera C, Shibata D, Forrester K, Martin J, Arnheim N, and Perucho M. Most human carcinomas of the exocrine pancreas contain mutant c-K-ras genes, *Cell,* **53** (1988) 549–554.

92. Capella G, Cronauer-Mitra S, Peinado MA, and Perucho M. Frequency and spectrum of mutations at codons 12 and 13 of the c-K-ras gene in human tumors, *Environ. Health Perspect.,* **93** (1991) 125–131.

93. Brentnall TA, Chen R, Lee JG, et al. Microsatellite instability and K-ras mutations associated with pancreatic adenocarcinoma and pancreatitis, *Cancer Res.,* **55** (1995) 4264–4267.

94. Bos JL. Ras oncogenes in human cancer: a review, *Cancer Res.,* **49** (1989) 4682–4689.

95. Stokoe D, Macdonald SG, Cadwallader K, Symons M, and Hancock JF. Activation of Raf as a result of recruitment to the plasma membrane, *Science,* **264** (1994) 1463–1467.

96. Leevers SJ, Paterson HF, and Marshall CJ. Requirement for Ras in Raf activation is overcome by targeting Raf to the plasma membrane, *Nature,* **369** (1994) 411–414.

97. Scarpa A, Capelli P, Mukai K, et al. Pancreatic adenocarcinomas frequently show p53 gene mutations, *Am. J. Pathol.,* **142** (1993) 1534–1543.

98. Chin K-V, Ueda K, Pastan I, and Gottesman MM. Modulation of the activity of the promoter of the human MDR1 gene by ras and p53, *Science,* **255** (1992) 459–462.

99. Miller DW, Fontain M, Kolar C, and Lawson T. Expression of multidrug resistance-associated protein (MRP) in pancreatic adenocarcinoma cell lines, *Cancer Lett.,* **107** (1996) 301–306.

100. Verovski VN, Van den Berge DL, Delvaeye MM, Scheper RJ, De Neve WJ, and Storme GA. Low-level doxorubicin resistance in P-glycoprotein-negative human pancreatic tumor PSN1/ADR cells implicates a brefeldin A-sensitive mechanism of drug extrusion, *Br. J. Cancer,* **73** (1996) 596–602.

101. Johnston PG, Lentz HJ, Leichman CG, et al. Thymidylate synthase gene and protein expression correlate and are associated with response to 5-fluorouracil in human colorectal and gastric tumors, *Cancer Res.,* **55** (1995) 1407–1412.

102. Lenz HJ, Leichman CG, Danenberg KD, et al. Thymidylate synthase mRNA level in adenocarcinoma of the stomach: a predictor for primary tumor response and overall survival, *J. Clin. Oncol.,* **14** (1996) 176–182.

103. Spears CP, Gustavsson BG, Berne M, Frosing R, Bernstein L, and Hayes AA. Mechanisms of innate resistance to thymidylate synthase inhibition after 5-fluorouracil, *Cancer Res.,* **48** (1988) 5894–5900.

104. Eckman WW, Patlak CS, and Fenstermacher JD. Critical evaluation of principles governing the advantages of intra-arterial infusions, *J. Pharmacokinet. Biopharm.,* **2** (1974) 257–285.

105. Chen H-SG and Gross JF. Intra-arterial infusion of anticancer drugs: theoretic aspects of drug delivery and review of responses, *Cancer Treat. Rep.,* **64** (1980) 31–40.

106. Collins JM and Dedrick RL. Pharmacokinetics of anticancer drugs, In Chabner B (ed), *Pharmacologic Principles of Cancer Treatment,* WB Saunders, Philadelphia, 1982, pp. 77–99.

107. Collins JM. Pharmacokinetics and clinical monitoring, In Chabner BA, Collins JM (eds), *Cancer Chemotherapy: Principles and Practice,* Lippincott, Philadelphia, 1990, pp. 16–31.

108. Green RF, Collins JM, Jenkins JF, Speyer JL, and Mycers CE. Plasma pharmacokinetics of adriamycin and adriamycinol: implications for the design of in vitro experiments and treatment protocols, *Cancer Res.,* **43** (1983) 3417–3421.

109. Weiss AJ, Metter GE, Fletcher WAS, Wilson WL, Grage TB, and Ramirez G. Studies on adriamycin

using a weekly regimen demonstrating its clinical effectiveness and lack of cardiac toxicity, *Cancer Treat. Rep.,* **60** (1976) 813–822.

110. Chan KK, Cohen JL, Gross JF, et al. Prediction of adriamycin disposition in cancer patients using physiologic, pharmacokinetic model, *Cancer Treat. Rep.,* **62** (1978) 1161–1171.

111. Erttmann R, Erb N, Steinhoff A, and Landbeck G. Pharmacokinetics of doxorubicin in man: dose and schedule dependence, *J. Cancer Res. Clin. Oncol.,* **114** (1998) 509–513.

112. Matsushima Y, Kanazawa F, Hoshi A, et al. Time-schedule dependency of the inhibiting activity of various anticancer drugs in the clonogenic assay, *Cancer Chemother. Pharmacol.,* **14** (1985) 104–107.

113. Mitchell RB, Ratain MJ, and Vogelzang NJ. Experimental rationale for continuous infusion chemotherapy, In Lokich JJ (ed), *Cancer Chemotherapy by Infusion,* 2nd ed., Precept, Chicago, 1990, pp. 3–34.

114. Ensminger WD and Gyves JW. Clinical pharmacology of hepatic arterial chemotherapy, *Semin. Oncol.,* **10** (1983) 176–182.

115. Ensminger WD and Gyves JW. Regional cancer chemotherapy, *Cancer Treat. Rep.,* **68** (1984) 101–115.

116. Curt GA and Collins JM. Clinical pharmacology of infusional chemotherapy, In Lokich JJ (ed), *Cancer Chemotherapy by Infusion,* 2nd ed., Precept, Chicago, 1990, pp. 35–41.

117. Garnick MB, Ensminger WD, and Israel M. Clinical-pharmacological evaluation of hepatic arterial infusion of adriamycin, *Cancer Res.,* **39** (1979) 4105–4110.

118. Hu E and Howell SB. Pharmacokinetics of intraarterial Mitomycin C in humans, *Cancer Res.,* **43** (1983) 4474–4477.

119. Ballet F, Vrignaud P, Robert J, Rey C, and Poupon R. Hepatic extraction, metabolism and biliary excretion of doxorubicin in the isolated perfused rat liver, *Cancer Chemother. Pharmacol.,* **19** (1987) 240–245.

120. Theodors A, Bukowski R, Hewlett J, Livingston R, and Weick J. Intermittent regional infusion of chemotherapy for pancreatic adenocarcinoma, *Am. J. Clin. Oncol.,* **5** (1982) 555–558.

121. Bengmark S and Andren-Sandberg A. Infusion chemotherapy in inoperable pancreatic carcinoma, *Rec. Res. Cancer Res.,* **86** (1983) 13–4.

122. Aigner KR, Muller H, and Bessermann R. Intra-arterial chemotherapy with MMC, CDDP and 5-FU for non-resectable pancreatic cancer. A phase II study, *Reg. Cancer Treat.,* **3** (1990) 1–6.

123. Link KH, Aigner KR, Kuehn W, Schwemmle K, and Kern DH. Prospective correlative chemosensitivity testing in high-dose intra-arterial chemotherapy for liver metastases, *Cancer Res.,* **46** (1986) 4837–4840.

124. Park J, Kramer BS, Steinberg SM, et al. Chemosensitivity testing of human colorectal carcinoma cell lines using a tetrazolium-based calorimetric assay, *Cancer Res.,* **47** (1987) 5875–5879.

125. Dedrick RL. Arterial drug infusion: pharmacokinetic problems and pitfalls, *JNCI,* **80** (1988) 84–89.

126. Link KH. Basics concepts for the application of mitomycin C in regional cancer treatment, In Taguchi T and Aigner KR (eds), *Mitomycin C in Cancer Chemotherapy.* Excerpta Medica, Tokyo, 1991, pp. 62–71.

127. Bold R and McConkey D. Gemcitabine-induced apoptotic cell death of human pancreatic carcinoma is determined by bcl-2 content. 51st Annual Cancer Symposium, *Society of Surgical Oncology,* 1998, p. 57 (Abstract).

128. Ohigashi H, Ishikawa O, Imaoka S, et al. New method of intra-arterial regional chemotherapy with more selective drug delivery for locally advanced pancreatic cancer, *Hepato-Gastroenterology,* **43** (1996) 338–345.

129. Cantore M, Bassi C, Tumulo S, et al. Intra-arterial chemotherapy for Stage III/IV pancreatic cancer. Anti-Cancer Treatment, Sixth International Congress, 1997, p. 133 (Abstract).

130. Ohigashi H, Ishikawa O, Sasaki Y, et al. Case report of preoperative intra-arterial infusion chemotherapy for pancreatic head carcinoma, *Jpn. J. Cancer Chemother.,* **24** (1997) 1825–1828.

131. McCracken JD, Olson M, Cruz AB Jr, Leichman L, and Oishi N. Radiation therapy combined with intra-arterial 5-FU chemotherapy for treatment of localized adenocarcinoma of the pancreas: a Southwest Oncology Group Study, *Cancer Treat. Rep.,* **66** (1982) 549–551.

132. Wiley AL Jr, Wirtanen GW, Mehta MP, Ramirez G, and Shahabi S. Treatment of probable subclinical liver metastases and gross pancreatic carcinoma with hepatic artery 5-fluorouracil infusion and radiation therapy, *Acta. Oncol.,* **27** (1988) 377–381.

133. Aigner KR and Gailhofer S. Regional chemotherapy for nonresectable, locally metastasized pancreatic cancer: four studies including 164 cases, *Reg. Cancer Treat.,* **1(Suppl)** (1993) A2.

134. Link KH, Gansauge F, Gorich J, Leder GH, Rilinger N, and Beger HG. Palliative and adjuvant regional chemotherapy in pancreatic cancer, *Eur. J. Surg. Oncol.,* **23** (1997) 409–414.

135. Ishikawa O, Ohigashi H, Sasaki Y, et al. Liver perfusion chemotherapy via both the hepatic artery and portal vein to prevent hepatic metastasis after extended pancreatectomy for adenocarcinoma of the pancreas, *Am. J. Surg.,* **168** (1994) 361–364.

136. Lygidakis NJ and Stringaris K. Adjuvant therapy following pancreatic resection for pancreatic duct carcinoma: a randomized prospective study, *Hepato-Gastroenterology,* **43** (1996) 671–680.

137. Dedrick RL, Oldfield EH, and Collins JH. Arterial drug infusion with extracorporeal removal. Theoretical basis with particular reference to the brain, *Cancer Treat. Rep.,* **68** (1984) 373–380.

138. Oldfield EH, Dedrick RL, Yeager RL, et al. Reduced systemic drug exposure by combining intra-arterial chemotherapy with hemoperfusion of regional venous drainage, *J. Neurosurg.,* **63** (1985) 726–732.

139. Muchmore JH. Treatment of advanced pancreatic cancer with regional chemotherapy plus hemofiltration, *Semin. Surg. Oncol.,* **11** (1995) 154–167.

140. Aigner KR, Thiller H, Walther H, and Link KH. Drug filtration in high-dose regional chemotherapy, *Contr. Oncol.,* **29** (1988) 261–280.

141. Muchmore JH, Krementz ET, Carter RO, Meyer GM, Preslan JE, and George WJ. Management of advanced intra-abdominal malignancy using high-dose intra-arterial chemotherapy with concomitant hemofiltration, *Reg. Cancer Treat.,* **3** (1990) 211–215.

142. Muchmore JH, Krementz ET, Carter RD, Preslan JE, and George WJ. Treatment of abdominal malignant neoplasms using regional chemotherapy with hemofiltration, *Arch. Surg.,* **126** (1991) 1390–1396.

143. Aigner KR and Gailhofer S. Celiac axis infusion for locally metastasized pancreatic cancer using spherex/mitoxantron microembolization and mitomycin C/chemofiltration, *Reg. Cancer Treat.,* **4** (1991) 3.

144. Winchester JF, Rahman A, Tilstone WJ, et al. Sorbent removal of adriamycin in vitro and in vivo, *Cancer Treat. Rep.,* **63** (1979) 1787–1793.

145. Winchester JF, Rahman A, Tilstone WJ, et al. Will hemoperfusion be useful for cancer chemotherapeutic drug removal?, *Clin. Toxicol.,* **17** (1980) 557–569.

146. Kihara T, Nakazawa H, Agishi T, Honda H, and Ota K. Superiority of selective bolus infusion and simultaneous rapid removal of anticancer agents by charcoal hemoperfusion in cancer treatment, *Trans. Am. Soc. Artif Intern. Organs,* **34** (1988) 581–584.

147. Ku Y, Saitoh M, Iwaasaki T, et al. Intra-arterial infusion of high-dose adriamycin for unresectable hepatocellular carcinoma using direct hemoperfusion under hepatic venous isolation, *Eur. J. Surg. Oncol.,* (1993) 387–392.

148. Ku Y, Fukumoto T, Tominaga M, et al. Single catheter technique of hepatic venous isolation and extracorporeal charcoal hemoperfusion for malignant liver tumors, *Am. J. Surg.,* **173** (1997) 103–109.

149. Ravikumar TS, Pizzorno G, Bodden W, et al. Percutaneous hepatic vein isolation and high-dose hepatic arterial infusion chemotherapy for unresectable liver tumors, *J. Clin. Oncol.,* **12** (1994) 2723–2736.

150. Tominaga M, Ku Y, Iwasaki T, Suzuki Y, and Saitoh Y. Pharmacological evaluation of portal venous isolation and charcoal haemoperfusion for high-dose intra-arterial chemotherapy of the pancreas, *Br. J. Surg.,* **84** (1997) 1072–1076.

151. Myers CE Jr and Chabner BA. Anthracyclines, In Chabner BA, Collins JM (eds), *Cancer Chemotherapy,* Lippincott, Philadelphia, 1990, pp. 356–381.

152. Drewinko B, Yang L-Y, Barlogie B, and Trujillo JM. Comparative cytotoxicity of bisantrene, mitoxantrone, ametantrone, dihydroxyanthracenedione, dihydroxyanthracenedione diacetate, and doxorubicin on human cells in vitro, *Cancer Res.,* **43** (1983) 2648–2653.

153. Fountzilas G, Gratzner H, Lim LO, and Yunis AA. Sensitivity of cultures human pancreatic carcinoma cells to dihyroxyanthracenedione, *Int. J. Cancer,* **33** (1984) 347–353.

154. Chan KK, Cohen JL, Gross JF, et al. Prediction of adriamycin disposition in cancer patients using physiologic, pharmacokinetic model, *Cancer Treat. Rep.,* **62** (1978) 1161–1171.

155. Skibba JL, Jones FE, and Condon RE. Altered hepatic disposition of doxorubicin in the perfused rat liver at hyperthermic temperatures, *Cancer Treat. Rep.,* **66** (1982) 1357–1363.

156. Chaudhuri PK, Arrendondo MA, Crist KA, and Thomford NR. Method of isolated perfusion of pancreas-duodenum in humans, *Reg. Cancer Treat.,* **3** (1990) 7–9.

157. Crist KA, Arrendondo MA, Chaudhuri B, Thomford NR, and Chaudhuri PK. Pharmacokinetics and

toxicity of isolated perfusion of human pancreas-duodenum with mitomycin C, *Reg. Cancer Treat.,* **3** (1991) 305–307.

158. Tomikawa M, Kubota T, Matsuzaki SW, et al. Mitomycin C and cisplatin increase survival in a human pancreatic cancer metastatic model, *Anticancer Res.,* **17** (1997) 3623–3625.

159. Yang L, Hwang R, Pandit L, Gordon EM, Anderson WF, and Parekh D. Gene therapy of metastatic pancreas cancer with intraperitoneal injections of concentrated retroviral herpes simplex thymidine kinase vector supernatant and ganciclovir, *Ann. Surg.,* **224** (1996) 405–417.

8 National Cancer Institute Experience with Regional Therapy for Unresectable Primary and Metastatic Cancer of the Liver or Peritoneal Cavity

H. Richard Alexander, David L. Bartlett, and Steven K. Libutti

CONTENTS

INTRODUCTION
ISOLATED HEPATIC PERFUSION
CONTINUOUS HYPERTHERMIC PERITONEAL PERFUSION
REFERENCES

1. INTRODUCTION

Patients who have unresectable primary or metastatic cancers of the liver or peritoneal carcinomatosis are rarely curable. The large number of regional treatments for the liver or peritoneal cavity that are under clinical evaluation underscore the difficulty in treating these conditions. In general, the rationale for regional therapies to intensify therapy, while minimizing unnecessary systemic toxicity, has been well established *(1–3)*. Over the past 6 yr, regional treatment protocols, using specialized surgical techniques to deliver regional therapy to the peritoneal cavity or liver, have been under clinical evaluation in the Surgery Branch of the National Cancer Institute (NCI). These include isolated hepatic perfusion (IHP) for the treatment of unresectable primary or metastatic cancers confined to the liver, and continuous hyperthermic peritoneal perfusion (CHPP) for the treatment of, or prophylaxis against, peritoneal carcinomatosis.

2. ISOLATED HEPATIC PERFUSION

2.1. Treatment of Unresectable Primary or Metastatic Cancers to the Liver

IHP was first used in the clinical setting almost 40 yr ago, at Roswell Park Cancer Institute in Buffalo, NY. Ausman et al. *(4)* reported results in five patients treated with nitrogen mustard administered via a normothermic IHP. Although no response data were given, survival data did suggest that 2 of 5 patients may have derived some benefit from treatment (Table 1). Twenty-three yr later, Aigner et al. *(5,6)* reported results in

From: *Current Clinical Oncology: Regional Chemotherapy: Clinical Research and Practice*
Edited by: M. Markman © Humana Press Inc., Totowa, NJ

Table 1
Summary of Previous IHP Chemotherapy Trials

Author, yr (ref.)	n	Agent(s)	Dose	Duration (h)	Temperature (°C)	Results
Ausman, 1961 (4)	5	Nitrogen mustard	0.2–0.4 mg/kg	NA	37	Two apparent long-term survivors, no response data
Aigner et al., 1984 (5)	32	5-FU	700–1100 mg	1 h	39.5–40	Median survival: 8 mo
Skibba and Quebbeman, 1986 (7)	8	Hyperthermia	–	4 h	42.0–42.5	5/6 responders[a]
Schwemmle et al., 1987 (9)	50	5-FU mitomycin C (14) cisplatin (4)	300–1250 mg 5–50 mg 50 mg	1 h	39.0–39.5	Median survival: 14 mo CR:9 (18%); PR:28 (50%)[a]
Hafstrom 1994 (9a)	29	Melphalan Cisplatin	0.5 mg/kg 0.5 mg/kg	1 h	40.0	PR: 20%; five survived 3 yr
Marinelli et al. 1996 (10)	9	Mitomycin C	30 mg/m²	1 h	37	1 PR; 1 CR (28% RR)
Van de Velde 1996 (11)	24	Melphalan	0.5–4 mg/kg	1 h	37	1 CR; 6 PR (41% RR)

[a]Using nonstandard criteria.
Used with permission from ref. 38.

32 patients treated with 700–1100 mg 5-fluorouracil, (5-FU) administered as a 1 h hyperthermic IHP. Again, no response data were reported, and the therapeutic effect of IHP was not conclusively demonstrated, because the median survival was only 8 mo after IHP alone, and 12 mo after IHP plus intra-arterial chemotherapy. Skibba and Quebbeman *(7)* and Skibba et al. *(8)* reported results in eight patients treated with a 4-h IHP, using hyperthermia alone, at 42.5°C. Although standard response criteria were not used, radiographic evidence of central tumor necrosis was evident in 5 of 6 evaluable patients. In 1987, Schwemmle et al. *(9)* reported results in 50 patients treated with a 1-h IHP, using 5-FU alone or in combination with mitomycin C (MMC) and cisplatin. Although the complete response (CR) was reported to be 18%, and the overall response rate was 68%, responses were scored using nonstandard radiographic criteria or decreased circulating carcinoembryonic antigen levels. In the 1990s, only two centers in Europe have reported significant clinical experience with IHP. Hafström from Sweden treated 29 patients with melphalan and cisplatin for 1 h at 40°C, and reported a partial response (PR) rate of 20% *(9a)*. Van de Velde et al. *(10,11)* reported results in over 30 patients treated with either melphalan or MMC for 1 h, using normothermic IHP, with response rates of 20% for the former and 41% for the latter agent (Table 1).

Treatment-related and operative mortality in these series was between 8 and 25%. However, most reports of IHP represented the initial institutional experience with this specialized surgical technique, often in limited numbers of patients with very advanced tumor burden. Because of the specialized nature of the IHP procedure, the attendant morbidity and potential mortality associated with it, and the lack of documented efficacy, this regional treatment strategy has not gained widespread or consistent clinical evaluation. Nevertheless, these data suggest that IHP may have the capacity to cause clinically meaningful regression of advanced cancers confined to the liver.

2.2. Technical Aspects

IHP, like other regional liver treatments, is a method of delivering dose-intensive therapy directly to the liver, while limiting unnecessary systemic exposure of the therapeutic agents. IHP has several potential advantages over other established regional treatments. In contrast to local ablative techniques such as cryotherapy, IHP can treat numerous and bulky (>5 cm) metastases; potentially, it may treat occult or microscopic disease in other regions of the liver. Hepatic artery infusion of chemotherapeutics, using an implantable pump, or embolic agents via percutaneously placed catheters, have been refined to optimize dose delivery of the therapeutic agents to the tumor *(3)*. IHP has the capacity to completely isolate the vascular supply of the liver from the systemic circulation; therefore, dose intensification is limited only by the tissue tolerance of the normal liver to the therapeutic agents being delivered. IHP can deliver uniform and potentially clinically relevant amounts of hyperthermia to the liver that may take advantage of the potential direct tumoricidal effects of hyperthermia alone *(12,13)*, as well as the established synergistic effects with various chemotherapeutics or biological agents *(14,15)*. In addition, at the completion of IHP, the liver is flushed with several liters of normal saline, which effectively removes any residual perfusate containing the therapeutic agents from the hepatic vascular bed.

On the other hand, there are several disadvantages to IHP, compared to other regional treatments. First, it is a technically complex treatment to administer, and there is attendant morbidity associated with the operative procedure, as described above. In addition, the therapeutic agents being administered must have sufficient efficacy, with

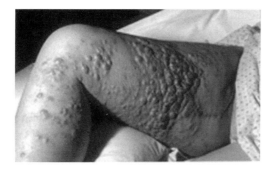 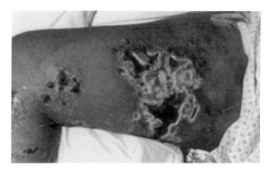

Pre-op   **14 days post-ILP**

Fig. 1. Pre- and 14-d post-ILP results in a 34-yr-old female with metastatic eccrine gland adenocarcinoma that arose originally from the heel, and had diffusely spread throughout the right lower extremity. After a hyperthermic ILP with TNF and melphalan, the patient had a significant response. Note the eschar formation and sparing of adjacent skin, reminiscent of the antitumor effects observed with TNF in experimental murine models. The patient had failed prior intra-arterial and systemic chemotherapy.

a single brief exposure to the tumor, to warrant such an aggressive approach. The efficacy of previously used agents in IHP has not been established.

In 1992, Lienard et al. *(16)* published their initial results, using a combination of interferon (IFN)-γ, tumor necrosis factor (TNF), and melphalan, administered via isolated limb perfusion (ILP), for patients with in-transit melanoma or unresectable high-grade sarcoma of the extremity. In this initial trial, 21 of 23 evaluable patients had a CR (89%), and two others had a PR to treatment. Based on these remarkable initial results, a number of institutions, including the Surgery Branch at the NCI, initiated clinical trials to confirm the efficacy of this ILP treatment regimen for in-transit melanoma or unresectable extremity sarcoma. Although the response rates in subsequent series have not been as high, CR rates between 70 and 80%, and overall response rates between 90 and 100%, have been reported *(17–19)*. During that time, a patient was evaluated, at this institution, who had a refractory eccrine gland adenocarcinoma originally arising from the foot, which had extensively spread throughout the leg. This patients was treated, under a compassionate exemption, with ILP using TNF and melphalan, and had a dramatic, albeit transient, near CR in the perfusion field (Fig. 1). This result prompted us to evaluate the potential utility of TNF and melphalan with IHP for adenocarcinoma or other tumor histologies confined to the liver. Therefore, in 1993, clinical trials were initiated to evaluate the feasibility of TNF-based regimens administered via IHP for patients with unresectable primary or metastatic cancers confined to the liver.

The operative setup for IHP is shown in Fig. 2. The extracorporeal bypass circuit consists of a roller pump, oxygenator, heat exchanger, and reservoir. The components of the perfusate include 700 mL balanced salt solution, 300 mL packed red blood cells, and 2000 U heparin. Sodium bicarbonate is added to the perfusate during the procedure, in order to maintain an arterial perfusate pH between 7.2 and 7.3. Temperature probes placed percutaneously in the right and left hepatic lobes, as well as a central hepatic thermister probe advanced into the portal vein to the liver, document prompt and uniform heating of the liver parenchyma to the desired temperature of 39.5–40°C during IHP. The typical perfusion parameters are shown in Table 2.

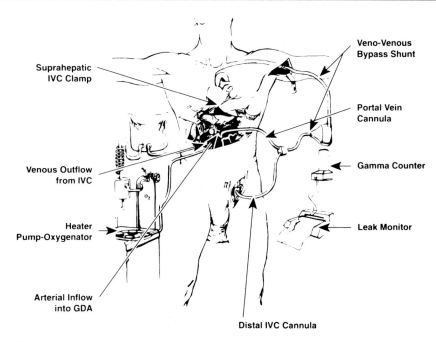

Fig. 2. Illustration of the operative setup during isolated liver perfusion. The extracorporeal bypass circuit, containing a reservoir, heat exchanger, oxygenator, and roller pump, is shown on the patient's right. Venous outflow is collected via a cannula positioned in an isolated segment of retrohepatic IVC. Inflow is via the gastroduodenal artery. The external veno-veno bypass circuit, which shunts portal venous and IVC blood flow back to the heart, is shown on the patient's left. The continuous intraoperative leak monitoring system consists of a gamma counter positioned over the centrifugal pump housing to detect radioactivity in the systemic blood, which is connected to a stripchart recorder.

Table 2
Treatment and Perfusion Parameters Used During IHP

Duration:	1 h
Agents:[a]	
TNF	1.0 mg
Melphalan	1.5 mg/kg
Hepatic tissue temperature	39.5–40.0°C
Flow rates:	600–1200 mL/min
Perfusate volume:	1 L
Perfusate composition:	700 mL crystalloid
	300 mL PRBC[b]
	2000 U heparin
	20–40 mEq $NaHCO_3$[c]
Postperfusion flush:	
Hepatic artery	1.5 L crystalloid
	1.5 L colloid
Portal vein	1.0 L crystalloid

[a]Used in a phase II trial.
[b]Packed red blood cells.
[c]$NaHCO_3^-$ is titrated to maintain arterial perfusate pH at 7.2–7.3.
   Alexander et al. Isolated hepatic perfusion: a potentially effective treatment for patients with metastatic or primary cancers confined to liver. Cancer J. Sci. Am.
   Adapted with permission from *ref. 38.*

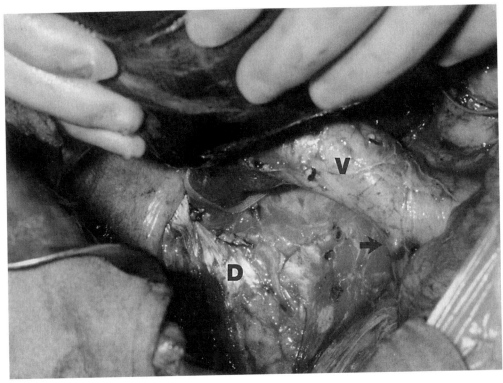

Fig. 3. Intraoperative photograph of the retrohepatic IVC dissection (V), showing complete mobilization of the IVC from the level of the renal veins (arrow) to the diaphragm (D), including ligation and division of the right adrenal vein, to prevent leak of perfusate into the systemic circulation during treatment.

The authors have made several modifications in the technique, in order to improve the safety and potentially the efficacy of IHP. During IHP, blood flow through the retrohepatic inferior vena cava (IVC) is temporarily occluded with vascular clamps above and below the liver, so that venous outflow from the hepatic veins can be collected from an isolated segment of retrohepatic IVC, and delivered to the outflow line of the extracorporeal bypass circuit. Inflow to the liver is via the hepatic artery, using a cannula positioned in the gastroduodenal artery (Fig. 2). During this time, arterial inflow is occluded with a vascular clamp placed across the proximal hepatic artery, and the portal vein flow to the liver is also temporarily occluded. In previous reports, IVC and portal venous flow were shunted to the heart during IHP with a passive internal shunt system, using a double-lumen cannula positioned in the retrohepatic IVC. The authors use an external active veno-veno bypass circuit to shunt venous blood flow back to the heart, using a centrifugal pump similar to that used in hepatic transplantation procedures (20); (Fig. 2). This may be the optimal method for ensuring adequate venous return and hemodynamic stability during IHP. A thorough dissection and preparation of the liver prior to IHP is routinely done, in order to ensure that all potential arterial and venous collateral blood flow from the liver to the systemic circulation is controlled. This involves extensive mobilization of the liver, including mobilization of the retrohepatic IVC from the retroperitoneum. The right adrenal vein, phrenic veins, and direct small venous tributaries from the IVC to the retroperitoneum are all ligated and divided (Fig. 3). The gallbladder is removed prophylactally, in order to prevent a chemical

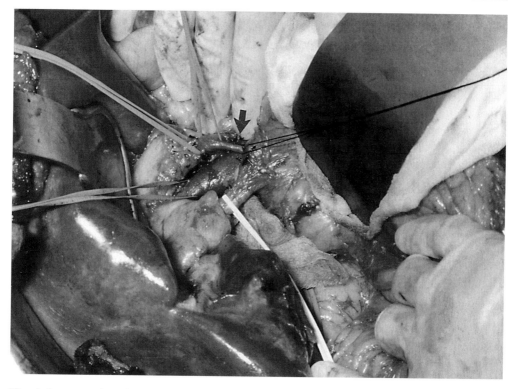

Fig. 4. Intraoperative photograph showing the extent of the periportal dissection prior to IHP. The portal structures have been skeletonized to prevent leak of perfusate during treatment, and to facilitate cannulation of the portal vein and gastroduodenal artery (arrow).

cholecystitis in the early postoperative period. An extensive dissection of the portahepatis is done, to prevent leak of perfusate through small vascular channels in the connective tissue around the common bile duct, portal vein, or hepatic artery (Fig. 4). A continuous intraoperative leak monitoring system, adapted from the leak monitoring system, which has been described for ILP, is utilized *(21)*. In 100 patients treated on various clinical IHP protocols in the Surgery Branch, all have been able to successfully complete the 60-min perfusion, and have had stable hemodynamic parameters during this time, in some measure, because of the external veno-veno bypass circuit. In addition, using the standardized operative approach and the leak monitoring system, the authors have been able to confirm that complete vascular isolation can be achieved consistently in these patients, and have experienced only three measurable leaks of perfusate (all less than 4%). All were correctable with various small technical maneuvers during IHP.

2.3. Clinical Results

The initial clinical trials with IHP in the Surgery Branch were designed to define the safe maximum-tolerated doses (MTDs) of, initially, TNF with IFN-γ and subsequently TNF in combination with melphalan (Table 3). Assessment of regional and systemic toxicity in these trials deserves some comment. Because the treatment is being administered in the context of a major operative procedure, and the liver is undergoing significant manipulation, with some brief periods of relative ischemia, a toxicity scoring system was used in an attempt to discriminate between true treatment-related toxicity and that occurring as a consequence of the operative procedure itself. Therefore, systemic

Table 3
Summary of Surgery Branch IHP Protocols

Study	n	Agent	Doses	Overall Response Rate (%)	Clinical Outcome
Phase I	16	TNF IFN	0.3–2.0 mg 0.2 mg	20	Coagulopathy was dose-limiting toxicity
Phase I	14	TNF Melphalan	1.0–1.5 mg 1.0–2.0 mg/kg	50	Hepatic VOD was melphalan dose-limiting toxicity
Phase II	43	TNF Melphalan	1.0 mg 1.5 mg/kg	75	One (3%) VOD fatality; majority of patients had undergone previous treatment
Pilot	9	Melphalan Post-IHP FUDR LV	1.5 mg/kg .2 mg/kg/d 15 mg/m^2/d	78	FUDR/LV given as 14 d infusion every 28 d
Phase I	Open	Melphalan	1.5–3.0 mg/kg	NA	For noncolorectal histologies
Phase I	Open	Melphalan Post-IHP FUDR LV	1.5–3.0 mg/kg 0.2 mg/kg/d 15 mg/m^2/d	NA	For colorectal histology FUDR/LV given as 14 d infusion every 28 d

NA = not available; LV = Leucovorin; VOD = veno-occlusive disease.

toxicities were scored as those that persisted beyond 24 h after the IHP procedure. Hepatic transaminases and bilirubin are elevated within the first 36–72 h after IHP, and returned toward baseline by 7 d after the procedure. In order to distinguish between the effects of physical and vascular manipulation of the liver and those related to treatment, regional toxicities were scored as abnormalities on liver function tests that persisted beyond 7 d after the procedure. Approximately 75% of patients experience reversible grade III or IV hepatic toxicity after IHP.

In the initial clinical trial at the Surgery Branch, using 0.3–2.0 mg TNF administered with a fixed low dose of IFN-γ (200 µg) within the perfusion circuit, dose-limiting coagulopathy was observed at 2 mg TNF, and, therefore, the safe MTD was determined to be 1.5 mg. This dose is substantially lower than the 3–4 mg TNF administered via ILP with IFN and melphalan, and highlights the highly variable tissue tolerances of this agent. Subsequently, 14 patients were treated with an alternating dose escalation of TNF and melphalan, again administered via a 1-h hyperthermic IHP. Hepatic veno-occlusive disease secondary to melphalan was observed in patients receiving 2 mg/kg melphalan in combination with 1 mg TNF. Therefore, in a subsequent phase II study, 1 mg TNF and 1.5 mg/kg melphalan were used.

In the phase II study, 43 patients with various tumor histologies were treated. Perfusion parameters are outlined in Table 4, from a cohort of 34 of these patients. The overall response rate was 74%, including two patients who had radiographic CR to treatment (Table 5). Responses were seen across all histologies treated, including patients with colorectal cancer (CRC), ocular melanoma, adenocarcinoma of unknown

Table 4
Isolated Hepatic Perfusion
Treatment Parameters in 34 Patients

	Mean ± SEM (range)
Flow rate:	844 ± 117 mL/min (600–1200)
Central hepatic temperature:	39.9 ± 0.4°C (39.0–41.8)
Perfusion arterial line pressure:	159 ± 33 mm Hg (103–255)
Melphalan dose:	102 ± 5 mg (75–135)
TNF dose:	1 mg
% leak	
0:	32 (94%)
<4:	2 (6%)
Veno-veno bypass flow rate:	1807 ± 316 mL/min (1200–2600)
MAP[a]	81 ± 5 mg (60–108)

[a]MAP = mean arterial pressure during IHP.
Alexander et al. Isolated hepatic perfusion with tumor necrosis factor and melphalan for unresectable cancers confined to liver, *J. Clin. Oncol.,* **16** (1998) 1479–1489.
Modified from *ref. 21a.*

Table 5
Response Data in 43 Evaluable Patients Treated with TNF and Melphalan IHP

Histology	n	Overall (%)	PR (%)	CR (%)
All	43	32 (74)	30 (70)	2 (4)
Colon adenocarcinoma	31	24 (77)	24 (77)	0
Ocular melanoma	7	4 (57)	2 (28)	2 (28)
Other	5	4 (80)	4 (80)	0

CR = complete radiographic response; PR = partial radiographic response. Adapted with permission from *ref. 38.*

primary, and hepatocellular carcinoma. In 33 patients who have had pretreatment factors evaluated, such as the number of lesions, diameter of largest lesion, and percent hepatic replacement, the response rates appeared to remain consistent, despite increasing numbers of large lesions or advanced hepatic disease (Table 6). At a median potential follow-up of 15 mo, the mean duration of response in these 33 evaluable patients is 9 mo and ranges from 2 to 30 mo *(21a).*

The majority of patients treated had metastatic CRC to the liver. Three patients who had previously failed intra-arterial infusional chemotherapy had a response to IHP (Fig. 5). Some of the more durable and significant responses were observed in patients with metastatic ocular melanoma to the liver (Fig. 6). One patient had a radiographic CR of 11 mo duration, who was appreciated to have multiple radiographically visible

Table 6
Response to IHP[a]

	n	PR or CR[b]	%
Overall	33	25	75
Number[c]			
1–4	9	7	78
5–19	13	9	69
≥20	11	9	81
Diameter largest lesion (cm)			
<5	4	2	50
5–9.9	12	9	75
≥10	17	14	82
Hepatic replacement (%)			
<20	6	5	83
20–49	15	10	66
≥50	12	10	83

[a]Based on number of lesions, diameter of largest tumor, or percent hepatic replacement in 33 evaluable patients.

[b]Partial (PR) or complete (CR) response.

[c]Radiographically imageable lesions.

Adapted with permission from *ref. 21a*.

Alexander et al. Isolated hepatic perfusion with tumor necrosis factor and melphalan for unresectable cancers confined to liver. *J. Clin. Oncol.*, **16** (1998) 1479–1489.

Pre IHP CT CEA = 35.4 µg/L

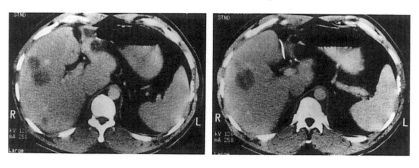

5 Months Post IHP CT CEA = 13.7 µg/L

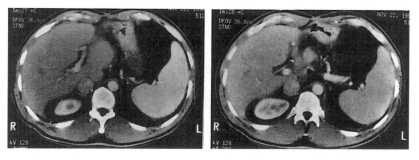

Fig. 5. Pre- and post-IHP CT scan of the liver in a 38-yr-old male with metastatic CRC. The patient had previously failed systemic and intra-arterial chemotherapy, and has an ongoing PR in the liver 11 mo after treatment.

Pre-IHP

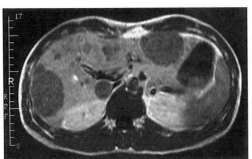 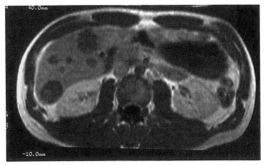

1 year post-IHP

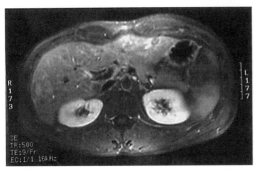 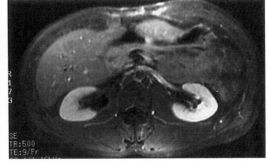

Fig. 6. Pre- and 1-yr post-IHP T_1 gadolinium-enhanced MRI of the liver in a 30-yr-old male with metastatic ocular melanoma. The patient has an ongoing and significant PR in the liver 2½-yr after treatment.

bilobar hepatic metastasis, and literally hundreds of occult, small pigmented nodules diffusely present in the liver, recognized at the time of laparotomy. A second patient, with a large metastatic deposit in the liver on the right side, was initially explored at another institution, in contemplation of resection. However, at that time, she was noted to have multiple deposits diffusely present throughout the liver, and subsequently had a 60-min hyperthermic perfusion with TNF and melphalan, with a radiographic PR that persisted for 30 mo.

In 98 patients who have been treated on various IHP protocols at this institution, the authors have had three treatment-related and three operative mortalities. The three treatment-related mortalities were a result of melphalan-induced veno-occlusive disease in two patients and TNF-induced multisystem organ failure in another. Two of these occurred in the setting of dose levels of melphalan and TNF that defined dose-limiting toxicity. One patient developed irreversible progressive veno-occlusive disease on the phase II study, and at autopsy was noted to have chronic iron deposition in the liver, suggesting some underlying occult hepatocellular abnormality that may have predisposed him to the veno-occlusive disease. One patient was treated with a 75-min perfusion, and developed immediate and profound multisystem organ failure postoperatively.

Of the three perioperative deaths, one patient, who had metastatic renal cell carcinoma isolated to the liver, was treated early in the authors' experience, and had a fatal pulmonary tumor embolism develop after IHP. At autopsy, it was noted that the tumor had invaded the hepatic veins. Two other patients had ischemic injury to the liver, resulting from cannulation difficulties and the setting of scar tissue around the hepatic artery, secondary to previous treatment.

2.4. Future Directions

Based on the initial encouraging results with IHP, further refinements in technique appear warranted. It is important to consider overall response rates, duration of response, and patterns of recurrence in patients treated with IHP. In addition, one must consider the profile of regional (liver) and systemic toxicities following IHP, and what other regional or systemic therapies might be considered, based on the histology of the tumor.

Despite high initial response rates, the median duration of response has been unacceptably short, considering the nature of the treatment. Initial sites of recurrence in 25 patients who had a response was liver in one-third, systemic in 40%, and both in 10%. However, the high incidence of systemic failure may reflect the fact that these patients were at high risk of harboring occult systemic disease. The protocol allows patients with minimal resectable extrahepatic disease to be treated with IHP, if the liver was the clear dominant site of life-threatening tumor progression. In fact, a number of patients had metastatic regional lymph nodes in the periportal area that were resected and not considered a contraindication for IHP. Because early systemic failure should decrease with more careful patient selection, and because the liver was the initial site of recurrence alone or with systemic disease in almost half the patients treated, further regional therapies designed to prolong the duration of response within the liver would seem appropriate.

Another question is whether TNF is a significant contributing factor to the efficacy of the therapy. It is likely that TNF is contributing to toxicity. When TNF levels are measured in the perfusate, and systemically, there are no consistently detectable levels in the systemic circulation, and the concentration of TNF appears to remain fairly constant in the perfusion circuit, indicating minimal tissue absorption or degradation of the protein (Fig. 7). However, systemic concentrations of proinflammatory cytokines, such as interleukin (IL)-6 and IL-8, are high following IHP, and may cause some of the cardiovascular effects that are observed during the first 24 h after treatment. These cytokines may be produced primarily by the secondary effects of TNF on one of the resident cell types of the liver. Therefore, although TNF may be tolerated in the liver during IHP, it may be inducing production of secondary mediators, which cause subsequent systemic toxicities, once the native blood flow through the liver has been reestablished. There are prospective random assignment trials in Europe and the United States, in which ILP perfusion, using TNF and melphalan, is compared to melphalan alone, for in-transit melanoma of the extremity. Early analyses of the U.S. trial did not show any significant difference in the overall response rates between the groups (22). In the authors' phase I IHP trial with escalating-dose TNF, the overall response rate was only 20%, and the few patients who did respond were in the group of patients that received the lowest doses of TNF. This suggests that TNF alone has virtually no significant antitumor effects in IHP, and this has also been observed in a limited number of patients undergoing ILP with TNF alone (23).

The question as to whether or not the dose of melphalan within the perfusion could be increased significantly, when used without TNF, and still produce comparable response rates, has not been determined. Van de Velde et al. (personal communication) have used doses up to 200 mg within the perfusion circuit (about 3–4 mg/kg), and have seen no dose-limiting regional toxicity. However, severe postperfusion neutropenia has been seen in some patients, suggesting that complete vascular isolation during the

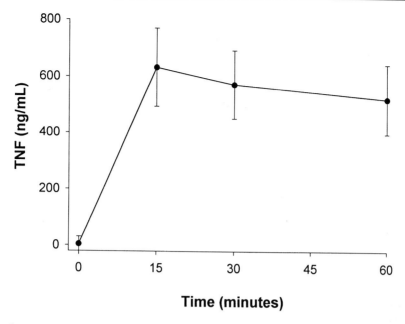

Fig. 7. Perfusate TNF concentrations in 34 patients undergoing a 60-min hyperthermic IHP with 1 mg TNF and 1.5 mg/kg melphalan. The initial concentration value of 0.6 mg/L is consistent with the dilutional effect of 1 mg TNF administered in a circuit containing 1 L perfusate and approx 400–500 mL blood in the liver. The concentration remains fairly stable over the treatment interval, indicating minimal tissue uptake or degradation. Adapted with permission from *ref. 21a.*

perfusion may not be consistently achieved. These data also suggest that the liver will tolerate higher doses of melphalan in the perfusion circuit, when used without TNF.

A small number of patients with CRC have been treated in a pilot study combining IHP with melphalan alone, at a dose of 1.5 mg/kg, followed by intra-arterial infusional floxuridine (FUDR) and leucovorin. At the completion of the IHP, an intra-arterial gastroduodenal artery port is left in place. Patients are allowed to convalesce for 6 wk, and are then treated with 0.2 mg/kg/d FUDR and 15 mg/m²/d leucovorin, administered as a constant infusion over 14 d, followed by a 14-d rest period. Nine patients with metastatic CRC confined to the liver were treated on that protocol between January and September, 1997. The overall response rate in patients, following hepatic perfusion and FUDR, is 78%. Although follow-up is extremely short, only two patients have failed within the liver, and other responses are ongoing between 3 and 12 mo following perfusion. These early data suggest that hepatic perfusion, followed by intra-arterial FUDR, is feasible, and may prolong the duration of hepatic response.

Currently, a phase I trial is being conducted for patients with metastatic CRC to the liver, in which the dose of melphalan administered in the perfusate is being gradually increased (Table 3). At 6 wk after perfusion, patients are being treated with intra-arterial FUDR, as outlined above.

For patients with other histologies for which regional chemotherapy has not had established efficacy, the technique of hepatic perfusion has been modified slightly, in order to optimize tissue delivery of the therapeutic agent during IHP. The cannulation procedure has been modified to include a double-inflow system, so that the portal vein and hepatic artery are perfused, using an escalating melphalan dose schedule identical to the one used for patients with CRC. Based on recent data reporting a 40% response rate in patients with metastatic ocular melanoma to the liver treated with continuous infusion arterial fotemustine *(24)*, the use of this agent following IHP may be useful in patients with ocular melanoma, in order to prolong the duration of hepatic response.

2.5. Summary

Data indicate that IHP can be done safely in patients with metastatic disease confined to the liver, and can cause clinically meaningful regression of unresectable cancers confined to the liver of various histologies. Complete vascular isolation of the liver can be consistently achieved, and further refinements in this treatment technique are warranted, based on the authors' initial results. Combining IHP with other regional treatment strategies may prove optimal for durable control of unresectable liver cancers.

3. CONTINUOUS HYPERTHERMIC PERITONEAL PERFUSION

3.1. Treatment or Prophylaxis of Peritoneal Carcinomatosis

Peritoneal carcinomas from gastrointestinal (GI) malignancies is a clinical condition that has an extremely grave prognosis, and for which there is no satisfactory therapeutic intervention. For many patients with gastric, appendiceal, small bowel, pancreatic, or colorectal cancers, peritoneal carcinomatosis may develop, and, when present, is the sole or major contributing cause of morbidity and mortality. A variety of innovative strategies have been devised that deliver treatment directly to the peritoneal cavity, in an attempt to intensify regional dose delivery and minimize systemic toxicity. Such therapies include intraperitoneal (ip) photodynamic therapy, ip immunotherapy using monoclonal antibodies, adoptive cellular immunotherapy, and ip administration of cytokines, such as TNF. In addition, there has been considerable clinical application of single-agent or combination-agent therapy administered as an ip dwell in patients with carcinomatosis from GI or ovarian malignancies *(25)*.

CHPP is an attractive treatment option, because it is technically straightforward to administer, and may be an effective method of distributing a therapeutic agent to a complex surface, such as the peritoneal cavity. In addition, it can deliver significant hyperthermia to the peritoneal cavity, which takes advantage of its direct tumoricidal activity, as well as its established synergy with chemotherapeutic or biological agents. Treatment can be administered at the time of laparotomy, when small-volume peritoneal carcinomatosis is identified, or could be used as a prophylactic treatment in patients with high-risk primary tumors, such as those penetrating through serosa (Table 7).

3.2. Previous History

The first clinical report of CHPP, in which hyperthermia and chemotherapy were delivered into the peritoneal cavity via a recirculating infusion system, was published in 1980 by Spratt et al. *(26)*. This case report involved a highly motivated 35-yr-old man with pseudomyxoma peritoneii, who had performed extensive research on his diagnosis, and traveled to Louisville and insisted on being the first person to undergo this treatment at his own expense.

The vast majority of initial clinical series evaluating CHPP were from Japan (Table 8). A number of multiarm studies evaluating the efficacy of prophylactic or therapeutic CHPP, after resection for gastric cancer (GC), have been conducted. Koga et al. *(27)* reported results in 60 patients undergoing gastric resection with curative intent, selected to receive either CHPP with 8–10 mg/L perfusate of MMC administered via CHPP, or no further treatment. In a subset analysis of 47 patients who had histopathologic evidence of serosal invasion, the trend was toward better survival in the CHPP-treated

Table 7
Considerations in Use of CHPP for Treatment of Carcinomatosis

Parameter	Favorable	Unfavorable
Patient	Opportunity to apply therapy early. CHPP can be done in conjunction with major procedures.	Most suitable patients are those with small-volume or microscopic disease.
Tumor	Peritoneal implants are surface malignancies: Do not invade peritoneal surface deeply.	Topically applied treatment may have variable tumor penetration.
Peritoneal cavity	Acts as a barrier: Drug permeability should be less than plasma clearance; amenable to delivery of hyperthermia.	Complete and uniform distribution of perfusate is critical.
Chemotherapy	Much higher regional concentrations possible, compared with systemic administration	May have dose-limiting regional toxicity.
Hyperthermia	Neoplastic tissue is very sensitive to the lethal effects; synergizes with chemotherapy.	Difficult to uniformly heat tumors in vivo.

Adapted with permission from *ref. 25.*

group at 3 yr (83%) than in the control group (67%). Five-yr survival in CHPP-treated patients was significantly better, compared to historically matched controls. Fujimoto et al. *(28)* reported a comparable trial in 59 patients undergoing resection for GC, who were treated with 10 mg/L perfusate of MMC administered via CHPP, vs no further treatment following resection for GC *(28)*. Overall survival was significantly better for patients who received CHPP, and, in an unplanned subgroup analysis, the beneficial effect was seen in patients with and without documented peritoneal seeding. It is remarkable that the median postoperative survival in patients with peritoneal carcinomatosis was 12 mo, and the median survival of 20 patients with peritoneal implants treated with CHPP had not been reached, with a maximum potential follow-up of 3 yr. Fujimura et al. *(29)* reported results using a combination of 200 mg/m^2 cisplatin and 20 mg/m^2 MMC administered for between 40 and 60 min via CHPP, with target temperatures ranging between 41 and 43°C. All patients had documented peritoneal carcinomatosis, and, in 12 patients treated with CHPP, a second-look laparotomy was performed. Of these, 41% were assessed to have had either a CR (four of 12) or PR (1 of 12). In a three-arm random assignment trial comparing the results of CHPP with continuous normothermic peritoneal perfusion or surgery alone, in patients with GC with T3 lesions (serosal invasion) undergoing resection with curative intent, survival was significantly better in the treatment groups, compared to those receiving surgery alone *(30)*. Hamazoe et al. *(31)* reported comparable results in 82 patients with GC who had gross serosal invasion without evidence of peritoneal metastases. In the 42 patients randomly assigned to receive prophylactic CHPP with MMC, there was a lower incidence of peritoneal recurrence, compared to untreated controls ($P_2 = 0.08$), but no significant difference in overall survival.

Table 8
Clinical Results of Multi-Arm Studies Evaluating Efficacy of Prophylactic or Therapeutic CHPP Immediately After Resection for GC

Author (ref.)	n	Treatment Arm	Agents	Dose	Duration (Min)	Temperature (°C)	Follow-up (Yr)	Survival (%)	P_2
Koga et al. (27)	26	CHPP	MMC	8–10 mg/L	60	44–45	2½	83	NS
	21	Control	–	–			–	67	
Koga et al. (27)	38	CHPP	MMC	8–10 mg/L	60	44–45	3	74	<0.04
	55	Control[a]	–	–			–	53	
Fujimoto et al. (28)	30	CHPP	MMC	10 mg/L	120	44–47	1	80	<0.001
	29	Control	–	–			–	34	
Fujimura et al. (30)	22	CHPP	MMC and cisplatin	30 mg	60	41–42	3	68	<0.01[b]
	18	CHPP		300 mg/kg	60	37–38		51	
	18	Control	–	–			–	23	
Hamazoe et al. (31)	42	CHPP	MMC	10 mg/L	60	48–50	5	64	NS
	40	Control	–	–			–	53	

[a]Historical control group.
[b]CHPP or CNPP vs control.
CHPP = continuous hyperthermic peritoneal perfusion; CNPP = continuous normothermic peritoneal perfusion; MMC = mitomycin C; NS = not significant.
Adapted with permission from ref. 25.

Based on these results, a number of centers in Europe and the United States have initiated clinical trials evaluating CHPP for the treatment or prophylaxis of peritoneal carcinomatosis, using, primarily, MMC, cisplatin, or a combination of the two. Several centers have reported that malignant ascites can be effectively palliated with CHPP. Fujimoto et al. *(32)* reported that 5 of 6 patients with malignant ascites secondary to recurrent GI cancer had resolution of ascites after undergoing tumor resection and CHPP at a mean follow-up of 13 mo. Gilley et al. *(33)* reported that 9 of 10 patients had no evidence of recurrent ascites on ultrasound 2 mo after CHPP. Taken together, these data indicate there may be some palliative, therapeutic, or prophylactic efficacy for the use of CHPP.

3.3. Technical Considerations

Because the perfusate must deliver tumoricidal doses of the therapeutic agents to the center of the peritoneal implants primarily via diffusion, data would suggest that tumors greater than 6 mm in diameter will not get tumoricidal doses of the therapeutic agents at their center. Dikhoff et al. *(34)* showed that concentrations of platinum in tumor after ip administration remained relatively constant and high, up to a distance of 3 mm from the surface of the tumor. However, at a distance of 5 mm from the surface of the tumor tissue, concentrations of platinum dropped to only 20% of that seen at the tumor surface. Platinum concentrations in tumor and intra-abdominal organs were severalfold higher with ip delivery, compared to an equivalent iv dose. Therefore, patients with small-volume disease would theoretically be best suited for CHPP.

The peritoneal cavity should be thoroughly explored at the time of laparotomy, and attempts should be made to reduce the tumor burden to levels at would be consistent with a potential therapeutic effect using CHPP. Once this has been accomplished, inflow and outflow catheters are positioned at either end of the peritoneal cavity (Fig. 8). Typically, an inflow catheter is placed over the dome of the liver or in the lesser sac of the abdomen, and the outflow catheter is placed in the pelvis. Although some have advocated the use of a Y connector to infuse the perfusate to both upper abdominal quadrants, the benefit of more infusion catheters vs one has not been demonstrated. Once the inflow and outflow catheters are positioned, several ip temperature probes are placed in the peritoneal cavity to document uniform and sufficient heating of the peritoneal surfaces during treatment. The abdominal fascia is then temporarily closed, and the catheters are connected to a perfusion circuit, which consists of a reservoir bag, roller pump, and heat exchanger (Fig. 8). Because the peritoneal cavity is a complex surface, all ip adhesions should be divided, and the peritoneal surfaces should be completely mobilized, theoretically, in order to allow adequate distribution of the therapeutic agent and hyperthermia to all the peritoneal surfaces. Initially, the perfusion circuit contains only saline, until a satisfactory perfusion circuit has been established, and the peritoneal cavity has been warmed; the therapeutic agent is then administered into the reservoir bag, and CHPP is continued for 90 min.

Because the peritoneal cavity can act as a heat sink, it is necessary to have rapid flow rates through the peritoneal cavity (1.5–2 L/min) to achieve uniform and adequate ip hyperthermia. The patient should be positioned on a cooling blanket prior to the procedure, and the arms should be abducted on arm boards, to allow the head, neck, and axilla to be packed with icebags, as necessary, to maintain a core (esophageal) temperature less than 40°C. In addition, a cisplatin-binding agent, sodium thiosulfate, is administered as a continuous systemic infusion during the CHPP, as described by Howell *(35)*, and urine output is increased using iv hydration and diuretics, in order

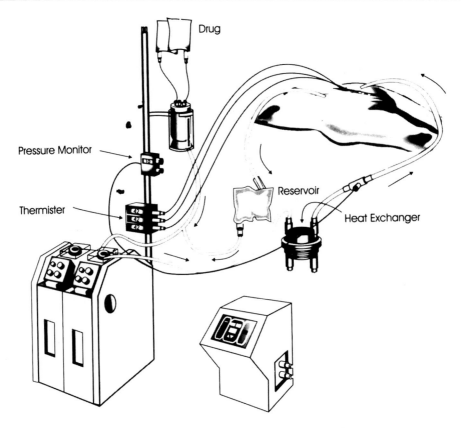

Fig. 8. Illustration of the intraoperative setup during CHPP. The inflow and outflow cannulae are connected with a closed recirculating circuit consisting of a reservoir bag, roller pump, and heat exchanger.

to minimize renal exposure to high concentrations of platinum that may diffuse through the peritoneal membrane. Platinum is a large hydrophilic compound that is less permeable across the peritoneal cavity than small lipophilic compounds, and the estimated clearance across the peritoneal cavity during CHPP has been calculated at approx 18 mL/min, which compares quite favorably to the observed plasma clearance of platinum of 329 mL/min (*36*).

During CHPP, the peritoneal cavity should be slightly distended with perfusate, which facilitates the circulation of the perfusate through the cavity (Fig. 9). During perfusion, the patient's position is periodically changed slightly, and there is a continuous manual agitation of the abdominal wall, to prevent streaming of the perfusion fluid through the peritoneal cavity. Once the perfusion has been completed, the abdominal cavity is opened, the perfusate is evacuated and the catheters and temperature probes are removed.

3.4. Clinical Results at Surgery Branch of NCI

In 1992, a phase I dose-escalation trial, using cisplatin administered via CHPP, at a temperature of 41–42°C, was initiated for patients with peritoneal carcinomatosis from any histology. In that trial, dose-limiting renal toxicity was observed at a dose of 350–400 mg/m² cisplatin. Based on data indicating that ip TNF administered as a dwell resulted in favorable regional pharmacokinetics and palliation of malignant ascites,

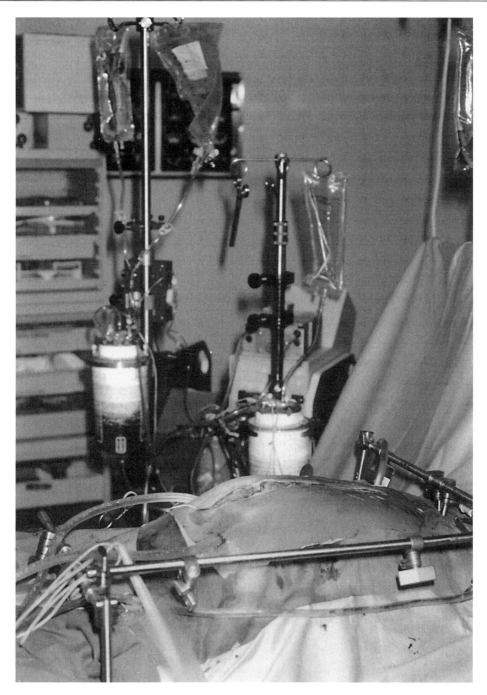

Fig. 9. Intraoperative photograph of a patient undergoing CHPP. The fascia has been temporarily closed, to prevent leak of perfusate during the treatment period. Note the mild distention of the abdominal wall.

and on data that established synergy between TNF, cisplatin, and hyperthermia in experimental models *(14,37)*, a subsequent phase I CHPP trial of escalating doses of TNF, administered with a fixed 250 mg/m^2 dose of cisplatin, was conducted. TNF was administered initially at a dose of 0.1 mg/L perfusate. At the first escalation to 0.3 mg/

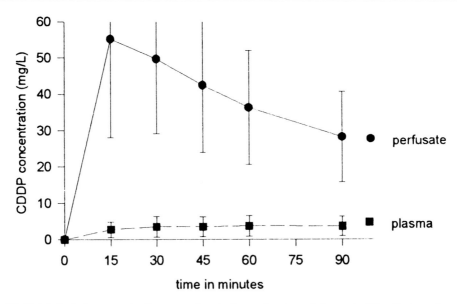

Fig. 10. Total cisplatin concentrations over time in the perfusate and plasma in 27 patients undergoing a 90-min hyperthermic CHPP for established carcinomatosis. Adapted with permission from *ref. 39.*

L perfusate, severe dose-limiting nephrotoxicity was encountered. Therefore, the safe MTD of cisplatin and TNF, given in combination, was 250 mg/m^2 and 0.1 mg/L, respectively.

The pharmacologic advantage of cisplatin administered via CHPP is demonstrated in Fig. 10. In data from 27 patients, the area under the concentration over time curve (AUC) of total cisplatin in the perfusate over 90 min was 3518 ± 1402 mg/min/mL, compared to 287 ± 212 mg/min/mL in plasma. The ratio of perfusate AUC to plasma AUC ranged from 4.6 to 119, with a median of 14 (Fig. 10). There was even a more marked pharmacologic advantage with ip TNF. The perfusate AUC was more than 4000-fold higher than plasma AUC for TNF (Fig. 11). Figure 12 shows the AUC of plasma cisplatin administered at various doses of TNF. There is a 1.6-fold higher plasma cisplatin AUC in the two patients who received 0.3 mg/L TNF, compared to seven patients receiving 0.1 mg/L TNF. There was a 2.5-fold higher plasma cisplatin AUC in the two patients receiving 0.3 mg/L, compared to the four patients receiving no TNF, but an equivalent dose of platinum.

Currently, two CHPP trials are being conducted in the Surgery Branch of the NCI. A phase II trial of neoadjuvant CHPP, using cisplatin and MMC for patients with high-risk resectable GCs, is being conducted. The primary end points of this treatment modality are to determine the feasibility of a neoadjuvant perfusion administered laparoscopically approx 2–3 wk prior to definitive resection, in patients with a disease process that has a known propensity for peritoneal dissemination. Once the feasibility of this treatment approach can be demonstrated, further components of therapy may be added, in order to intensify the ip therapy. A second trial for patients with established peritoneal carcinomatosis has been initiated to determine the feasibility and safe maximum-tolerated doses of 5-FU and paclitaxel administered via an ip dwell, following laparotomy tumor debulking and CHPP with cisplatin.

One subset of patients, who appear to have benefitted from a strategy of aggressive

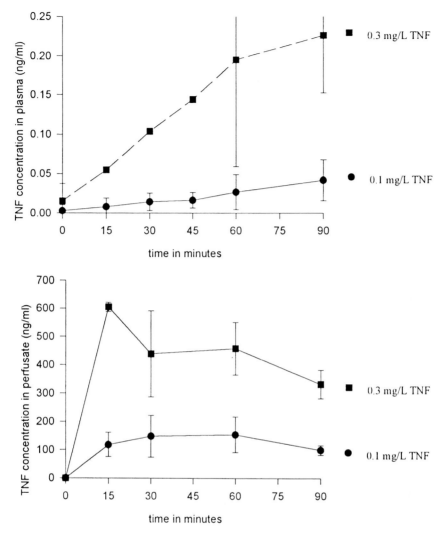

Fig. 11. Plasma (top) and perfusate (bottom) concentrations of TNF by dose in patients undergoing a 90-min hyperthermic CHPP. Adapted with permission from *ref. 39.*

debulking and CHPP, are those with malignant primary peritoneal mesothelioma. Sixteen patients have undergone 17 CHPPs with biopsy-proven primary peritoneal mesothelioma. Fourteen patients have been treated with 150–400 mg/m² cisplatin alone, and three have been treated with 250 mg/m² cisplatin and 0.1–0.3 mg/L perfusate of TNF. Operations performed included omentectomy and debulking in 15, splenectomy and omentectomy in one, and a small bowel resection with debulking in one. The median perfusate volume in these patients was 6 L, and median ip temperature was 41°C (range 39.5–43°C). In this cohort, there was no operative or treatment-related mortality. With a median potential of 20 mo (range 2–45), three patients are dead of disease, three are alive with disease at 16, 24, and 34 mo after treatment, and 10 are free of disease, with a median duration of progression-free survival of 16 mo (range 8–24 mo). Thirteen patients had symptomatic ascites prior to treatment, of which 11 (85%) have had complete palliation following CHPP (Fig. 13).

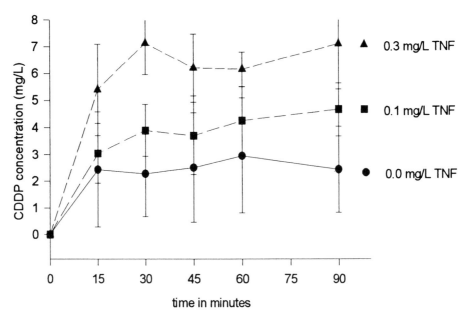

Fig. 12. Total plasma cisplatin concentrations over time by TNF dose in patients undergoing CHPP. Adapted with permission from *ref. 39.*

15 year old female with refractory Malignant Mesothelioma

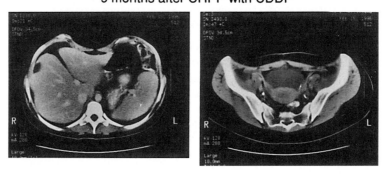

9 months after CHPP with CDDP

Fig. 13. CT scans of a 15-yr-old female with refractory malignant peritoneal mesothelioma, who had previously been treated with systemic chemotherapy before (top panels) and 9 mo after (bottom panels) CHPP with cisplatin. The patient remains radiographically and clinically free of disease 2.5 yr after treatment.

3.5. Summary

Aggressive surgical debulking, combined with CHPP, using agents at the safe MMDs was determined in phase I studies, demonstrating that there is no significant regional or systemic toxicity. The procedure can be performed in conjunction with major operative procedures, with no apparent increase in perioperative morbidity. These data indicate that CHPP with platinum may represent an effective means of palliating malignant ascites and improving the outlook, particularly for patients with malignant peritoneal mesothelioma. Its role in the treatment of peritoneal carcinomatosis from other histologies, including the GI tract, is under continued evaluation.

REFERENCES

1. Dedrick RL. Theoretical and experimental bases of intraperitoneal chemotherapy, *Semin. Oncol.,* **12** (1985) 1–6.
2. Markman M. Intraperitoneal 'Belly Bath' chemotherapy, In T. Lokich (ed), *Cancer Chemotherapy by Infusion,* 1990, pp. 552–574.
3. Alexander HR, Bartlett DL, Fraker DL, and Libutti SK. Regional treatment strategies for unresectable primary or metastatic cancer confined to the liver, PPO Updates, Lippincott, Philadelphia, **10** (1996) 1–19.
4. Ausman RK. Development of a technic for isolated perfusion of the liver, *NY State J. Med.,* **61** (1961) 3393–3397.
5. Aigner KR, Walther H, Tonn JC, Link KH, Schoch P, and Schwemmle K. Die isolierte leberperfusion bei fortgeschrittenen metastasen kolorektaler karzinome, *Onkologie,* **7** (1984) 13–21.
6. Aigner K, Walther H, Tonn J, et al. First experimental and clinical results of isolated liver perfusion with cytotoxics in metastases from colorectal primary, *Recent Results Cancer Res.,* **86** (1983) 99–102.
7. Skibba JL and Quebbeman EJ. Tumoricidal effects and patient survival after hyperthermic liver perfusion, *Arch. Surg.,* **121** (1986) 1266–1271.
8. Skibba JL, Quebbeman EJ, Komorowski RA, and Thorsen KM. Clinical results of hyperthermic liver perfusion for cancer in the liver, In KR Aigner, et al. (eds), *Regional Cancer Treatment,* Karger, Basel, 1988, pp. 222–228.
9. Schwemmle K, Link KH, and Rieck B. Rationale and indications for perfusion in liver tumors: current data, *World J. Surg.,* **11** (1987) 534–540.
9a. Hafström LR, Holmberg SB, Naredi PJ, et al. Isolated hyperthermic liver perfusion with chemotherapy for liver malignancy, *Surg. Oncol.,* **3** (1994) 103–108.
10. Marinelli A, de Brauw LM, Beerman H, et al. Isolated liver perfusion with mitomycin C in the treatment of colorectal cancer metastases confined to the liver, *Jpn. J. Clin. Oncol.,* **26** (1996) 341–350.
11. van Zuidewign DBW, de Brauw LM, Marinelli A, Keijzer HJ, van Bockel JH, and Van de Velde CJH. Isolated liver perfusion with mitomycin-C or melphalan in patients with hepatic metastases, *Soc. Surg. Oncol.,* **46** (1993) 198 (Abstract).
12. Dudar TE and Jain RK. Differential response of normal and tumor microcirculation to hyperthermia, *Cancer Res.,* **44** (1984) 605–612.
13. Cavaliere R, Ciogatto EC, Giovanelli BC, et al. Selective heat sensitivity of cancer cells, *Cancer,* **20** (1967) 1351–1387.
14. Buell JF, Reed E, Lee KB, et al. Synergistic effect and possible mechanisms of tumor necrosis factor and cisplatin cytotoxicity under moderate hyperthermia against gastric cancer cells, *Ann. Surg. Oncol.,* **4** (1997) 141–148.
15. Klostergaard J, Leroux E, Siddik ZH, Khodadadian M, and Tomasovic SP. Enhanced sensitivity of human colon tumor cell lines *in vitro* in response to thermochemoimmunotherapy, *Cancer Res.,* **52** (1992) 5271–5277.
16. Lienard D, Ewalenko P, Delmotte JJ, Renard N, and Lejeune FJ. High-dose recombinant tumor necrosis factor alpha in combination with interferon gamma and melphalan in isolation perfusion of the limbs for melanoma and sarcoma, *J. Clin. Oncol.,* **10** (1992) 52–60.
17. Alexander HR, Fraker DL, and Bartlett DL. Isolated limb perfusion for malignant melanoma, *Semin. Surg. Oncol.,* **12** (1996) 416–428.
18. Fraker DL, Alexander HR, Andrich M, and Rosenberg SA. Treatment of patients with melanoma of

the extremity using hyperthermic isolated limb perfusion with melphalan, tumor necrosis factor, and interferon-gamma: results of a TNF dose escalation study, *J. Clin. Oncol.,* **14** (1996) 479–489.

19. Eggermont AMM, Koops HS, Klausner JM, et al. Isolated limb perfusion with tumor necrosis factor and melphalan for limb salvage in 186 patients with locally advanced soft tissue extremity sarcomas, *Ann. Surg.,* **224** (1996) 756–765.
20. Diebel LN, Wilson RF, Bender J, and Paules B. Comparison of passive and active shunting for bypass of the retrohepatic IVC, *J. Trauma,* **31** (1991) 987–990.
21. Barker WC, Andrich MP, Alexander HR, and Fraker DL. Continuous intraoperative external monitoring of perfusate leak using I-131 human serum albumin during isolated perfusion of the liver and limbs, *Eur. J. Nucl. Med.,* **22** (1995) 1242–1248.
22. Fraker DL, Alexander HR, Bartlett DL, and Rosenberg SA. Prospective randomized trial of therapeutic isolated limb perfusion (ILP) comparing melphalan (M) versus melphalan, tumor necrosis factor (TNF) and interferon-gamma (IFN): an initial report, *Soc. Surg. Oncol.,* **49** (1996) 6, (Abstract).
23. Posner MC, Lienard D, Lejeune FJ, Rosenfelder D, and Kirkwood J. Hyperthermic isolated limb perfusion with tumor necrosis factor alone for melanoma, *Cancer J. Sci. Am.,* **1** (1995) 274–280.
24. Leyvraz S, Spataro V, Bauer J, et al. Treatment of ocular melanoma metastatic to the liver by hepatic arterial chemotherapy, *J. Clin. Oncol.,* **15** (1997) 2589–2595.
25. Alexander HR, Buell JF, and Fraker DL. Rationale and clinical status of continuous hyperthermic peritoneal perfusion for the treatment of peritoneal carcinomatosis, In DeVita VT Jr, Hellman S, and Rosenberg SA (eds), *Principles and Practice of Oncology: PPO updates.* Lippincott, Philadelphia, 1995, pp. 1–9.
26. Spratt JS, Adcock RA, Muskovin M, Sherrill W, and McKeown J. Clinical delivery system for intraperitoneal hyperthermic chemotherapy, *Cancer Res.,* **40** (1980) 256–260.
27. Koga S, Hamazoe R, Maeta M, Shimizu N, Murakami A, and Wakatsuki T. Prophylactic therapy for peritoneal recurrence of gastric cancer by continuous hyperthermic peritoneal perfusion with mitomycin C, *Cancer,* **61** (1988) 232–237.
28. Fujimoto S, Shrestha RD, Kokuban M, et al. Positive results of combined therapy of surgery and intraperitoneal hyperthermic perfusion for far-advanced gastric cancer, *Ann. Surg.,* **212** (1990) 592–596.
29. Fujimura T, Yonemura Y, Fushida S, et al. Continuous hyperthermic peritoneal perfusion for the treatment of peritoneal dissemination in gastric cancers and subsequent second-look operation, *Cancer,* **65** (1990) 65–71.
30. Fujimura T, Yonemura Y, Muraoka K, et al. Continuous hyperthermic peritoneal perfusion for the prevention of peritoneal recurrence of gastric cancer: randomized controlled study, *World J. Surg.,* **18** (1994) 150–155.
31. Hamazoe R, Maeta M, and Kaibara N. Intraperitoneal thermochemotherapy for prevention of peritoneal recurrence of gastric cancer, *Cancer,* **73** (1994) 2048–2052.
32. Fujimoto S, Shrestha RD, Kokubun M, et al. Pharmacokinetic analysis of mitomycin C for intraperitoneal hyperthermic perfusion in patients with far-advanced or recurrent gastric cancer, *Reg. Cancer Treat.,* **2** (1989) 198–202.
33. Gilly FN, Carry PY, Sayag AC, et al. Regional chemotherapy (with mitomycin C) and intraoperative hyperthermia for digestive cancers with peritoneal carcinomatosis, *Hepato-gastroenterology,* **41** (1994) 124–129.
34. Dikhoff T, van der Heider J, Dubbelman R, and ten Bokkel Huinink WW. Tissue concentration of platinum after intraperitoneal cisplatin administration in patients, *Proc. AACR,* **26** (1985) 162.
35. Howell SB, Pfeifle CG, Wung WE, et al. Intraperitoneal cisplatin with systemic thiosulfate protection, *Ann. Intern. Med.,* **97** (1982) 845–851.
36. Flessner MF and Dedrick RL. Intraperitoneal chemotherapy, In Gokal R and Nolph KD (eds), *Textbook of Peritoneal Dialysis.* Kluwer, The Netherlands, 1994, pp. 769–789.
37. Kitamura K, Kuwano H, Matsuda H, Toh Y, Masuda H, and Sugimachi K. Synergistic effects of intratumor administration of cis-diamminedichloroplatinum(II) combined with local hyperthermia in melanoma bearing mice, *J. Surg. Oncol.,* **51** (1992) 188–194.
38. Alexander HR, Bartlett DL, and Libutti SK. Isolated hepatic perfusion: A potentially effective treatment for patients with metastatic or primary cancers confined to the liver, *Cancer J. Sci. Amer.,* 4 (1998) 2–11.
39. Bartlett DL, Buell JF, Libutti SK, et al. A phase I trial of continuous hyperthermic peritoneal perfusion with tumor necrosis factor and cisplatin in the treatment of peritoneal carcinomatosis, *Cancer,* **83** (1998) 1251–1261.

9 Surgical Considerations in Intraperitoneal Chemotherapy

Donald W. Wiper and Alexander W. Kennedy

CONTENTS

INTRODUCTION AND HISTORICAL PERSPECTIVE
PATIENT SELECTION AND TIMING OF CATHETER PLACEMENT
INSERTION TECHNIQUES
CATHETER CHOICES
COST ANALYSIS
CATHETER USE AND MAINTENANCE
COMPLICATIONS
SUMMARY
REFERENCES

1. INTRODUCTION AND HISTORICAL PERSPECTIVE

Carcinoma of the ovary and peritoneum typically spreads in a diffuse, intra-abdominal fashion, often limited to the peritoneal cavity, and not metastasizing via hematogenous or lymphatic routes. The development of intraperitoneal (ip) chemotherapy sought to deliver extraordinarily high concentrations of cytotoxic agents into the peritoneal cavity, to take advantage of ovarian cancer remaining confined to the peritoneal cavity during much of its natural history. The pharmacokinetics and pharmacodynamics of ip therapy, first studied by Dedrick and Myers *(1)* working at the National Cancer Institute (NCI) in the 1970s, have been well studied by a number of other investigators *(2–8)*, and it is clear that high ip concentrations of many chemotherapeutic agents can be obtained. In addition, numerous authors *(9–15)* have demonstrated effective tumoricidal activity using ip therapy, particularly in the setting of superficially invasive, small-volume disease. Table 1 summarizes the current clinical situations in which ip therapy may be considered *(10)*.

Given the numerous clinical settings in which ip therapy may be appropriate, the logistics of safe ip access, drug delivery, and patient selection are of prime consideration.

2. PATIENT SELECTION AND TIMING OF CATHETER PLACEMENT

The ideal candidate for ip therapy has small-volume disease, is a low-risk surgical candidate for catheter placement, and has had no prior surgeries or radiation. Many

From: *Current Clinical Oncology: Regional Chemotherapy: Clinical Research and Practice*
Edited by: M. Markman © Humana Press Inc., Totowa, NJ

Table 1
Clinical Situations in Which IP Therapy May Be Considered

1. Small-volume residual disease (microscopic disease or largest remaining tumor <0.5cm) following initial systemic therapy.
2. Initial treatment of patients with high-grade, low-volume stage I–II cancers.
3. Consolidation treatment for high-grade, stage III–IV cancers that have had a surgically defined complete response or microscopically positive residual disease.
4. Initial therapy of selected advanced cancers, e.g., optimally debulked stage III with combination iv therapy.
5. Initial treatment of advanced disease after a limited number (≤3) of courses of systemic therapy, i.e., chemical debulking via iv route, followed by IP.

patients, however, have more challenging clinical situations, such as obesity, prior radiotherapy, and multiple prior abdominal surgeries, many with bowel resections and anastomoses. IP therapy may be inappropriate in these patients, because safety must be a prime concern. Additionally, ip therapy may not be practical in these patients: ip distribution of dialysate is often asymmetric, and thus treatment efficacy is compromised in patients with intra-abdominal adhesions. Nonetheless, many patients have some of these risk factors, and may still be candidates for ip therapy. The literature does not provide clear data on patient selection or timing of catheter insertion. Jenkins et al. *(16)* commented on less-consistent catheter function when placed at the time of laparotomy, because of the formation of adhesions, fibrin clots, and subsequent catheter obstruction. However, this problem was not common: In their report on 78 Tenckhoff (Quinton Instruments, Seattle, WA) catheters, only two developed inflow obstruction. Davidson, et al. *(17)* reported that the risk of complications was unrelated to the timing of catheter placement, i.e., at the time of laparotomy or in a separate procedure. Their analysis did indicate, however, a clear trend toward increased catheter complication if bowel surgery was performed concomitantly with catheter placement, or if subsequent bowel surgery was performed in patients with catheters *in situ*. In total, catheter-related infections occurred in 4% of small bowel procedures, 16% of large bowel procedures, and 15% of appendectomies. Although not statistically significant, because of small sample size, these rates are 2–3× those reported in noncontaminated cases, and certainly warrant consideration. Braly et al. *(18)* did not report any infectious complications in their small group of patients (*n* = 6), who had concomitant catheter placement and bowel surgeries. However, one patient developed a sigmoid colon perforation, with an intraluminal catheter tip found on laparotomy. Davidson et al. *(17)*, on the basis of their own findings, recommend delayed catheter placement for several weeks, in cases of large bowel entry. The authors follow a similar policy at this institution. They also recommend radiographic studies in any cases of suspected bowel perforation, profuse diarrhea immediately following initiation of ip infusion, or with problematic flow. This problem-oriented use of dye studies is also in agreement with the authors' approach to catheter management. One study by Smith et al. *(19)* assessed the risk of bowel perforation by number of prior laparotomies. These authors were inserting single-use, No. 5 French central venous catheters at bedside, with local anesthesia and no radiographic or ultrasound guidance, in 25 patients to be treated with ^{32}P. In 11 patients with one prior laparotomy each, one large bowel perforation was documented (9%). Nine patients had successful catheter placement on the first attempt, and a total of 14 attempts were made. In 14 patients with two or more prior laparotomies, four small bowel perforations were documented (29%). Nine patients had successful catheter placement on the first attempt, and a total of 29 attempts were made. Although limited by small numbers, this study underscores the risk of blind, percutaneous catheter placement in patients with prior abdominal surgeries.

The selection of patients for ip therapy must be done carefully, and the timing of catheter insertion should be thoughtfully considered. In uncomplicated, clean cases, catheters may be inserted at the time of initial laparotomy, or in a later, limited procedure. It seems clear that catheter insertion, combined with simultaneous or subsequent bowel surgery, adds additional risk for eventual catheter failure.

3. INSERTION TECHNIQUES

Given the demonstrated efficacy of ip therapy in certain settings, the development of safe, tolerable, ip delivery systems has been of prime practical consideration. Three basic approaches are in use: single-use percutaneous catheter, transcutaneous semipermanent catheter, and implanted semipermanent catheter with indwelling portal. Despite the development and widespread use of semipermanent trans- or subcutaneous (sc) delivery systems, there remains support for single-use-only paracentesis technique, usually using a peritoneal dialysis catheter, which is placed just prior to each chemotherapy course. Runowicz et al. (20) and Morales (21) both advocate this approach, and have reported markedly lower complication rates. Runowicz et al. studied 28 patients, using 12 Tenckhoff catheters and 21 No. 5 French central venous catheters, or No. 11 French peritoneal catheters. Tenckhoff catheters were placed at the time of laparotomy. The single-use catheters were placed percutaneously, under local anesthesia, without ultrasound guidance. Some patients required multiple attempts to establish adequate inflow. This exact number was not stated. The authors reported complications in 67% of patients with Tenckhoff catheters during the course of therapy, compared with 19% using single-use catheters. This lower rate was reduced to just 3.8%, when the number of insertions, not patients, was used as the denominator. Each patient had an average of five percutaneous treatments, and no bowel perforations were clinically evident in either the percutaneous or transcutaneous techniques. In this small series, among patients in whom a Tenckhoff catheter was used ($n = 12$), half required removal because of peritonitis, hematoma, abscess, and tumor progression. Despite the small sample size and lack of statistical significance, this trend guided the authors to exclusively employ the percutaneous method. Other authors have not reported such high complication rates with the Tenckhoff catheter (16–18). A clear disadvantage of the single-use method is the unquantifiable toll it may take on patients: It is repetitive, painful, and, no doubt, anxiety-provoking. Also, as mentioned, Smith et al. (19) reported a 29% bowel perforation rate, using the percutaneous method in patients with two or more prior laparotomies. Nonetheless, in some settings, it may be preferable. Patient comfort and satisfaction were not specifically addressed in these reports, but must remain a priority for practitioners.

Review of the peritoneal dialysis literature reveals division of thought on this same issue. Rubin et al. (22,23) and Olcott et al. (24) reported that peritonitis is the major problem with the Tenckhoff catheter, citing rates of 18–56%. A countervailing concern was expressed by Leehey et al. (25), whose data concurred with Smith et al. (19), both of whom reported unacceptably high rates of abdominal viscous perforation with the single-use percutaneous approach. Leehey et al. concluded that indwelling systems, such as the Tenckhoff, were safer. The authors have generally opted for indwelling systems, for a number of reasons, including safety concerns raised in the literature, experience, and patient comfort.

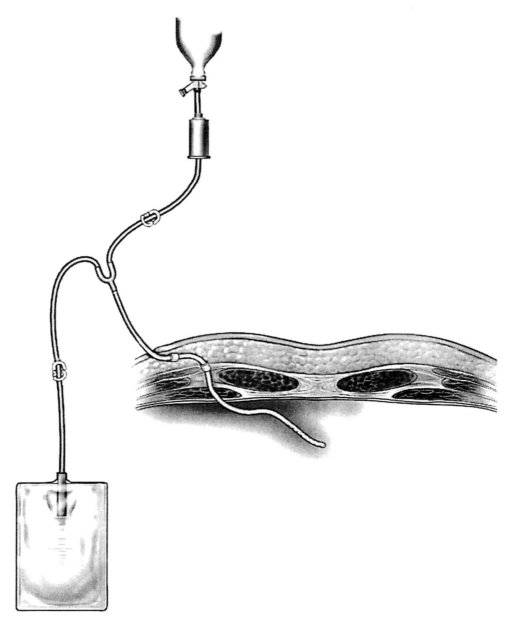

Fig. 1.

4. CATHETER CHOICES

There are several choices available for semipermanent catheters. Most experience has been obtained with the Tenckhoff system *(26,27)*. As seen in Fig. 1, this consists of a 42-cm-long, implanted catheter with a sc tunnel and exteriorized proximal end. The ip end is a curved tip, with 26 perfusion holes in the distal 12 cm. There are two dacron cuffs, one placed adjacent to the fascia and the other in midposition within a sc tunnel. These fibrose into place, which serves three functions: as a positional stabilizer; to help retard retrograde flow of ip fluid; and as an infection barrier. The separate peritoneal entry and skin exit sites via a sc tunnel also serve to reduce peritoneal

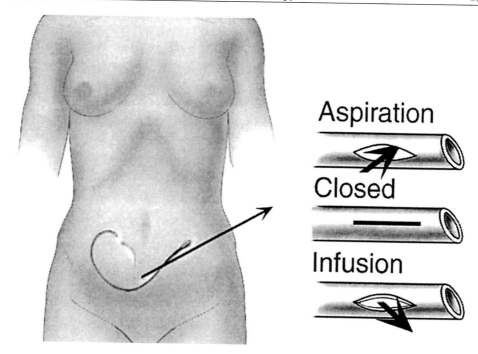

Fig. 2.

infection rates. Removal at the completion of therapy usually requires a minilaparotomy with adhesiolysis. In several patients with Tenckhoff catheters placed at the time of hysterectomy, the authors have encountered adherence of the catheter to the vaginal vault, with subsequent prompt flow of dialysate from the vagina, once ip use was attempted. This prompted several modifications: The 42-cm catheter may be shortened to 25–30 cm, so that it cannot reach the vaginal cuff; the catheter may also be sutured out of the pelvis, arcing from one pericolic gutter to another; last, if appropriate, the cervix may be left *in situ*.

A different modification of the Tenckhoff has been employed by Nguyen et al. *(28)*. In an attempt to reduce the incidence of inflow obstruction, and to improve distribution in obese patients, in whom much of the catheter length is consumed in traversing the abdominal wall, those authors increased the number of perfusion holes from 26 to 44 in the distal tip, and lengthened the catheter to 54 cm. The incidence of inflow obstruction, although showing a slightly less frequent trend, compared to historical controls using a standard Tenckhoff, was not statistically significant. The issue of dialysate distribution was not documented with any radiographic studies.

The Groshong catheter (R. Bard, Inc., Salt Lake City, UT) is similar to the Tenckhoff, as shown in Fig. 2. This catheter is 40-cm long, soft, silastic, and has a unique, pressure-sensitive, vocal-cord-type valve modification at the distal end. This design prevents fluid influx, and thus flushing is not required. The catheter is slightly thinner and more pliable than the Tenckhoff, and was initially designed for long-term iv access for chemotherapy, total parenteral nutrition, and antibiotics. In a combined series, Malviya et al. *(29)* and Delmore et al. *(30)* used the Groshong in 105 gynecologic oncology patients for iv access. All catheters were inserted and removed at bedside with minimal complications. This success prompted its use in ip chemotherapy, as first reported by Hrozencik and Ness in 1991 *(31)*. Groshong catheter use was further studied and

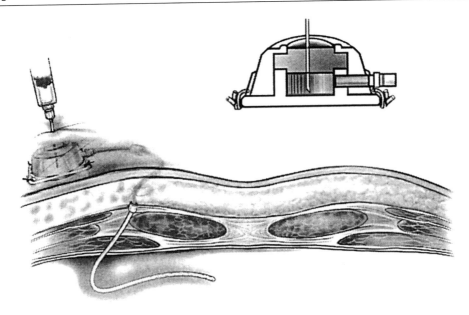

Fig. 3.

validated by Naumann et al. *(32)* in 1993 and Waggoner et al. *(33)* in 1994, who reported on their experience with a total of 47 Groshong catheters used for ip drug delivery. This externally accessed catheter is available with single or multiple lumens, in multiple calibers, and is straightforward to insert. The technique, as described by Waggoner, employs a 14-gage needle, placed through the abdominal wall into the peritoneal cavity at the conclusion of a laparotomy. A guidewire is then threaded through the needle, the needle is removed, and a dilator and tearaway sheath are inserted over the guidewire. The dilator is then removed, and the catheter is passed through the sheath, followed by sheath removal. The proximal catheter is tunneled subcutaneously to an exit site. Skin sutures are placed and removed 10–14 d later. Catheter removal is done at bedside.

The Port-a-Cath (Pharmacia, Frieburg, Germany) system is newer, and, as seen in Fig. 3, is an implantable version of the Tenckhoff system. The impetus to its design was to decrease the rate of exit site infections and catheter dislodgment seen with the Tenckhoff catheter, by not having an externally exposed component. Insertion can take place either at the time of exploratory laparotomy or as a separate, limited procedure, utilizing two small incisions: one over the lower anterior rib cage, just above the costal margin; and another lateral to the umbilicus, for ip placement of the catheter under direct visualization. The incision over the anterior rib cage is carried down to the fascia, and a pocket large enough to house the port is created bluntly within the sc space. The port is sutured to the fascia with four permanent sutures. Once the port is secured, a Tenckhoff catheter within the peritoneal cavity is tunneled through the sc tissues and attached to the port, which features a self-sealing membrane, as depicted in Fig. 4. Use of delayed absorbable sutures, to anchor the port to the fascia, is not advised. There are reports of such sutures having eventual inadequate adherence to the fascia, and ports then becoming mobile within the sc space, and being accessible only with fluoroscopic guidance. This has been a particular problem in obese patients, when the port is not easily located by palpation. In addition, ports may become completely inaccessible after flipping over 180 degrees, and having the access membrane facing

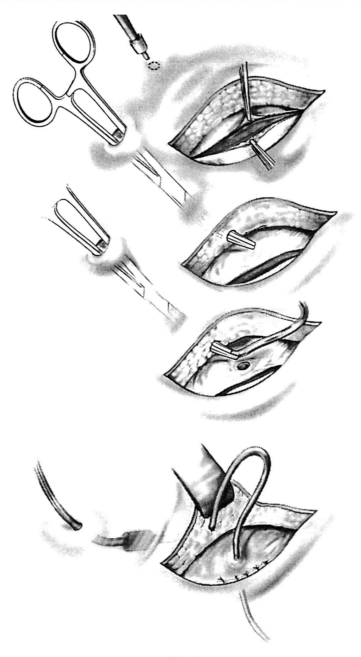

Fig. 4.

the fascia. However, provided that the port is in stable position, this system is accessed transcutaneously for each use. Experience with this system has shown three major advantages over exteriorized devices: There may be a slightly lower rate of intra-abdominal infection or peritonitis; once the immediate postoperative period is over, there are few maintenance demands; patient anxiety is less, and satisfaction is higher with the totally implanted system. The patient's daily activities are less encumbered, and the freedom from maintenance requirements of an external catheter are popular.

Table 2
Catheter Type

Catheter	Tenckhoff	Port-a-Cath	Groshong	
Expense	$80.50	$520.00	$80.50	
Other (total hospitalization, surgeon, anesthesia)	$2000–5000	$2000–5000	$2000–5000	
Total cost				
Low estimate	$2080.50	$2520.00	$2080.50	$2080.50
High estimate	$5080.50	$5520.00	$5080.50	$5050.00

There remain some clear advantages to the Tenckhoff or Groshong catheters. In some patients, the indwelling port feature of the Port-a-Cath, which rests just above the costal margin, can be bothersome as it rubs against clothing. The implanted system is more costly than the Groshong or Tenckhoff, and requires two surgical procedures for placement and removal. Some oncologists will remove the externalized catheters at bedside, and avoid a second operative procedure. The authors' experience with frequent adhesion formation from bowel and peritoneum to catheter has led to intraoperative removal of these catheters for safety and comfort reasons. Infusion times are shorter with the Tenckhoff catheter, because this system is not limited by flow into and out of a portal. Inflow obstruction and the one-way valve effect occur with equal frequency with the transcutaneous or Port-a-Cath systems, but troubleshooting is somewhat easier with an exteriorized component. High-pressure infusion may be performed, or a stylet may be introduced with extreme caution, in an attempt to dislodge fibrin clots, or to straighten a kinked catheter.

5. COST ANALYSIS

As seen in Table 2, most of the cost for catheter placement is in the hospital stay, and in surgeon and anesthesia fees. Although the Port-a-Cath is much more expensive than the nonimplanted systems, this difference is nearly irrelevant when total cost is viewed, and thus may not be a factor in choosing a catheter. The strongest argument for bedside, percutaneous placement of catheters prior to each ip delivery may be a financial one, because the cost in this setting is mostly for the catheter itself. However, as already noted, this technique has safety and satisfaction issues that must be considered over cost. As reported by Waggoner et al. *(33)*, some catheters placed at the time of initial laparotomy will subsequently not be used, because of protocol randomization to non-ip treatment arms or nonqualifying tumor types. However, this is rare, and, given that there are no currently ongoing Gynecologic Oncology Group protocols employing ip therapy, may not be relevant. In any event, if, at the time of laparotomy, it is reasonable to believe ip therapy is appropriate, it is prudent, from a cost standpoint, to insert the catheter simultaneously. The cost of unused catheters would be easily offset by the cost not incurred for separate catheter placements.

The choice of delivery system remains personal, to be mutually agreed upon by physician and patient. The complications of each system, though somewhat different, are comparable in frequency and severity. A system must be chosen for each patient individually. A comprehensive summary of published complications is shown in Table 3.

Table 3
Summary of Literature By Catheter Type and Number of Complications Reported (% of Trial)

Catheter type	Author, yr (ref.)	No. catheters	Skin infection	Peritonitis abscess	Hematoma bleeding	Viscous perforation	Inflow obstruction	Outflow obstruction	SBO ileus
Port-a-cath	Pfeifle et al., 1984 (44)	54	2	1	—[a]	0	3	—	—
	Piccart et al., 1985 (45)	145	0	12	0	2	3	67	0
	Braly et al., 1986 (46)	37	2	4	0	1	0	—	1
	Rubin et al., 1989 (23)	136	4	3	0	0	7	—	—
	Davidson et al., 1991 (17)	227	10	2	—	8	20	—	—
	Totals	599	18 (3.0)	22 (3.6)	0	11 (1.8)	33 (5.5)	67 (45)	1 (21.0)
Tenckhoff	Jenkins et al., 1982 (16)	78	3	3	—	3	2	—	—
	Myers 1983 (47)	71	0	3	6	2	3	—	—
	Braly et al., 1985 (46)	8	0	1	0	0	0	—	—
	Ozols 1985 (48)	78	3	3	0	3	0	—	—
	Piccart et al., 1985 (45)	143	9	8	18	5	6	63	7
	Runowicz et al., 1986 (20)	12	0	4	1	0	1	—	7
	Totals	390	15 (3.8)	22 (5.6)	25 (6.4)	13 (3.3)	12 (3.0)	63 (43)	7 (1.7)
Modified Tenckhoff	Nguyen et al., 1993 (28)	116	4 (3.4)	3 (2.5)	—	3 (2.5)	4 (3.4)	—	—
Groshong	Hrozenick and Ness, 1991 (31)	25	1	0	0	0	0	—	—
	Naumann et al., 1993 (32)	20	1	0	0	0	0	—	—
	Waggoner et al., 1994 (33)	27	1	0	0	0	0	—	—
	Totals	72	3 (4.2)	0 (0)	0 (0)	0 (0)	0 (0)	—	—
Single-Use	Runowicz et al., 1986 (20)	21	0	2	1	1	0	—	—
	Smith et al., 1994 (19)	25	0	1	—	5	—	—	—
	Totals	46	0	3 (6.5)	—	6 (13.0)	—	—	—

[a]Dash indicates not reported.

6. CATHETER USE AND MAINTENANCE

6.1. IP Fluid Distribution

Once a catheter is placed, the issues of function and maintenance become critical. Much attention has been devoted to radiographic studies used to document adequacy of ip fluid distribution. Dunnick et al. *(34)*, at the NCI, demonstrated that 2 L of fluid given intraperitoneally will be distributed evenly throughout the abdominal cavity in 90% of patients, despite the presence of extensive adhesions from prior laparotomies or bulky abdominal tumors. Radiologic evaluation of ip fluid distribution using such techniques as 25% Hypaque in 2 L of 1.5% Inpersol (Abbott, North Chicago, IL) and Dianeal (Travenol Labs., Deerfield, IL) followed by computed tomography (CT) scan, has been used intermittently in the past *(18,34)*. Other methods using radioisotopes, such as technicium 99, have been employed *(35,36)*. Rosenshein et al. *(37)*, working with primates, demonstrated that small volumes of infused fluid (50–200 mL) tend to pool in the peritoneum near the infusion site. Manual manipulation of subjects failed to redistribute the fluid, and uniform distribution was seen only when the volume of infused fluid was sufficient to distend the abdomen, which was approx 2000 mL. Braly et al. *(18)* routinely used CT scan and a 25% Hypaque infusion protocol in all postoperative catheter placements. These studies were repeated after four and eight courses of chemotherapy. In this study of 37 catheters, 67% of patients who underwent catheter placement without exploratory laparotomy had suboptimal ip fluid distribution. In those undergoing laparotomy, 35% had suboptimal distribution. This difference was explained by the authors as the opportunity to perform adhesiolysis in the laparotomy group. The Braly study also attempted to correlate adequacy of fluid distribution and response to therapy, and the authors reported a trend toward more complete or partial responders in those with diffuse dialysate distribution. This part of the study was problematic, and does not allow any conclusions. The sample sizes were small, the treatment groups included previously untreated patients with advanced disease, as well as those with recurrent disease, and the untreated group received iv therapy along with ip. Most of the responders were in the previously untreated group (7 of 9): This is more likely to reflect inherent tumor response to cytotoxic agents given both iv and ip, and not the intracavitary fluid distribution pattern. Notably, three of five patients with poor distribution on CT had partial or complete responses to therapy. Despite the limitations on these latter conclusions, it is widely accepted, by virtue of numerous studies and clinical experience, that a minimum volume of approx 2 L is required for adequate ip distribution. The usefulness of routine radiologic evaluation to document ip fluid distribution has been questioned by numerous authors *(16,17)*. As experience with ip infusions in this patient population has grown, many oncologists increasingly rely on clinical signs and symptoms to assess the adequacy of the infusion *(17)*. At the authors' institution, no routine studies are performed; instead, reliance is on clinical signs and symptoms that may be indicative of nonuniform infusion: asymmetric distention with localized pain, resistance to infusion, or gastrointestinal (GI) complaints. Use of radiographic studies is reserved for these more worrisome cases.

6.2. Catheter Maintenance

The Port-a-Cath, once inserted, and once the immediate issues of wound care and healing are finished, is essentially maintenance-free. With each use, the portal is accessed with strict sterile technique, using the Huber needle. The port and catheter are flushed with normal saline, to assure patency. Once the setup is secured, about 300 mL saline is infused, followed by the dose of chemotherapy. A fluid loculation at the catheter tip, or asymmetric distribution, is usually apparent with the initial 300 mL saline or initial volume of chemotherapy. Abdominal discomfort is common, and frequently narcotics are required during infusions. Clinical experience helps to distinguish the normal discomfort that accompanies ip infusions from the pain of asymmetric distribution associated with adhesions. The authors intermittently place patients in Trendelenberg, and have them roll from side to side to assist in fluid distribution. Once the chemotherapy is infused, the balance of saline (usually about 1 L) is infused. The port and catheter are then flushed with 20 mL saline, followed by 20 mL heparinized (5000 U) saline. No nursing or patient maintenance is required between courses of chemotherapy.

The Tenckhoff and Groshong catheters require daily maintenance and an able and cooperative patient. Recommendations have been adopted from the chronic ambulatory peritoneal dialysis (CAPD) experience, and, though labor-intensive, have yielded excellent results. Following catheter placement, a series of dialysis exchanges must be performed to assure catheter patency. Typically, 1 L 1.5% Dianeal or Inpersol, plus 500 U heparin, are infused repeatedly, until fluid returns are clear of blood. Next, in efforts to evaluate capacity and patient tolerance for future treatments, dialysate volumes are progressively increased to 2 L, which, as mentioned above, is considered to be a minimum volume for uniform ip distribution. A typical regimen is 1 L exchanges every 6 h × 4, 1.5 L every 12 h × 2, then 2 L every 24 h until discharge. During this time, intensive patient and family education must take place for home catheter care. Instructions given patients *(49)* are similar to those given the CAPD patients:

1. Complete healing and stabilization of the catheter requires 4–6 wk.
2. Following placement, the exit site must be kept covered for 1 wk.
3. The catheter must be kept taped to the abdominal wall at all times.
4. Counterpressure should be applied with a pillow, when coughing, to protect the incision line.
5. Avoid constipation. Straining puts pressure on the newly placed catheter, and can cause leaks. Eat foods high in bulk, such as fruits and bran. Laxatives may be used.
6. Following placement, patients may not shower, take a tub bath, or swim for 6 wk.
7. Patients are asked to return for weekly irrigation.
8. Following placement, no lifting in excess of 25 lb.
9. Chronic exit-site care includes daily dressing changes, washing exit site with antibacterial soap and replacement of anchoring tape.
10. Additional precautions include covering the catheter while in the shower, to prevent water from accessing the catheter; cleaning the shower head after each shower with disinfectant spray; no bathing in a bathtub, to avoid dirty, stagnant water; and swimming only in chlorinated, private pools.

(Ohio Renal Care Group, Home Dialysis Instructions, CCF, *ref. 49.*)

6.3. Dialysate Considerations

Once ip chemotherapy commences, a number of decisions must be made regarding infusion dialysates. These vehicles for distribution vary regarding ion composition, pH, and osmolality, and selection depends on choice of cytotoxic agent to be delivered.

Lessons learned from the CAPD experience have shown that the dialysate composition and number of exchanges can have a significant impact on serum electrolytes. Hypokalemia is a common problem with prolonged exchanges; dialysates typically contain 4 mEq/L KCl, to prevent gradient-induced serum losses to the peritoneal fluid.

Fortunately, in the usual single exchange of ip chemotherapy, potassium losses are negligible *(38)*. Patients receiving cisplatin often have a baseline hypomagnesemia. As with potassium, gradient-driven losses into the dialysate within the peritoneum can lower magnesium levels even further, to a symptomatic range *(38)*. Plasma equivalent concentrations of magnesium should be added to dialysates to avoid this problem. An additional consideration is the avoidance of excessive fluid absorption from the peritoneal cavity. This issue is of more urgent concern in patients with chronic renal failure, but many oncology patients have less than optimal fluid balance, with marginal cardiac and pulmonary function, and cannot easily accommodate additional intravascular fluid volumes. In efforts to equilibrate the osmotic pressure of the dialysate and the hydrostatic pressure of the peritoneal fluid, it has become common to add 1.5% glucose to the dialysis fluid. At higher glucose concentrations, there is bulk flow of fluid from tissues into the peritoneal cavity. Conversely, dialysate composed of normal saline alone favors flow into tissues. This theoretically could aid in drug delivery and tissue/tumor penetration, but a clinical benefit to this strategy has not been shown.

Dialysate pH is another consideration with a number of drugs, such as 5-FU, which are poorly soluble at physiologic pH. The choice of acid or alkaline dialysates must be tailored to each chemotherapeutic agent.

7. COMPLICATIONS

7.1. Mechanical Obstruction

Table 3 summarizes the published data on ip therapy complications by catheter type and author (previously referenced, plus *44–46*). The types of complications can generally be grouped as mechanical malfunction, infectious, and GI. The most common problem, which is innocuous for the most part, is mechanical outflow obstruction, i.e., drainage from the peritoneal cavity to the exterior. This is typically caused by the well-described valve effect on the catheter tip, probably secondary to fibrin deposition. Fortunately, drainage of chemotherapeutic dialysate after a given dwell time is not usually necessary, and most protocols leave instilled fluids within the cavity to be resorbed over time.

Another potential use of the catheter as a drainage device is in the removal of ascites, but the merits of this practice continue to be debated, and loss of this capability with indwelling catheters is of secondary concern. Inflow obstruction is a less frequent problem with the cumulative incidence rates seen in Table 3. A summary of the literature reporting on 599 Port-a-Cath catheters reveals an incidence of 5.5%. This compares to a 3% incidence on reports of 390 Tenckhoff catheters. This difference is small, but statistically significant. The comparatively small published experience with 72 Groshong catheters revealed no inflow obstructions. Maneuvers to correct inflow obstructions may be performed. These can often be overcome by high-pressure infusion of saline, or cautious stylet placement. Davidson et al. *(17)* reported on 15 cases of inflow obstruction. Twelve of these were caused by distal fibrin deposition, two by intraluminal catheter obstruction, and one by implanted port rotation, which prevented access. Eleven attempted surgical corrections were performed, either by lysis of adhesions or catheter replacement. Eight of 11 patients went on to have uncomplicated ip therapy. The authors noted that surgical success seemed more likely, if the adhesions were localized to the catheter tip, and not to a diffuse intra-abdominal process. There is no evidence that choice of chemotherapy can modify the incidence of obstruction.

7.2. Infectious Complications

Catheter-associated infections remain the most problematic complication, and the main reason for catheter removal. As can be seen in Table 3, when total experience is evaluated, rather than single author reports, there is no clear advantage to any one system in avoiding infectious morbidity. The cumulative data show equivalent rates of cutaneous infection for all systems, with each total in the 3–4% range. There was a slightly lower rate of peritonitis or abscess formation in the Port-a-Cath group, with a total incidence of 3.6% in 599 catheters used, compared to a rate of 5.6% in 390 Tenckhoff catheters. As with the inflow obstruction data, this difference is small, but statistically significant. The data on the Groshong catheter, although demonstrating no intra-abdominal infections, must be interpreted with caution, because the sample size is quite small, compared to the experience with the Tenckhoff and Port-a-Cath. Similar caution must be used in interpreting the single-use catheter data, with only 46 patients reported. Among these, there were no cutaneous infections, but 6.5% intra-abdominal infections. One prospective, randomized study by Mueller et al. *(39)* demonstrated equivalent cutaneous and intra-abdominal infectious complication rates with sc and transcutaneous devices.

One trend, mentioned previously and noted by a number of authors *(17,40,41)*, and supported by experimental data *(42)*, reveals that catheter placement, coinciding with or preceding subsequent bowel resections, significantly raises infectious morbidity and eventual catheter failure. The baseline infection rate, either exit site or peritonitis, ranges from 2 to 6%, but this risk increases to 9–23% when the bowel is entered.

7.3. Management of Catheter Infections

Infectious peritonitis complicating continuous ambulatory peritoneal dialysis has been well studied, but considerably less is published on infectious morbidity in ip chemotherapy populations. Kaplan et al. *(43)* provided considerable insight into this problem. They reported on 32 episodes of infectious peritonitis that developed in 90 patients receiving ip chemotherapy. *Staphylococcus epidermidis* accounted for 66% of cultured organisms, followed by *S. aureus*, 17%, and *S. viridans*, 9%. Physical findings were varied: 63% demonstrated fever; 69% had either abdominal pain or tenderness. Peritoneal fluid Gram stains were positive in just 35% of peritonitis cases. White blood cell counts rose from 5400/mm^3 preinfection to 7300/mm^3—a significant, but small difference.

The treatment for catheter-related infections included iv and occasionally ip antibiotics. Cefazolin was most commonly used, 1 g iv every 6 h, and 125–250 mg/L every 6 h ip. 74% of cases were cleared of infection; 26% failed to clear. The indications for catheter removal were summarized as a persistently positive peritoneal fluid culture, an exit-site tunnel infection, recurrent infections with the same organism in less than 4 wk, and failed clinical improvement. Kaplan et al.'s study *(43)* failed to reveal improved outcome in those receiving ip and iv antibiotics, compared to iv alone. There was also no advantage to multiagent antibiotic regimens in the small number studied. The duration of treatment, provided there is prompt clinical improvement and negative peritoneal cultures, should be 10–14 d, the first seven iv. If a catheter is removed, and then replaced once infection is cleared, the recurrent complication rate, either as another infection or flow obstruction, ranges from 36 to 50% *(17)*. The authors' management policy at the Cleveland Clinic includes prompt removal in the setting of suspected sepsis or obviously ill patient. In less worrisome situations, a course of both iv and ip antibiotics is attempted, to salvage the catheter. Indications for removal are similar to those published by Kaplan.

7.4. GI Complications

GI complications are the last source of major morbidity. The incidence of bowel perforation was consistently low, ranging from 1.8% with the Port-a-Cath to 3.3% with the Tenckhoff. Whether this slightly higher rate of perforation correlates with the higher intra-abdominal infection rate is unknown. The data on 46 patients receiving therapy by single-use technique insertions revealed a total bowel perforation incidence of 13%. This rate jumped to 28% when single-use catheters were placed in patients with multiple previous laparotomies.

Perforations may be noted early, at the time of insertion, documented by the withdrawal of feculent material, or by profuse diarrhea with the instillation of dialysate. Perforations may also occur in a delayed or late time-frame, from weeks to many months after insertion. As described by Davidson et al. *(17)* these perforations present with evidence of catheter infection such as a purulent exit site, and signs and symptoms of peritonitis. Davidson et al. *(17)* reported on eight such patients: Three were asymptomatic and diagnosed on reassessment laparotomy; the five with symptoms presented with a range of findings: a colocutaneous fistula, purulent port site, fever and abdominal pain, feculent material in the catheter aspirate, leakage from a port incision at the time of catheter use, and profuse watery diarrhea immediately following chemotherapy infusion. The authors have mentioned experience with several patients with catheter–vaginal fistulae. The risk of this with the unmodified catheter is less than 1%.

As mentioned earlier, in addition to bowel perforation, wandering catheters may also erode through the vaginal cuff, evidence of which is promptly noted with catheter usage. A few authors *(45,46)* have commented on the incidence of ileus or partial small bowel obstruction, but there is too little data to draw conclusions regarding this. In addition, this nonspecific diagnosis encompasses many complaints of patients with intra-abdominal cancer who are receiving toxic chemotherapy, and the catheters may be wrongly blamed for symptoms that are part of the natural history of these diseases.

8. SUMMARY

The role of ip chemotherapy continues to be defined. Over the past 15 yr, it has become evident that common to any strategy employing ip therapy must be the requirement of small-volume disease. Bulky disease, requiring deep tissue penetration, is a clear limitation on the ip modality. Numerous options for administration of ip therapy exist, and extensive analysis reveals that no one system is superior to another. Multiple technological advances allow ip chemotherapy to be administered to most patients in a safe and acceptable fashion.

REFERENCES

1. Dedrick RL, Myers CE, Bungay PM, et al. Pharmacokinetic rationale for peritoneal drug administration in the treatment of ovarian cancer, *Cancer Treat. Rep.*, **62** (1978) 1–11.
2. Speyer JL, Collins JM, Dedrick RL, et al. Phase I pharmacological studies of 5-fluorouracil administered intraperitoneally, *Cancer Res.*, **40** (1980) 567–572.
3. Ozols RF, Young RC, Speyer JL, et al. Phase 1 and pharmacological studies of adriamycin administered intraperitoneally to patients with ovarian cancer, *Cancer Res.*, **42** (1982) 4265–4269.

4. Ozols RF, Corden BJ, Jacob J, et al. High-dose cisplatin in hypertonic saline, *Ann. Intern. Med.*, **100** (1984) 19–24.

5. Howell SB, Chu BCF, Wung WE, et al. Long-duration intracavitary infusion of methotrexate with systemic leucovorin protection in patients with malignant effusion, *J. Clin. Invest.*, **67** (1981) 1161–1170.

6. Casper ES, Kelsen DP, Alcock NW, et al. Ip cisplatin in patients with malignant ascites: pharmacokinetic evaluation and comparison with the iv route, *Cancer Treat. Rep.*, **67** (1983) 325–328.

7. Jones RB, Collins JM, Myers CE, et al. High-volume intraperitoneal chemotherapy with methotrexate in patients with cancer, *Cancer Res.*, **41** (1981) 55–59.

8. Alberts DS, Young L, Mason N, et al. In vitro evaluation of anticancer drugs against ovarian cancer at concentrations achievable by intraperitoneal administration, *Semin. Oncol.*, **12(suppl 4)** 38–42.

9. Markman M. Intraperitoneal antineoplastic agents for tumors principally confined to the peritoneal cavity, *Cancer Treat. Rev.*, **13** (1986) 219–242.

10. Markman M. Intraperitoneal chemotherapy, In *Cancer of the Ovary*, Markman M, and Hoskins WJ (eds), Raven, New York, 1993.

11. Los G, Mutsaers PHA, van der Vijgh, et al. Direct diffusion of cis-platinum in intraperitoneal rat tumors after intraperitoneal chemotherapy: a comparison with systemic chemotherapy, *Cancer Res.*, **49** (1989) 3380–3384.

12. Los G, Verdegaal EME, Mutsaers PHA, et al. Penetration of carboplatin and cisplatin into rat peritoneal tumor nodules after intraperitoneal chemotherapy, *Cancer Chemother. Pharmacol.*, **28** (1991) 159–165.

13. Reichman B, Markman M, Hakes T, et al. Intraperitoneal cisplatin and etoposide in the treatment of refractory/recurrent ovarian carcinoma, *J. Clin. Oncol.*, **7** (1989) 1327–1332.

14. Alberts DS, Liu PY, Hannigan EV, et al. Phase III study of intraperitoneal cisplatin/intravenous cyclophosphamide vs. IV cisplatin/IV cyclophosphamide in patients with optimal disease stage III ovarian cancer: a SWOG-GOG-ECOG intergroup study, *Proc. Am. Soc. Clin. Oncol.*, **14** (1995) 273.

15. Levin L and Hryniuk WM. Dose-intensity analysis of chemotherapy regimens in ovarian carcinoma, *J. Clin. Oncol.*, **5** (1987) 756–767.

16. Jenkins J, Sugarbaker PH, Gianola FJ, et al. Technical considerations in the use of intraperitoneal chemotherapy administered by Tenckhoff catheter, *Surg. Gynecol. Obstet.*, **154** (1982) 858–864.

17. Davidson SD, Rubin SC, Markman M, et al. Intraperitoneal chemotherapy: analysis of complications with an implanted subcutaneous port and catheter system, *Gynecol. Oncol.*, **41** (1991) 101–106.

18. Braly P, Doroshow J, and Hoff S. Technical aspects of intraperitoneal chemotherapy: introduction of a new "single use" delivery system: A preliminary report, *Gynecol. Oncol.*, **35** (1989) 47–49.

19. Smith HO, Gaudette DE, Goldberg GL, et al. Single-use percutaneous catheters for intraperitoneal P32 therapy, *Cancer*, **73** (1994) 2633–2637.

20. Runowicz CD, Dottino PR, Shafir MK, et al. Catheter complications associated with intraperitoneal chemotherapy, *Gynecol. Oncol.*, **24** (1986) 41–50.

21. Morales M and Dorta J. Use of acute peritoneal dialysis catheters for intraperitoneal chemotherapy instead of the semipermanent/permanent Tenckhoff catheters, *Support. Care Cancer*, **2** (1994) 132–133.

22. Rubin J, Adair CM, Raju S, et al. Tenckhoff catheter for peritoneal dialysis, *Nephron*, **32** (1982) 370–374.

23. Rubin S, Hoskins W, Markman M, et al. Long-term access to the peritoneal cavity in ovarian cancer patients, *Gynecol. Oncol.*, **33** (1983) 46–48.

24. Olcott C, Feldman CA, Coplon NS, et al. Continuous ambulatory peritoneal dialysis, *Amer. J. Surg.*, **146** (1982) 98–102.

25. Leehey DJ, Daugirdas JT, Ing TS, et al. Case against the temporary peritoneal dialysis catheter, *Int. J. Artif. Organs*, **5** (1982) 334–335.

26. Tenckhoff H. *Manual for Chronic Peritoneal Dialysis*, University of Washington School of Medicine, Seattle, 1974.

27. Tenckhoff H and Schechter H. Bacteriologically safe peritoneal access device, *Am. Soc. Artif. Organs*, **12** (1968) 181.

28. Nguyen HN, Averette HE, Wyble L, et al. Preliminary experience with a modified Tenckhoff catheter for intraperitoneal chemotherapy, *J. Surg. Oncol.*, **52** (1993) 237–240.

29. Malviya VK, Deppe G, Gove N, et al. Vascular access in gynecologic cancer using the Groshong right atrial catheter, *Gynecol. Oncol.*, **33** (1989) 313–316.

30. Delmore JE, Horbelt DV, Jack BL, et al. Experience with the Groshong long-term central venous catheter, *Gynecol. Oncol.*, **34** (1989) 216–218.

31. Hrozenick SP and Ness EA. Intraperitoneal chemotherapy via the Groshong catheter in the patient with gynecologic cancer, *Oncol. Nurs. Forum*, **18** (1991) 1245–1246.

32. Naumann RW, Alvarez RD, Partridge EE, et al. Groshong catheter as an intraperitoneal access device in the treatment of ovarian cancer patients. *Gynecol. Oncol.*, **50** (1993) 291–293.

33. Waggoner SE, Johnson J, Barter J, et al. Intraperitoneal therapy administered through a Groshong catheter, *Gynecol. Oncol.*, **53** (1994) 320–325.

34. Dunnick NR, Jones RB, Doppman JL, et al. Intraperitoneal contrast infusion for assessment of intraperitoneal fluid dynamics, *Am. J. Roentgenol.*, **133** (1979) 221.

35. Howell S, Pfeifle C, Wung W, et al. Intraperitoneal cisplatin with systemic thiosulfate protection, *Ann. Intern. Med.*, **97** (1982) 845–851.

36. Gyves J, Ensminger W, Stetson P, et al. Constant intraperitoneal 5-fluorouracil infusion through a totally implanted system, *Clin. Pharmacol. Ther.*, **35** (1984) 83–89.

37. Rosenshein N, Blake D, McIntyre PA, et al. Effect of volume on the distribution of substances instilled into the peritoneal cavity, *Gynecol. Oncol.*, **6** (1978) 106–110.

38. Meyer C. Use of intraperitoneal chemotherapy in the treatment of ovarian cancer, *Semin. Oncol.*, **11** (1984) 275–284.

39. Mueller BU, Skelton J, Callendar, et al. Prospective randomized trial comparing the infectious and noninfectious complications of an externalized catheter versus a subcutaneously implanted device in cancer patients, *J. Clin. Oncol.*, **10** (1992) 1943.

40. Markman M. Intraperitoneal chemotherapy in the treatment of ovarian cancer, *Ann. Med.*, **28** (1996) 293–296.

41. Vaccarello L and Hoskins WJ. Central venous and intraperitoneal access, In Markman M, Hoskins W (eds), *Cancer of the Ovary*. Raven, New York, 1993.

42. Fumagalli U, Trabucchi E, Soligo M, et al. Effects of intraperitoneal chemotherapy on anastomotic healing in the rat, *J. Surg. Res.*, **50** (1991) 182.

43. Kaplan RA, Markman M, Lucas W, et al. Infectious peritonitis in patients receiving intraperitoneal chemotherapy, *Am. J. Med.*, **76** (1985) 49–53.

44. Pfeifle CE, Howell SB, Markman M, et al. Totally implantable system for peritoneal access, *J. Clin. Oncol.*, **2** (1984) 1277–1280.

45. Piccart MJ, Speyer JL, Markman M, et al. Intraperitoneal chemotherapy: technical experience at five institutions, *Semin. Oncol.*, **12** (1985) 90–96.

46. Braly P, Doroshow J, and Hoff S. Technical aspects of intraperitoneal chemotherapy in abdominal carcinomatosis, *Gynecol. Oncol.*, **25** (1986) 319–333.

47. Myers CE and Collins JM. Pharmacology of intraperitoneal chemotherapy, *Cancer Invest.* **I**(5) (1983) 395–407.

48. Ozoos RF, Ostchga Y, Curt G, et al. High dose carboplatin in hypertonic saline in retractory ovarian cancer. *T. Clin. Oncol.*, **3** (1985) 1246.

49. Ohio Renal Care Group, Home Dialysis Instructions, (1998) Cleveland Clinic Foundation, Cleveland, OH.

10 Memorial Sloan-Kettering Cancer Center Experience with Intraperitoneal Chemotherapy of Ovarian Cancer

Richard R. Barakat and David R. Spriggs

CONTENTS

1. INTRODUCTION

In the past decade, there has been a large number of studies examining the potential role of intraperitoneal (ip) therapy in the treatment of ovarian cancer (OC). As it becomes clear that the theoretical advantages can be translated into survival advantages for patients, it is useful to examine the accumulated experience, to better understand the role of ip therapy in the treatment of OC. The Memorial Sloan-Kettering Cancer Center (MSKCC) group has been committed to the rational development of ip therapy for more than a decade. In the MSKCC experience outlined below, there is an unparalleled database of surgically documented responses to various ip regimens, and a novel consolidation therapy experience. Pilot data for both mitoxantrone (MTZ) and paclitaxel have also been accumulated. Currently, MSKCC has integrated ip therapy into the standard approach to the treatment of women with recurrent/persistent OC cancer.

From: *Current Clinical Oncology: Regional Chemotherapy: Clinical Research and Practice*
Edited by: M. Markman © Humana Press Inc., Totowa, NJ

2. TECHNICAL ASPECTS OF IP THERAPY: MSKCC EXPERIENCE

By far the largest experience with the technical aspects of ip chemotherapy has been the MSKCC experience with subcutaneously implanted port and catheter systems. In 1989, Rubin et al. *(1)* reported their preliminary experience with 136 catheters used to deliver 629 courses of chemotherapy in 130 patients. The system used consisted of a stainless steel or titanium port with a silicone septum, attached to a Silastic catheter with multiple side holes. The port is placed in a subcutaneous (SC) pocket over the lower rib cage, so that it is firmly supported, and sutured in place with permanent sutures. The catheter is passed through a SC tunnel to midabdominal level, where it is passed through the abdominal wall into the peritoneal cavity. Early versions of the catheter included a dacron cuff that was placed in the SC tunnel to anchor the catheter. More recently, this cuff has been eliminated, because catheter movement has not been a problem, and the cuff makes catheter removal considerably more difficult.

In a recent report from MSKCC, Davidson et al. *(2)* analyzed data on 249 catheters used to deliver 1331 courses of chemotherapy to 227 patients. These included 230 original catheters and 19 replacement catheters, which were analyzed separately. All patients were enrolled in one or more prospective clinical trials of ip therapy designed to deliver 3–24 treatment cycles over a 3–6-mo interval. Catheters were placed either at the time of laparotomy, with the abdomen open (181 catheters), or as a separate limited surgical procedure (68 catheters). In the latter instance, two small incisions were made: one over the lower anterior rib cage for port placement, and one lateral to the umbilicus for placement of the catheter into the peritoneal cavity. There were no complications associated with catheter placement by either of these techniques. Twenty (8%) of the original catheters developed blockage interfering with drug infusion. On reexploration, such blockage was generally caused by the formation of a dense sheath of fibrinous adhesions around the catheter. An additional 20 (8%) of the original catheters developed catheter-related infection. In eight of these cases, the infection developed in association with a late erosion of the catheter into the intestine. In some cases, the intestinal perforation was clinically occult, and was found incidentally at elective repeat laparotomy. None of these patients suffered permanent sequelae. Of the 12 remaining cases of catheter-related infection, 10 involved infection around the port, and two involved mild peritonitis. All responded to antibiotics and catheter removal.

The risk of catheter complication was unrelated to whether the catheter was placed at the time of exploratory laparotomy or as a separate procedure. There was no apparent relationship between the development of a complication and the interval from catheter implantation to first use, weeks of use, number of cycles of chemotherapy, or number of catheter accessions. This report also examined the risk of infection as it related to the performance of intestinal surgery at the time of catheter insertion, or at a subsequent operation, when a catheter was present and left in place. There was a trend toward increased infectious complications with large-bowel surgery and appendectomy, which did not reach statistical significance. The authors recommended avoiding catheter insertion at the time of these procedures.

3. INCORPORATION OF IP CISPLATIN INTO UPFRONT THERAPY: CYCLOPHOSPHAMIDE/PLATINUM WITH INTERVAL DEBULKING AND IP THERAPY

In the prepaclitaxel era, the authors had the opportunity to explore the role of upfront ip therapy in the management of advanced epithelial ovarian cancer (EOC)

(3). Treatment included a first laparatomy as primary debulking. Chemotherapy was begun 1–3 wk later, with iv 200 mg/m^2/d cyclophosphamide for 5 d and 30–40 mg/m^2/d cispatin for 4–5 d with hypertonic saline, which was repeated after 28 d, and followed in another 28 d. Twenty-eight d following the second cycle of chemotherapy, a second laparotomy was performed for placement of an ip catheter (not to be confused with a classic second-look laparotomy). During this interim surgery, further debulking was done, when possible, to reduce residual disease to 1 cm. At least 1 wk later, chemotherapy was resumed with ip cisplatin at 50–100 mg/m^2 administered in 2 L normal saline, and was repeated every 21 d for four cycles. A third laparotomy was done in all patients, except those who had a complete response (CR) at second laparotomy, to define response and plan for further therapy.

Forty patients were entered onto this study. Most patients had advanced-stage (III/IV) and poorly differentiated histology, with large-diameter residual disease after initial laparotomy. Eighty-five percent of patients had stage IIIC or IV disease, 63% had poor histology, and 68% had >1 cm residual disease after first laparotomy. Thirty-six patients were evaluable.

The surgically defined CR rate was 47%. Seven of these CRs were documented at the second laparotomy, and 10 at the third laparotomy. Nineteen percent (7 of 36) of patients had surgically defined partial responses, of whom 5% (2 of 36) had only microscopic residual disease found at third laparotomy. The additional debulking surgery performed at the second laparotomy was an important determinant of final response. CRs were equally likely among those who arrived at the second laparotomy with <1 cm maximum-diameter residual disease, or those who were able to be debulked to ≤1 cm residual (53 vs 47%). Eighty-three percent of patients had ≤1 cm residual at the conclusion of the second laparotomy. No CRs were seen among the six patients with >1 cm maximum-diameter residual disease at the end of the second laparotomy. These findings concur with prior observations, which showed that ip therapy is relatively ineffective for tumor masses >1 cm in maximum diameter *(4)*. Median survival is 41.8 mo. Twelve of 17 patients (71%) achieving CR have recurred at a median of 19.5 mo, usually in the peritoneal cavity. Median survival among CRs is 68.3 mo. Like CRs, relapses and survival did not differ statistically among stage II/III vs stage IV disease, with a median survival of 44.5 vs 26.7 mo, respectively ($P = 0.68$). Survival after first laparotomy, according to residual disease ≤1 cm vs >1 cm, was not statistically different, with median survival of 50.6 vs 37.0 mo, respectively ($P = 0.60$). Nor was there a statistical difference between patients who arrived at second laparotomy with residual disease ≤1 cm and those who were debulked at second laparotomy to ≤1 cm, with median survival of 42.9 vs 49.1 mo, respectively ($P = 0.67$). However, although patients with grade 3 cancers were as likely as those with grades 1 or 2 to achieve a CR (50 vs 46%), relapses were more frequent (82 vs 50%), and survival was shorter (median 37.0 vs 72.0 mo) among the grade 3 tumors, compared to grades 1 or 2 ($P = 0.05$).

The results of this study suggest that a regimen of intensified surgery and chemotherapy improved interim measures of success, namely, surgically defined CR rate and short-term survival. These results were comparable to the current standard of care using cisplatin and paclitaxel *(5)*, which demonstrated a 14-mo survival advantage over cisplatin and cyclophosphamide. Recent data from large randomized trials supports the role of both ip therapy and interval surgical debulking. The authors do not advocate using this regimen, but fully support the concept of combining multimodality therapy in the treatment of advanced OC. Many of the concepts upon which this clinical trial was founded, including interval surgical debulking and ip cisplatin, have proven true in large randomized trials. The aspect of dose-intensity remains controversial. It appears that modest increases in dose-intensity are unlikely to produce clinical benefit; however, significant dose-intensity may only be accomplished using stem support. It appears that intensive multimodality therapy, with both intensive surgical and chemotherapeutic strategies, may help improve response rates and survival in this disease.

4. ROLE OF IP THERAPY IN SPECIAL CIRCUMSTANCES

The ideal candidate for ip therapy in OC needs to be defined. Clearly, patients with large-volume (>1 cm) disease residual at surgical reassessment are poor candidates for salvage ip therapy. Additionally, because a large pharmacokinetic advantage, described as the peak peritoneal drug level to plasma level, is achieved with ip therapy, the chief advantage would be to patients whose disease is confined to the peritoneal cavity. Those with stage IV or extra-abdominal disease are generally not considered good candidates for ip therapy. Because the benefit of ip therapy is secondary to increased local exposure, it is important that direct contact with tumor tissue occurs. Patients with dense adhesions are also not good candidates for ip therapy, because uniform drug distribution would be unlikely. The presence of disease in the retroperitoneal lymph nodes has been considered a relative contraindication to the use of ip treatment, although data addressing this issue is limited. It is uncertain whether these nodes may serve as a sanctuary site for tumor cells in patients receiving ip therapy. The authors, therefore, undertook a review of patients with advanced EOC involving the retroperitoneal nodes, who were treated with salvage ip therapy, and compared their outcome with a similar group of patients with surgically documented negative lymph nodes. In addition, the authors reviewed their own experience with salvage ip therapy for patients with stage IV disease. Finally, the authors had the opportunity to evaluate the response to ip cisplatin in patients previously treated with iv platinum.

4.1. Salvage IP Therapy of Advanced EOC: Impact of Retroperitoneal Nodal Disease

The authors retrospectively reviewed the records of 43 patients with advanced EOC treated between September 1983 and July 1995, who had undergone retroperitoneal nodal sampling prior to salvage/ip chemotherapy (6). Of these 43 patients with stage III ovarian adenocarcinoma treated with debulking surgery and platinum-based chemotherapy, 20 (47%) had disease noted in retroperitoneal lymph nodes at initial surgery or at reassessment laparotomy; 23 (53%) had biopsy-proven negative nodes. The mean age of the node-positive group was 49 yr. Thirteen patients had nodal disease detected at initial surgery, and seven at reassessment laparotomy. Histologic tumor grades were 1 (four pts), 2 (two pts), and 3 (14 pts). Residual disease prior to initiation of ip therapy was optimal (<2 cm) in 17 patients and suboptimal in three.

Twenty-three patients, with a mean age of 55 yr, were found to be node-negative. Five underwent nodal sampling at initial laparotomy; 18 were found to be node-negative at reassessment laparotomy. Histologic tumor grades were 1 (five pts), 2 (four pts), 3 (11 pts), and was not recorded for three patients. Residual disease prior to initiation of ip therapy was optimal (<2 cm) in all 23 patients. All patients received salvage ip chemotherapy. With a median follow-up of 39 mo, the median survival in the node-positive group is 44 mo, compared to 46 mo for the node-negative group. The authors concluded that the presence of retroperitoneal nodal disease did not appear to be a contraindication for the use of salvage ip chemotherapy in advanced OC.

4.2. Second-Line IP Chemotherapy in Patients with Stage IV EOC

In an attempt to determine the efficacy of second-line IP chemotherapy in patients with persistent/recurrent stage IV EOC, the authors retrospectively reviewed the medical records of 31 patients with stage IV EOC treated between 1985 and 1993, who received ip therapy following the documentation of persistent/recurrent disease. All patients had previously received systemic platinum-based therapy. The median age of the patients was 53 yr (range 35–72 yr). Classification of stage IV disease was based on positive pleural cytology alone (19 pts), skin/umbilical metastasis (five pts), parenchymal liver disease (four pts), and cervical/vaginal disease (three pts). Histologic tumor grades were 1 (one pt), 2 (seven pts), 3 (20 pts), and was not recorded for three cases. Residual disease prior to initiation of ip therapy was optimal (≤1.0 cm) in 23 patients and suboptimal in eight patients. Three patients were invaluable for response, secondary to catheter malfunction. The remaining 28 patients received a mean of six cycles of ip therapy, consisting of a platinum combination or MTZ. Twenty of the 28 patients had previously responded to systemic platinum-based therapy; eight had disease progression. During ip therapy, 19 of 28 (68%) experienced disease progression, 5 of 28 (18%) had a complete surgical or clinical response, 1 of 28 (4%) had a partial response, and 3 of 28 (10%) had stable disease. Eight of 23 (35%) patients had persistent/progressive disease following ip therapy involving the liver or extra-abdominal sites; the remaining patients had intra-abdominal disease alone. With a median follow-up of 26.7 mo, the median survival from the initiation of ip treatment was 17.9 mo. Second-line ip chemotherapy for patients with persistent/recurrent stage IV EOC resulted in a 21% overall response rate in patients who had previously received systemic platinum-based therapy. The high failure rate (35%) in extra-abdominal sites, however, should preclude the routine use of second-line ip therapy in these patients.

4.3. Effect of Prior Cisplatin

In order to examine the effect of prior iv cisplatin on response to ip cisplatin, the authors retrospectively reviewed the records of 89 patients treated with either ip cisplatin + etoposide or cisplatin + cytarabine (7). All of these patients had received ip therapy as treatment for persistent/recurrent disease after iv cisplatin therapy. Fifty-two of the 89 patients (58%) had previously had an objective response to platinum therapy. In this group of patients, 56% of patients had some response to ip therapy, and 33% achieved a surgical CR. In contrast, the 37 patients who did not respond to prior iv cisplatin had a 11% response rate, and only a 3% CR rate ($P < 0.0001$). Moreover, if patients with bulky residual disease were excluded, a group of 36 patients with prior responses to cisplatin showed a 42% CR rate. It is clear that patients with a history of platinum responsiveness are much more likely to benefit from ip cisplatin-based therapy than patients with platinum-refractory disease.

5. IP THERAPY AND SURVIVAL

To evaluate the impact on survival of the attainment of a surgically defined response to salvage ip chemotherapy, the authors previously examined patients treated on several phase II ip trials conducted at this institution. A total of 58 patients, whose largest residual tumor masses measured ≤0.5 cm in maximum diameter at the initiation of therapy, were evaluable for response. Twenty-eight of these 58 patients (48%) demonstrated a surgically defined response, including 19 (33%) who achieved a surgically defined CR. Median follow-up was 43+ mo. Median survival from initiation of therapy for patients with microscopic residual disease experiencing a surgical CR (10 pts), following development salvage ip therapy, had not been reached, but exceeded 4 yr, compared to a median survival of 25 mo for the nonresponding patients (13 pts) (*P* = 0.004). The median survival for the 18 patients with small-volume macroscopic disease responding to therapy was 40 mo, compared to 19 mo for the nonresponders (*P* = 0.009) *(8)*. A recent update on these patients reveals that seven of 10 of the surgical complete responders remain alive, with a median survival of 100 mo following ip treatment, suggesting a curative potential for ip therapy in select patients.

6. IP THERAPY WITH CARBOPLATIN

Because it is now well established that carboplatin is a less toxic, and probably therapeutically equivalent, platinum complex, the authors have also examined the efficacy of ip carboplatin *(9)*. Forty-six patients with persistent or refractory OC received carboplatin (200–300 mg/m^2) and etoposide (100 mg/m^2) intraperitoneally each month, followed by a surgical response assessment. Twelve of 32 patients evaluable for efficacy achieved some response, including eight (25%) patients with surgically documented CRs.

In order to better define efficacy, compared to cisplatin, a retrospective analysis was undertaken, comparing cisplatin vs carboplatin in patients with a prior platinum response, small-volume (<0.5 cm) disease, and a surgical response assessment *(10)*. In this analysis, patients received 100 mg/m^2 cisplatin with either ip cytarabine (600–900 mg/m^2) or ip etoposide (100 mg/m^2); all carboplatin patients (200–300 mg/m^2) received etoposide (100 mg/m^2) ip, as well. For patients with no visible disease (microscopic only), the surgical CR rate was 46% (6 of 13 pts) with the ip cisplatin-based regimens; it was 38% (6 of 16 pts) for the ip carboplatin-based regimen (*P* > 0.25). However, for patients with very small disease (<0.5 cm) at the time of therapy, the CR rate was 41% for the cisplatin group, and only 11% for the carboplatin therapy patients (*P* < 0.1). No survival effects were noted.

7. IP CISPLATIN AND ETOPOSIDE AS CONSOLIDATION THERAPY

The optimal management of patients with advanced (stages IIC–IV) EOC, who have achieved a surgically defined CR following cytoreductive surgery and platinum-based combination chemotherapy, is controversial. Although overall response rates of up to 80% are achieved in patients receiving cisplatin-based combination chemotherapy, only 47% of patients who are clinically free of disease will be found to have no evidence of disease at second-look laparotomy *(11)*. Almost half of these patients will eventually recur, with a mean interval of 24 mo from second-look surgery to recurrence, and with 60% of these recurrences occurring in the peritoneal cavity *(12)*. Therefore, it is reasonable to manage these patients with some form of consolidation therapy that will not only treat the peritoneal cavity, but will also provide a systemic level of chemotherapy.

Between September 1988 and April 1996, 40 patients with stage II–IV EOC, who had undergone a negative second-look surgical assessment, were entered prospectively on a protocol to evaluate the efficacy of ip cisplatin/VP-16 as consolidation therapy. Patients were considered ineligible for protocol treatment, if there was any histologic, cytologic, or clinical evidence of persistent OC. Other reasons for exclusion included any concomitant invasive malignancy, and moderate or severe (grade 3 or 4) neurotoxicity secondary to prior cisplatin administration. Three patients who received protocol treatment were deemed ineligible on review for the following reasons: concomitant breast cancer (one), probable stage I disease (one), and negative third-look assessment (one). One additional patient was considered inevaluable, because she never received any therapy secondary to a malfunctioning ip catheter. These patients were therefore excluded from further analysis.

All 36 eligible patients had undergone primary surgery and primary chemotherapy, which included cisplatin in 18 patients (50%), carboplatin in 17 (47%), and both cisplatin and carboplatin in one (3%); in addition, 16 patients (44%) also received paclitaxel. A negative surgical reassessment was performed within 8 wk of protocol entry; 28 patients had laparotomies (78%), and eight had reassessment laparoscopies (22%). Eligible patients had white blood cells (WBC) $\geq 3000/mm^3$; platelets $\geq 150,000/mm^3$; hemoglobin ≥ 10 gm/L; serum creatinine ≤ 1.8 mg/dL; and serum glutamic oxaloacetic transminase ≤ 45 IU/dL. A written informed consent was required prior to treatment.

Patients received vigorous prehydration, to achieve a urinary output of at least 100 mL/h prior to therapy. The cisplatin (100 mg/m^2) and etoposide (200 mg/m^2) were each administered in a volume of 1000 mL via a SC peritoneal catheter. Following administration of 2 L of medication, up to 2 L additional D5/NS were administered, to distend the abdomen and ensure adequate distribution. All patients received aggressive antiemetic therapy as premedication, depending on the best therapy available at the time. Most patients received Decadron, serotonin antagonists, and delayed emesis prophylaxis with metaclopramide. Patients with abdominal pain from distention received meperidine as required. Patients were treated at 4-wk intervals, and there were no treatment delays for hematologic toxicity.

Treatment modifications were required for nephrotoxicity or hematologic toxicity. A 50% reduction in cisplatin dose for renal toxicity was based on serum creatinine (>1.5 mg/dL) or creatinine clearance (<50 mL/min) on the day of treatment. Patients with creatinine >2.0 were removed from therapy. Both cisplatin and etoposide were dose-reduced 50% for myelosuppression (WBC $\leq 3,000$ or platelets <90 K) on the day of treatment.

Recurrence and survival data for the protocol patients were retrospectively compared to that for a contemporaneous group of 46 patients who met protocol eligibility requirements, but underwent observation alone. Following cytoreductive surgery, all patients in the untreated group received platinum-based combination therapy (56% cisplatin, 35% carboplatin, and 9% cisplatin and carboplatin), which included paclitaxel for 10 patients (22%). Thirty-four of these patients (74%) underwent second-look laparotomy; the remaining 12 underwent reassessment laparoscopically.

Thirty-six patients undergoing protocol treatment were evaluable for toxicity and efficacy. Their median age was 52 yr (range 30–70 yr). Distribution by stage reflects a predominance of patients with advanced-stage disease, with a low frequency of stage II disease. The majority of patients had undergone a complete surgical resection (36%) or optimal cytoreduction (≤ 1 cm) (31%), reflecting the higher likelihood of such patients achieving a pathological CR. The entire cohort received patinum-based chemotherapy, with 50% receiving cisplatin, 47% receiving carboplatin, and 3% receiving both drugs during their primary treatment period. Because the period of protocol activity spanned the clinical introduction of paclitaxel, only 16 patients entered (44%) received paclitaxel therapy. The number of chemotherapy courses given ranged from four to nine.

A total of 97 courses of therapy were administered. The toxicity of the therapy was substantial: Only 50% of the patients entered into the study were able to complete three cycles of therapy without dose modification. Eleven patients required dose reduction, and 19 courses of reduced-dose chemotherapy were given. Six patients received reduced doses of cisplatin, because of nephrotoxicity.

Other toxicity was typical of cisplatin therapy. Two patients required dose reductions for neutropenia, including one with grade 4 leukopenia and fever, who required hospitalization for antibiotic therapy. One patient, admitted after the third cycle with grade 2 neutropenia and urosepsis, was treated successfully with antibiotics. Prophylactic hematopoietic growth factors were not routinely employed in this study. Nausea and vomiting (grade 1–2) were commonly observed, despite aggressive antiemetic prophylaxis, and led to dose reductions in three patients. One patient was rehospitalized for dehydration and inability to maintain adequate oral intake. One patient refused cycles 2 and 3, because of severe nausea. Increases in baseline neuropathy were common, but no patient experienced grade 3 or 4 peripheral neuropathy. One patient experienced grade 2 neuropathy after one cycle of therapy, and refused further treatment.

Technical problems with the peritoneal catheters were uncommon, and no episode of bacterial peritonitis during treatment was observed. One patient developed fever and abdominal tenderness after the peritoneal catheter was removed. On computerized tomography scan, it was discovered that a piece of the catheter remained, and it was removed surgically. The patient developed a pelvic abscess and a probable small-bowel fistula, which were treated with antibiotic therapy and bowel rest. This patient had a prolonged hospitalization, but, at last follow-up, has no evidence of disease, and no long-term sequelae. Two patients experienced catheter malfunction, and could not receive more than one cycle of ip therapy. Abdominal pain, reported as bloating and discomfort, was commonly observed after ip drug administration; only seven patients had grade 2 pain, which was controlled with meperidine. No patient died of chemotherapy-related complications.

The primary efficacy end point for this study was time to treatment failure. A third surgical procedure to confirm disease status postconsolidation therapy was not performed. With a median follow-up of 36 mo, 61% (22 of 36) of the treated patients are without evidence of recurrent disease. If one examines the risk of relapse as a function of actual therapy received, the results are even more striking: Only 5 of 18 (28%) of the patients who received three cycles of cisplatin–etoposide at full doses have relapsed. In contrast, 9 of 18 (50%) of the patients who either required dose reduction or did not receive three cycles of therapy have had disease recurrence.

These results of a nonrandomized pilot study were superior to published results. In order to assess the experience further, the authors reviewed the medical records of all patients with negative surgical reassessments since 1988. A group of patients was identified, treated during this time period, who received no therapy after a negative surgical reassessment. Forty-six of these patients were eligible for protocol entry, but were not treated because of patient or physician choice. The characteristics of this group are very similar to that of the protocol group. Median age and follow-up are identical. The observation-only group included more stage II patients (18 vs three), consistent with a bias toward observation in this group with a better overall prognosis following primary therapy. Conversely, more suboptimally debulked patients were present in the consolidation treatment group (33 vs 20%). A lower percentage of the observation group received paclitaxel (22 vs 44%). In this group, 54% of the patients have recurred, with a median disease-free survival (DFS) of 28.5 mo.

The results of the observation group were consistent with the authors' own prior results, and those from the literature *(12)*. When the observation group's DFS was compared (using the log-rank test) to the DFS in the consolidation therapy group, there was a significant improvement ($P \leq 0.03$). In a multivariate analysis of the two groups, the only significant predictor of DFS was consolidation therapy.

The risk of recurrent disease, following primary therapy for EOC, remains very high. In this phase II trial of ip consolidation, with three cycles of cisplatin and etoposide following negative second-look reassessment in patients with advanced EOC, the authors demonstrated a significant increase in DFS, compared to that of patients undergoing observation alone. Although this was not a randomized trial, these data do suggest that the role of ip consolidation warrants further evaluation.

8. IP SALVAGE THERAPY WITH NONPLATINUM AGENTS

Although platinum agents remain the most important agents, the authors have also examined a variety of other antineoplastics for this condition. The MSKCC group has utilized MTZ, fluoropyrimidines, and, more recently, paclitaxel as ip therapy. The results, although not as mature as the platinum data, are promising.

8.1. Mitoxantrone

The anthracyclines have substantial activity in the treatment of OC and remain an important part of the therapy in many institutions. MTZ is a dihydroxyquinone with an activity profile similar to that of doxorubicin, but is less irritating to tissues. The authors examined MTZ as an ip agent for the treatment of persistent and refractory OC. The initial trial at 20 mg/m^2 was marked by significant local complications *(13)*. Nearly three-quarters (74%) of patients required narcotics for abdominal pain at the time of drug administration. Six of 31 patients treated had episodes of symptomatic bowel obstruction during or after therapy (one required surgical intervention). However, 6 of 18 patients with small-volume disease (<1.0 cm) had surgically documented responses. The response rate in large-volume disease (>1.0 cm) was much lower (9%). In order to decrease the local toxicity, a lower dose of MTZ (10 mg/m^2) was tested on an every-other-week basis *(14)*. The toxicity was substantially diminished. Four of 13 surgically assessed patients with small-volume disease (<1.0 cm) had response, but only one CR was noted. The high frequency of adhesion formation with MTZ may impair efficacy by limiting distribution of drug.

8.2. IP Paclitaxel

When the activity of paclitaxel in OC became known, it was reasonable to examine the effect of ip paclitaxel *(15)*. The initial phase I study of paclitaxel incorporated a once-every-3-wk schedule. The recommended phase II dose was 125 mg/m^2, based on the same type of abdominal pain observed with MTZ. Lower doses of ip paclitaxel were very well tolerated. It was also encouraging that the paclitaxel concentrations in the peritoneal cavity seemed to be up to 10,000-fold higher than achievable plasma concentrations, and appeared to persist for more than 24 h. A second schedule was then examined under the auspices of the Gynecologic Oncology Group (GOG) *(16)*. When the dose of paclitaxel was decreased to 50–65 mg/m^2, patients could be treated each week with ip paclitaxel, achieving high paclitaxel exposures with acceptable toxicity. A phase II dose of 60 mg/m^2 was recommended. Several CA-125 responses were observed on this trial, but no surgical responses were documented, because only two patients underwent surgical evaluation after therapy. A phase II trial of this regimen is underway in the GOG, and ip paclitaxel has been incorporated into the investigational arm for primary chemotherapy of patients with small-volume residual disease.

9. CURRENT STATUS OF IP THERAPY AT MSKCC

In 1998, the authors did not utilize ip therapy as part of the primary chemotherapy treatment of OC, except as part of an investigational approach. For patients with small-volume (<0.5 cm) residual disease at the time of second-look surgical assessment, the authors currently recommend investigational therapy. However, for those patients unwilling to have investigational therapy, 5–6 cycles of ip cisplatin at 75–100 mg/m^2 are often employed. Based on experience in the consolidation of patients with negative second-look procedures, the authors now recommend three cycles of ip cisplatin (100 mg/m^2). In the recurrent disease setting, the authors restrict use of ip therapy to patients with platinum-sensitive disease and small-volume (<0.5 cm) disease.

REFERENCES

1. Rubin SC, Hoskins WJ, Markman M, Hakes T, and Lewis JL Jr. Long-term access to the peritoneal cavity in ovarian cancer patients, *Gynecol. Oncol.*, **33** (1989) 46–48.
2. Davidson SA, Rubin SC, Markman M, et al. Intraperitoneal chemotherapy: analysis of complications with an implanted subcutaneous port and catheter system, *Gynecol. Oncol.*, **41** (1991) 101–106.
3. Shapiro F, Schneider J, Markman M, et al. High-intensity cyclophosphamide and cispatin, interim surgical debulking, and intraperitoneal cisplatin in advanced ovarian carcinoma: a pilot trial with ten-year follow-up, *Gynecol. Oncol.*, **67** (1997) 39–45.
4. Reichman B, Markman M, Hakes T, et al. Intraperitoneal cisplatin and etoposide in the treatment of refractory/recurrent ovarian carcinoma, *J. Clin. Oncol.*, **7** (1989) 1327–1333.
5. McGuire WP, Hoskins WJ, Brady MF, et al. Cyclophosphamide and cisplatin compared with paclitaxel and cisplatin in patients with stage III and stage IV ovarian cancer, *N. Engl. J. Med.*, **334** (1996) 1–6.
6. Barakat RR, Fennelly D, Pizzuto F, Venkatraman ES, Brown C, and Curtin JP. Salvage intraperitoneal therapy of advanced epithelial ovarian cancer: impact of retroperitoneal nodal disease, *Eur. J. Gynaecol. Oncol.*, **18** (1997) 161–163.
7. Markman M, Reichman B, Hakes T, et al. Responses to second-line cisplatin-based intraperitoneal therapy in ovarian cancer: influence of a prior response to intravenous cisplatin, *J. Clin. Oncol.*, **9** (1991) 1801–1805.
8. Markman M, Reichman B, Hakes T, et al. Impact on survival of surgically defined favorable responses to salvage intraperitoneal chemotherapy in small-volume residual ovarian cancer, *J. Clin. Oncol.*, **10** (1992) 1479–1484.
9. Markman M, Reichman B, Hakes T, et al. Phase 2 trial of intraperitoneal carboplatin and etoposide as salvage treatment of advanced epithelial ovarian cancer, *Gynecol. Oncol.*, **47** (1992) 353–357.
10. Markman M, Reichman B, Hakes T, et al. Evidence supporting the superiority of intraperitoneal cisplatin compared to intraperitoneal carboplatin for salvage therapy of small-volume residual ovarian cancer, *Gynecol. Oncol.*, **50** (1993) 100–104.
11. Ozols RF, Rubin SC, and Thomas G. Epithelial ovarian cancer. In Hoskins WJ, Perez CA, Young RC (eds), *Principles and Practice of Gynecologic Oncology*, 2nd ed. JB Lippincott Co., Philadelphia, 1996, p. 960.
12. Rubin SC, Hoskins WJ, and Saigo PE. Prognostic factors for recurrence following negative second-look laparotomy in ovarian cancer patients treated with platinum-based chemotherapy, *Gynecol. Oncol.*, **42** (1991) 137–141.
13. Markman M, George M, Hakes T, et al. Phase II trial of intraperitoneal mitoxantrone in the management of refractory ovarian cancer, *J. Clin. Oncol.*, **8** (1990) 146–150.
14. Markman M, Hakes T, Reichman B, et al. Phase II trial of weekly or biweekly intraperitoneal mitoxantrone in epithelial ovarian cancer, *J. Clin. Oncol.*, **9** (1991) 978–982.

15. Markman M, Rowinsky E, Hakes T, et al. Phase I trial of intraperitoneal Taxol: a Gynecologic Oncology Group study, *J. Clin. Oncol.,* **10** (1992) 1485–1491.
16. Francis P, Rowinsky E, Schneider J, Hakes T, Hoskins W, and Markman M. Phase I feasibility and pharmacologic study of weekly intraperitoneal paclitaxel: a Gynecologic Oncology Group pilot study, *J. Clin. Oncol.,* **13** (1995) 2961–2967.

11 Southwest Oncology Group Experience with Intraperitoneal Chemotherapy of Ovarian Cancer

David S. Alberts, Dava J. Garcia, Emily Fisher, and P.Y. Liu

CONTENTS

1. INTRODUCTION

Ovarian cancer (OC) is the leading cause of gynecologic cancer death in the United States, and over 14,000 women will die of this disease in 1999 *(1)*. During the past two decades, median survival has improved dramatically with the advent of platinum- and paclitaxel-based chemotherapy. In the early 1970s, the median survival of a woman with stage III disease was approx 12 mo *(2)*. With currently available therapies, median survival has been extended to longer than 45 mo for patients with stage III disease and optimal surgical resections during the initial exploratory laparotomy *(3,4)*. Unfortunately, despite significant gains in therapeutic efficacy and high response rates to primary chemotherapy regimens, the majority of women with advanced OC develop drug-resistant tumors, and eventually succumb to their disease.

One approach to circumventing inherent drug resistance in advanced OC involves the administration of chemotherapeutic agents directly into the peritoneal cavity. The pioneering work of Dedrick et al. *(5)* established a strong pharmacokinetic rationale

From: *Current Clinical Oncology: Regional Chemotherapy: Clinical Research and Practice*
Edited by: M. Markman © Humana Press Inc., Totowa, NJ

for intraperitoneal (ip) drug therapy. Howell et al. *(6)* and Goel et al. *(7)* have documented that ip administration of cisplatin results in a peritoneal exposure that is 12–15× greater than plasma exposure. The pharmacologic advantage (defined as the ratio between the peritoneal drug area under the curve (AUC) and the plasma drug AUC) of ip administration is even greater for paclitaxel (1000-fold) and a variety of other chemotherapeutic agents with activity against OC *(8,9)*.

Beginning in the mid-1980s, the Gynecologic Cancer Committee of the Southwest Oncology Group (SWOG), in a collaborative effort with the Gynecologic Oncology Group (GOG), Eastern Cooperative Oncology Group (ECOG), and National Cancer Institute of Canada (NCIC), has undertaken a number of phase II and III studies to evaluate the efficacy of ip chemotherapy in women with optimal (<1–2 cm residual tumor) disease, epithelial ovarian cancer (EOC). Table 1 provides a brief summary of these ip studies.

SWOG-8501 (INT-0051, GOG-104, EST-3885) was a phase III study that compared iv cisplatin + iv cyclophosphamide (CY) vs ip cisplatin + iv CY as primary chemotherapy for patients with stage III, optimal disease. SWOG-8790 (INT-0083, GOG-133) was a phase III randomized study of observation vs ip interferon-α therapy in patients with stage III disease who achieved a pathologically verified complete response (CR) to primary platinum-based chemotherapy (with or without paclitaxel). SWOG-8835 was a randomized phase II study of ip floxuridine (FUDR) and ip mitoxantrone (MTZ) in patients with minimal residual disease following second-look surgery. SWOG-9227/GOG-114/ECOG GO114, was a GOG-led phase III trial that compared iv cisplatin + iv paclitaxel to iv carboplatin followed by iv paclitaxel and ip cisplatin as primary chemotherapy in stage III disease. SWOG-9619, a joint study among SWOG, ECOG, and NCIC, has recently completed accrual. This phase II trial utilized ip cisplatin and iv and ip paclitaxel as frontline therapy in women with optimally debulked stage III OC. Available results of these studies support the continued research focus of the SWOG Gynecologic Cancer Committee on the use of ip chemotherapy in OC patients who have minimal residual disease after primary or secondary exploratory laparotomies.

2. SWOG STUDIES OF IP THERAPY AS PRIMARY CHEMOTHERAPY FOR STAGE III, OPTIMAL DISEASE OC

2.1. INT-0051 (SWOG-8501/GOG-104/EST-3885)

INT-0051, Phase III Intergroup Study of IP Cisplatin IV Cyclophosphamide vs IV Cisplatin/IV Cyclophosphamide in Patients with Non-Measurable (Optimal) Disease Stage III Ovarian Cancer, is the largest U.S. phase III study in OC published to date (*see* Fig. 1 for study schema). The results revealed that ip cisplatin is superior to iv cisplatin when administered as primary chemotherapy to the study patient population *(3)*. Patients on the ip arm survived significantly longer and experienced less toxicity. This study was open to patient accrual from June 1986 to July 1992. Eligibility criteria included previously untreated, stage III, histologically confirmed EOC, following thorough exploratory laparotomy, including bilateral salpingo-oophorectomy, total abdominal hysterectomy, omentectomy, and tumor debulking to ≤2 cm in maximum diameter of individual masses. Patients were randomly assigned to iv 100 mg/m^2 cisplatin + iv 600 mg/m^2 CY vs ip 100 mg/m^2 cisplatin + iv 600 mg/m^2 CY every 3 wk for six cycles. Prior to randomization, patients were stratified according to amount of residual disease (≤0.5 vs >0.5–2 cm), SWOG performance status (0–1 vs 2), timing of registration (intraoperative vs postsurgical), and cooperative group (SWOG vs GOG vs ECOG).

Table 1
Phase II and III Studies of IP Chemotherapy
Performed by SWOG with GOG, ECOG, and NCIC Participation

Study no.	Eligibility criteria	Regimen(s)	Findings
SWOG-8501/ INT-0051/ GOG-104 EST-3885	Stage III, epithelial ovarian cancer (EOC) Initial exploratory laparotomy with optimal (<2 cm) tumor debulking No prior chemotherapy or radiation	IV 100 mg/m^2 cisplatin + iv 600 mg/m^2 Cyclophosphamide every 3 wk × six cycles vs IP 100 mg/m^2 cisplatin + iv 600 mg/m^2 Cyclophosphamide every 3 wk × six cycles	IP arm associated with superior survival and toxicity profile
SWOG-8790/ INT-0083/ GOG-133	Stage III EOC Optimal debulking during first-look surgery Completion of platinum-based (± paclitaxel) chemotherapy Pathologic complete response at second-look surgery	Observation vs IP Interferon-α 50 × 10^6 IU weekly × six cycles	Closed early due to poor accrual
SWOG-8835	Stage II or III EOC ≤1 cm residual disease at end of second-look surgery 1 prior chemotherapy regimen	IP FUDR 3 gm/d × 3 d every 3 wk × six cycles vs IP 10 mg/m^2 mitoxantrone every 2 wk × nine cycles	IP FUDR was selected for further study on the basis of both efficacy and toxicity data
SWOG-9227/ GOG-114/ ECOG GO114	Stage III EOC Initial exploratory laparotomy with optimal (<1 cm) tumor debulking No prior chemotherapy or radiation	IV 135 mg/m^2 paclitaxel over 24 h then iv 75 mg/m^2 cisplatin every 21 d × six cycles vs IV carboplatin AUC = 9 every 28 d × two cycles, then IV 135 mg/m^2 paclitaxel over 24 h + IP 100 mg/m^2 cisplatin every 21 d × six cycles	IP arm associated with superior recurrence-free and overall survival
SWOG-9619 (with participation by ECOG and NCIC)	Stage III EOC Initial exploratory laparotomy with optimal (<1 cm) tumor debulking No prior chemotherapy or radiation	IV 135 mg/m^2 paclitaxel over 24 h on d 1–2 + IP cisplatin 100 mg/ m^2 on d 2 + IP 60 mg/m^2 paclitaxel on d 8 every 3 wk × six cycles	Regimen selected for further study in GOG-172 and planned SWOG trial

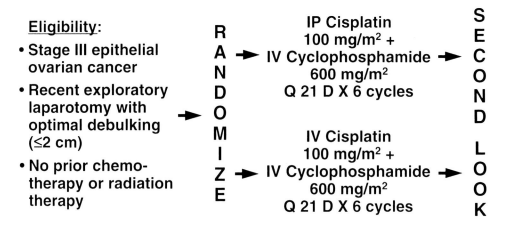

Fig. 1. Study schema for INT-0051, Phase III Intergroup Study of IP Cisplatin/IV Cyclophosphamide versus IV Cisplatin/IV Cyclophosphamide in Patients with Non-Measurable (Optimal) Disease Stage III Ovarian Cancer.

Table 2
Characteristics of Eligible Patients Enrolled in INT-0083/SWOG-8501

Eligible patient characteristics	IV Arm (n = 279)	IP Arm (n = 267)
Median age (range yr)	56 (21–85)	59 (24–84)
Residual diseases ≤0.5 cm	72%	73%
Performance status 0–1	86%	85%
Tumor histology other than clear cell or mucinous	95%	97%

Adapted from ref. *3.*

IV CY and iv cisplatin were administered according to standard clinical procedures. Patients who received ip cisplatin required surgical placement of a semipermanent catheter (Port-A-Cath™) which remained in place for the duration of the study, or insertion of a Tenckoff™-type catheter into the peritoneal cavity for each ip therapy administration. Cisplatin was administered in 2 L normal saline, as rapidly as possible (i.e., over 30–60 min). After instillation, no attempt was made to drain the peritoneal cavity. Patients on both study arms received iv hydration, with at least 1 L normal saline plus 3 gm magnesium sulfate and 40 gm mannitol concurrent with chemotherapy administration.

Six hundred and fifty-four patients were randomized to this study: 546 were eligible (279 on the iv arm and 267 on the ip arm). All eligible patients were included in efficacy analyses (based on the intent-to-treat principle); 20 eligible patients who did not receive study therapy were excluded from toxicity analyses. Patient characteristics for each of the study arms are provided in Table 2. There were no significant differences between the iv and ip study arms, with respect to important prognostic factors (i.e., age, amount of residual disease, performance status, and tumor histology).

As shown in Table 3, efficacy analysis revealed that survival of eligible patients on the ip arm (estimated median, 49 mo; 95% CI: 42–56) was significantly longer ($P = 0.02$) than on the iv arm (estimated median, 41 mo; 95% CI: 34–47). This survival advantage translated into an ip:iv death hazard ratio of 0.76 ($P = 0.02$). Thus, averaged

Table 3
Survival and Pathologic Complete Response Rates
in Eligible Patients Registered to INT-0083/SWOG-8501

	IV Arm	IP Arm
Survival		
Number at risk	279	267
Median survival (mo)	41	49
95% Confidence interval (mo)	34–47	42–56
IP/IV death hazard ratio	0.76	
P value	0.02	
Path CR rates		
Path CR in patients with no clinical evidence of disease after primary chemotherapy	57/158 (36%)	66/139 (47%)

Path CR = pathologic complete response.
Adapted from ref. *3*.

Table 4
Percentage of Toxicities Associated with Treatment on INT-0083/SWOG-8501

	IV Arm (n = 276)	IP Arm (n = 250)	P Value
≥ Grade 3 Hematologic Toxicity			
Anemia	25	26	0.84
Granulocytopenia	69	56	0.002
Leukopenia	50	40	0.04
Thrombocytopenia	9	8	0.64
≥ Grade 2 Nonhematologic Toxicity			
Abdominal pain	2	18	<0.001
Tinnitus	14	7	0.01
Clinical hearing loss	15	5	<0.001
Neuromuscular	21	16	0.18
Neuromuscular at end of study treatment	25	15	0.02
Pulmonary	0.4	3	0.002

Adapted from ref. *3*.

over the entire follow-up period, eligible patients on the ip arm were 24% less likely to die of their disease. This survival benefit is an important advance in gynecologic oncology, and is similar to that achieved with adjuvant therapy regimens for breast cancer *(10,11)*. There was also a trend toward improved pathologic CR rates associated with the ip arm. However, because of the substantial number of patients who failed to undergo second-look surgery, and the resulting potential for bias, statistical comparisons of pathologic CR rates were not conducted.

The percentage of patients who experienced grade 2 or greater neutropenia, tinnitus, clinical hearing loss, and neuromuscular toxicities was significantly less on the ip arm than the iv arm (Table 4). Grade 3 or greater neutropenia (neutrophil count <500/μL) was experienced by 56% of patients on the ip arm and 69% of patients on the iv arm (*P* = 0.002). Twice as many patients experienced grade 2–3 tinnitus on the iv arm (14%) as on the ip arm (7%, *P* = 0.01). Three times as many patients experienced grade 2–3 clinical hearing loss on the iv arm (15%) as on the ip arm (5%, *P* < 0.001).

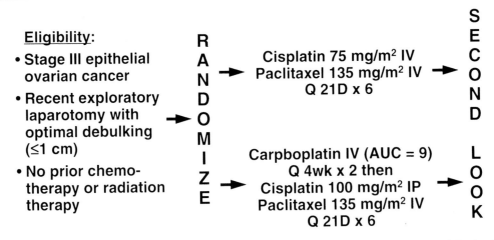

Fig. 2. Study schema for GOG-114/SWOG-9227/ECOG-G0114, A Phase III Randomized Study of IV Cisplatin and Cyclophosphamide versus IV Cisplatin and Taxol versus High Dose IV Carboplatin followed by IV Taxol and IP Cisplatin in Patients with Optimal Stage III Epithelial Ovarian Cancer.

Although the rates of peripheral neuropathy were similar between study arms during treatment, among those completing 5–6 courses of treatment (376 patients), there was significantly more grade 2–3 neuromuscular toxicity at the completion of study chemotherapy in patients on the iv arm (25 vs 15%, $P = 0.02$). As anticipated, grade 2 or greater abdominal pain was significantly more common in the ip cisplatin treated patients (2 vs 18%, $P < 0.001$), but the pain rarely lasted more than 24 h, and was controlled with nonopioid or mild opioid therapies. Grade 2 or greater pulmonary toxicity, typically transient dyspnea, also was experienced by more patients on the ip arm (3 vs 0.4%, $P = 0.002$), and was probably caused by lung base compression secondary to expansion of the ip cavity with ip fluid.

2.2. GOG-114/SWOG-9227

GOG-114/SWOG-9227/ECOG GO114, a Phase III Randomized Study of IV Cisplatin and Cyclophosphamide versus IV Cisplatin and paclitaxel versus High Dose IV Carboplatin followed by IV paclitaxel and IP Cisplatin in Patients with Optimal Stage III Epithelial Ovarian Cancer, was a GOG-led intergroup trial with participation by the SWOG and ECOG (4). Although originally designed as a three-arm study (*see* Fig. 2 for study schema), the iv cisplatin–CY arm was closed early, in response to the positive results of GOG-111, which revealed that iv paclitaxel–cisplatin was superior to iv cisplatin–CY. Eligible patients were required to have undergone a definitive exploratory laparotomy with maximum tumor resection to ≤1 cm residual disease, and to have adequate performance status and bone marrow, and hepatic and renal function. Patients could not have received prior chemotherapy or radiotherapy. Prior to randomization, patients were stratified on the basis of no gross residual disease vs gross disease. Regimen I consisted of 75 mg/m^2 cisplatin iv plus 750 mg/m^2 CY iv every 21 d for six courses. Regimen II administered 135 mg/m^2 paclitaxel by 24 h continuous iv infusion on d 1, followed by 75 mg/m^2 cisplatin iv on d 2, every 21 d for six courses. Patients on regimen III received carboplatin, AUC = 9 (as calculated by the Calvert formula), every 28 d for two courses, followed by 135 mg/m^2 paclitaxel iv on d 1 plus 100 mg/m^2 cisplatin ip on d 2, every 21 d for six courses. A total of 523 patients were registered to arms II and III of this study. Excluding the 60 patients who were later

Eligibility:

- **Recent initial laparotomy with optimal tumor debulking (≤1 cm)**

- **Histologically confirmed stage III epithelial ovarian cancer**

- **No prior chemotherapy, radiation or biologic therapy**

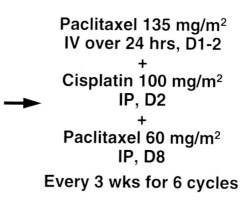

Paclitaxel 135 mg/m²
IV over 24 hrs, D1-2
+
Cisplatin 100 mg/m²
IP, D2
+
Paclitaxel 60 mg/m²
IP, D8
Every 3 wks for 6 cycles

Fig. 3. Study schema for SWOG-9619, Phase II Trial of IP Cisplatin and IV and IP Paclitaxel in Women with Optimally-Debulked Stage III Epithelial Cancer.

deemed to be ineligible, there were 228 evaluable patients on regimen II and 235 evaluable patients on regimen III.

Recurrence-free survival on the ip therapy arm was significantly better than on the iv cisplatin/paclitaxel arm (27.6 vs 22.5 mo, relative risk = 0.793, $P = 0.02$). Additionally, there was a borderline significant improvement in overall survival on the ip arm, compared to the iv cisplatin–paclitaxel arm (median survivals of 52.9 vs 47.6 mo, relative risk = 0.785, $P = .056$). The median survival of 52.9 mo on the ip arm is the longest reported to date in any phase III study of chemotherapy in patients with stage III EOC performed in the U.S.

Although the rationale for administering two courses of high-dose carboplatin in regimen III was to chemically debulk the residual tumor and potentially improve the efficacy of the ip cisplatin, the high-dose carboplatin treatments were associated with considerable myelosuppression, and hampered the administration of subsequent chemotherapy. Nineteen percent of patients on the ip arm received two or less cycles of ip therapy. Additional toxicity data are pending publication.

Because of an unacceptable toxicity profile, regimen III cannot be recommended for further use. However, the survival data strongly support further study of ip therapy in optimal disease OC. The GOG has initiated a follow-up phase III study of standard iv paclitaxel–iv cisplatin vs the ip cisplatin plus ip/iv paclitaxel regimen developed by the SWOG in SWOG-9619.

2.3. SWOG-9619

SWOG-9619, Phase II Trial of IP Cisplatin and IV and IP Paclitaxel in Women with Optimally-Debulked Stage III Epithelial Ovarian Cancer, was an intergroup trial with SWOG leadership and participation by the ECOG and the NCIC (*see* Fig. 3 for study schema). Patient accrual was completed on July 1, 1998, after enrollment of 85 patients. Eligible patients had stage III, optimal, histologically confirmed EOC. All patients had undergone an exploratory laparotomy with total abdominal hysterectomy, bilateral salpingo-oophorectomy, at least partial omentectomy, pelvic and periaortic lymph node sampling, and tumor debulking to ≤1 cm within 6 wk of study enrollment. Patients with prior chemotherapy or radiotherapy were excluded. The study regimen consisted of 135 mg/m² paclitaxel by continuous 24-h iv infusion on d 1–2 + 100 mg/ m² cisplatin ip on d 2 + 60 mg/m² paclitaxel ip on d 8, every 3 wk for six courses.

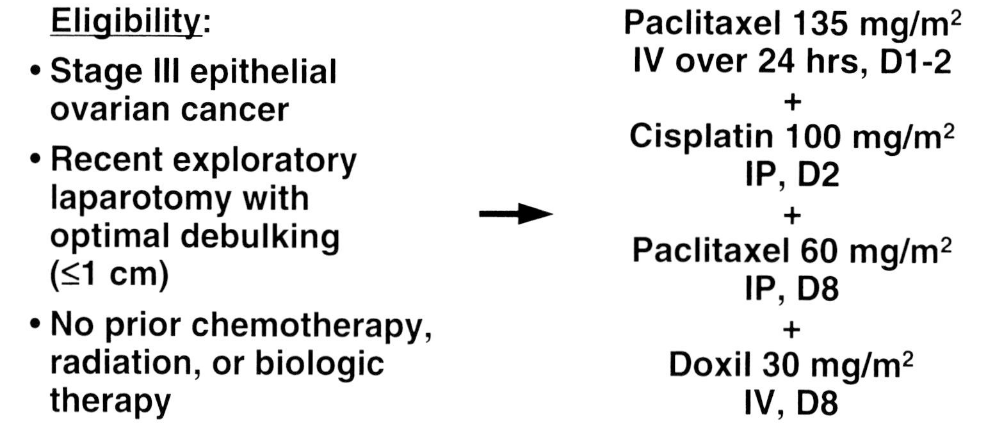

Eligibility:

- Stage III epithelial ovarian cancer
- Recent exploratory laparotomy with optimal debulking (≤1 cm)
- No prior chemotherapy, radiation, or biologic therapy

→

Paclitaxel 135 mg/m^2
IV over 24 hrs, D1-2
+
Cisplatin 100 mg/m^2
IP, D2
+
Paclitaxel 60 mg/m^2
IP, D8
+
Doxil 30 mg/m^2
IV, D8

Fig. 4. Study schema for follow-up study to SWOG-9619, Phase II Trial of IP Cisplatin, IV/IP Paclitaxel, and IV Doxil in Women with Optimally-Debulked Stage III Epithelial Ovarian Cancer.

Paclitaxel was selected for ip administration in SWOG-9619, because of a highly favorable pharmacokinetic profile when administered by this route. In two phase I and pharmacokinetic studies by Markman et al. *(8,9),* administration of paclitaxel by the ip route resulted in ip drug concentrations that were approx 1000-fold greater than concentrations that are cytotoxic in vitro. Additionally, ip paclitaxel exhibited a very slow clearance from the peritoneal space (mean clearance 0.42 ± 0.09 L/m^2/d) and a prolonged half-life of 73.4 ± 18.4 h. Indeed, at 24 and 48 h after administration, the ip concentrations of paclitaxel were several orders of magnitude greater than plasma concentrations that can be achieved with iv dosing of paclitaxel. Dose-limiting, delayed-onset abdominal pain was encountered at doses above 125 mg/m^2 every 3–4 wk. However, it was possible to administer ip paclitaxel at a dose of 60 mg/m^2/wk for 16 consecutive weeks without undue toxicity. Additionally, patients who had only microscopic disease prior to starting ip paclitaxel experienced a high pathologically proven CR rate at third-look surgery.

Final analysis of SWOG-9619 is pending maturation of survival data. However, the study regimen was well tolerated, and has been incorporated as the experimental ip study arm in comparison to iv paclitaxel–iv cisplatin in a recently activated GOG study in patients with optimally debulked, stage III disease (GOG-172).

The SWOG currently is developing a replacement study for SWOG-9619. The follow-up study will utilize 135 mg/m^2 paclitaxel by 24-h iv infusion on d 1–2 + 100 mg/m^2 cisplatin ip on d 2 + 60 mg/m^2 paclitaxel ip and 30 mg/m^2 liposomal encapsulated doxorubicin iv on d 8 *(see* Fig. 4 for study schema).

3. IP CHEMOTHERAPY FOR CONSOLIDATION OF PATHOLOGICALLY PROVEN CR AFTER SECOND-LOOK SURGERY (INT-0083/SWOG-8790/GOG-133)

INT-0083, a Randomized Trial of Adjuvant IP α-Interferon in Stage III Ovarian Carcinoma in Patients Who Have No Evidence of Disease After Surgery and Chemotherapy, was activated by SWOG in March, 1988 *(see* Fig. 5 for study schema). The study was developed to determine if ip interferon-α (IFN-α) consolidation therapy can reduce the approx 50% relapse rate in patients who have no pathologic evidence of disease

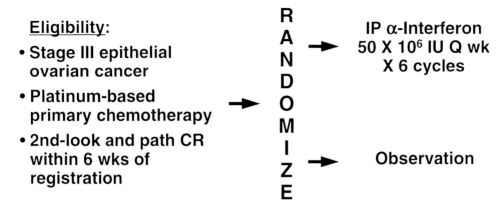

Fig. 5. Study schema for INT-0083/SWOG-8790/GOG-133, A Randomized Trial of Adjuvant IP α-Interferon in Stage III Ovarian Carcinoma in Patients Who Have No Evidence of Disease After Surgery and Chemotherapy.

at second-look surgery. Unfortunately, accrual to this study was inadequate, and it was closed in June, 1999. To be eligible, patients were required to have a histologically confirmed diagnosis of stage III EOC, been optimally debulked at their initial exploratory laparotomy, and were found to be free of disease at second-look surgery, after completion of one primary chemotherapy regimen with a cumulative cisplatin dose of ≥400 mg/m^2 or a cumulative carboplatin dose of ≥1200 mg/m^2, or AUC ≥20 mg × min/mL (other chemotherapeutic agents, including paclitaxel, may have been administered during primary chemotherapy). Patients were randomly assigned to either observation only or ip IFN-α2b recombinant 50×10^6 IU, administered weekly for 6 consecutive weeks.

4. IP THERAPY FOR PATIENTS WHO RESPONDED TO PRIMARY CHEMOTHERAPY, BUT HAVE MINIMAL RESIDUAL DISEASE AT SECOND-LOOK SURGERY (SWOG-8835)

SWOG-8835, a Randomized Phase II Study of IP Mitoxantrone versus IP Floxuridine (FUDR) in Ovarian Cancer Patients with Minimal Residual Disease After Second-Look Surgery, evaluated ip chemotherapy in patients with stage II or III EOC, who had completed initial platinum-based chemotherapy and were found to have residual disease at second-look surgery (*see* Fig. 6 for study schemas; *12*). To be eligible, patients were required to have ≤1 cm residual disease at the completion of the second-look surgery, and no extraperitoneal disease. Prior to randomization, patients were stratified on the basis of amount of residual disease (microscopic to 0.5 vs >0.5–1 cm) and serum CA-125 level (≤35 vs >35 U/mL). Patients were randomly assigned to either ip 3 gm FUDR (total dose)/d for 3 consecutive d, every 3 wk for six cycles, or MTZ. Initially, the MTZ dosing schedule was 20 mg/m^2 every 3 wk for six cycles, but, after an unacceptable level of severe abdominal pain in the first six patients treated on this arm, the MTZ dosing schedule was changed to 10 mg/m^2 every 2 wk for nine courses. It is important to note that this phase II randomized study was not designed to compare the study arms, but rather the primary goal of the study was to select the most promising of the two regimens for future phase III trials.

A total of 67 eligible patients were registered to SWOG-8835 between December 1988 and January 1994, with 39 evaluable patients on the MTZ arm and 28 on the FUDR arm. The results from both efficacy and toxicity analyses selected FUDR as the

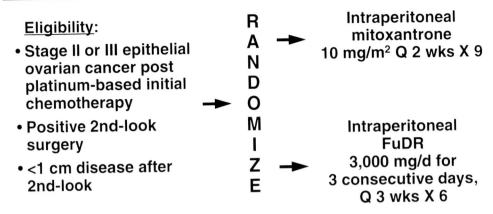

Fig. 6. Study schema for SWOG-8835, A Randomized Phase II Study of IP Mitoxantrone versus IP Floxuridine (FUDR) in Ovarian Cancer Patients with Minimal Residual Disease After Second-Look Surgery.

Table 5
Survival of Evaluable[a] Patients Enrolled in SWOG-8835

	IP MTZ (n = 39)	IP FUDR (n = 28)
Median progression-free survival (mo)	11	25
Median overall survival (mo)	21	38

[a]Eligible and received study therapy.
Data from ref. *12*.

most promising agent. Patients on the FUDR arm had a median progression-free survival of 25 mo, and median overall survival of 38 mo (progression-free and overall survival on the mitoxantrone arm were 11 and 21 mo, respectively) (Table 5). In addition to treatment assignment, the serum CA-125 level at the time of study entry appeared to be significantly associated with survival: Thirty-eight study patients with a serum CA-125 ≤35 U/mL had a median survival of 36 mo, compared to a median survival of 20 mo in 29 patients with a CA-125 >35 U/mL.

IP FUDR was tolerated better than ip MTZ therapy. Twelve patients (31%) on the MTZ arm discontinued treatment early, because of complications associated with ip therapy and/or gastrointestinal symptoms (pain, adhesions, nausea, vomiting, bowel obstruction, and vaginal spasm); 3 patients (11%) discontinued FUDR because of catheter-induced adhesions and pain. As shown in Table 6, grade 3/4 toxicities on the MTZ arm were abdominal pain (23%), infection (5%), nausea/vomiting (5%), diarrhea (3%), fever (3%), anemia (5%), and neutropenia (3%). Grade 3/4 toxicities on the FUDR arm were abdominal pain (14%), nausea/vomiting (14%), diarrhea (11%), headache (4%), infection (4%), mucositis (4%), neutropenia (18%), leukopenia (11%), thrombocytopenia (11%), and anemia (7%). Although the degree of bone marrow suppression on the FUDR arm appeared greater, it did not compromise the ability to deliver the nine cycles of the planned therapy.

Although the results of SWOG-8835 are promising, phase III study is needed to define the role of ip FUDR in the treatment of patients with minimal residual disease OC.

Table 6
Percent of ≥Grade 3 Toxicities
During Treatment on SWOG-8835

	IP MTZ (%)	IP FUDR (%)
Hematologic toxicities		
Anemia	5	7
Neutropenia	3	18
Leukopenia	0	11
Thrombocytopenia	0	11
Nonhematologic toxicities		
Abdominal pain	23	14
Diarrhea	3	11
Fever	3	0
Headache	0	4
Infection	5	4
Mucositis	0	4
Nausea/vomiting	5	14

Adapted with permission from ref. *12*.

5. DISCUSSION

IP cisplatin therapy for advanced EOC has been studied carefully in a series of preclinical studies and phase I, II, and III clinical trials. In the 1970s, Dedrick et al. *(5)* established the pharmacokinetic basis for ip chemotherapy by showing that ip administration of a cytotoxic agent in a large volume of fluid can achieve high drug concentrations within the ip space. In phase I and pharmacokinetic studies during the 1980s, Howell et al. *(6)* documented a ≥12–15-fold pharmacokinetic advantage for cisplatin, when administered by the ip route to OC patients. In the late 1980s, multiple researchers, including Howell and Markman *(13–16)*, demonstrated a >30% surgically verified response rate to salvage ip cisplatin therapy. In the mid-1990s, the results of a large phase III trial (Intergroup-0051) *(3)* documented a significant survival advantage and an improved toxicity profile with ip administration of cisplatin as primary chemotherapy for stage III, optimal disease OC. Initial results of a second phase III trial, GOG-114/SWOG-9227/ECOG-GO114, demonstrated disease-free and overall survival advantages in OC patients randomized to two courses of high-dose iv carboplatin, followed by six courses of iv pacitaxel and ip cisplatin *(4)*.

Phase I/II studies of ip paclitaxel have documented a profound ip pharmacokinetic advantage and high pathologically proven CR rates (in patients with only microscopic ip disease after second-look surgery) *(8,9)*. Accordingly, ip paclitaxel was incorporated into a primary chemotherapy regimen in a phase II study conducted by the SWOG, ECOG, and NCIC (SWOG-9619). Efficacy analysis is pending, but the regimen was well tolerated with respect to both myelosuppressive and nonmyelosuppressive toxicities. As a result, the GOG has initiated a definitive phase III trial of this experimental regimen vs iv paclitaxel-iv cisplatin, in stage III, optimal disease patients (GOG-172). Furthermore, the SWOG soon will initiate a phase II trial in which iv liposomal encapsulated doxorubicin (30 mg/m^2 iv on d 8) will be added to the SWOG-9619 regimen.

IP therapy also has been studied as a consolidation regimen in stage III OC patients who achieve a pathologic CR to primary chemotherapy (INT-0083/SWOG-8790/GOG-133). IP interferon-α has proven active as consolidation therapy in patients with minimal (i.e., <0.5 cm) residual ip tumor plaques after second-look surgery, with surgically documented response rates of >30% in at least one phase II study *(17)*. Unfortunately, despite these results and the recent positive results of other studies of ip therapy discussed in this review, INT-0083 was recently closed due to poor accrual.

Patients with an incomplete response to primary chemotherapy may also benefit from ip chemotherapy. SWOG-8835 documented that ip FUDR is well tolerated, can be administered in an outpatient setting, and may have important activity *(12)*. Its role in treating OC remains to be determined in a definitive phase III study.

The SWOG and other cooperative study groups continue to evaluate ip chemotherapy in the treatment of stage III, optimally debulked EOC. New agents, such as topotecan, irinotecan, gemcitabine, and docetaxel, undoubtedly will be considered for future phase I/II studies. However, considerable phase III clinical trials data from the SWOG and GOG have established ip cisplatin and ip paclitaxel as active therapies to be examined further in ongoing cooperative group studies.

REFERENCES

1. Parker SL, Tong T, Bolden S, and Wingo PA. Cancer statistics 1999, *CA Cancer J. Clin.,* **49** (1999) 8–31.
2. Nye EB. Ovarian carcinoma: improvement in survival time after chemotherapy, *J. Obstet. Gynaecol. Br. Commonw.,* **79** (1972) 550–554.
3. Alberts DS, Liu PY, Hannigan EV, et al. Intraperitoneal cisplatin plus intravenous cyclophosphamide versus intravenous cisplatin plus intravenous cyclophosphamide for stage III ovarian cancer, *N. Engl. J. Med.,* **335** (1996) 1950–1955.
4. Markman M, Bundy B, Benda J, et al. Randomized phase II study of intravenous (IV) cispatin (CIS)/ paclitaxel (PAC) versus moderately high dose IV carboplatin (CARB) followed by IV PAC and intraperitoneal (IP) CIS in optimal residual ovarian cancer (OC): an intergroup trial (GOG, SWOG, ECOG), *Proc. Am. Soc. Clin. Oncol.,* **17** (1998) 361a.
5. Dedrick RL, Myers CE, Bungay PM, De Vita VT Jr. Pharmacokinetic rationale for peritoneal drug administration in the treatment of ovarian cancer, *Cancer Treat. Rep.,* **62** (1978) 1–11.
6. Howell SB, Pfeifle CL, Wung WE, et al. Intraperitoneal cisplatin with systemic thiosulfate protection, *Ann. Intern. Med.,* **97** (1982) 845–851.
7. Goel R, Cleary SM, Horton C, et al. Effect of sodium thiosulfate on the pharmacokinetics and toxicity of cisplatin, *J. Nat. Cancer Inst.,* **81** (1989) 1552–1560.
8. Markman M, Rowinsky E, Hakes T, et al. Phase I trial of intraperitoneal Taxol: a Gynecologic Oncology Group Study, *J. Clin. Oncol.,* **10** (1992) 1485–1491.
9. Francis P, Rowinsky E, Schneider J, et al. Phase I feasibility and pharmacologic study of weeky intraperitoneal paclitaxel: a Gynecologic Oncology Group Study, *J. Clin. Oncol.,* **13** (1995) 2961–2967.
10. Early Breast Cancer Trialists' Collaborative Group. Systemic treatment of early breast cancer by hormonal, cytotoxic, or immune therapy. 133 randomized trials involving 31,000 recurrences and 24,000 deaths in 75,000 women, *Lancet,* **339** (1992) 1–15.
11. Early Breast Cancer Trialists' Collaborative Group. Systemic treatment of early breast cancer by hormonal, cytotoxic, or immune therapy. 133 randomized trials involving 31,000 recurrences and 24,000 deaths in 75,000 women, *Lancet,* **339** (1992) 71–85.
12. Muggia FM, Liu PY, Alberts DS, et al. Intraperitoneal mitoxantrone or floxuridine: effects on time to failure and survival in patients with minimal residual ovarian cancer after second-look laparotomy: a randomized phase II study by the Southwest Oncology Group, *Gynecol. Oncol.,* **61** (1996) 395–402.
13. Howell SB, Zimm S, Markman M, et al. Long-term survival of advanced refractory ovarian carcinoma patients with small-volume disease treated with intraperitoneal chemotherapy, *J. Clin. Oncol.,* **5** (1987) 1607–1612.
14. Kirmani S, Lucas WE, Kim S, et al. Phase II trial of intraperitoneal cisplatin and etoposide as salvage treatment for minimal residual ovarian carcinoma, *J. Clin. Oncol.,* **9** (1991) 649–657.

15. Reichman B, Markman M, Hakes T, et al. Intraperitoneal cisplatin and etoposide in the treatment of refractory/recurrent ovarian carcinoma, *J. Clin. Oncol.,* **7** (1989) 1327–1332.
16. Markman M. Current status of intraperitoneal therapy for ovarian cancer, *Curr. Opinion Obstet. Gynecol.,* **5** (1993) 99–104.
17. Berek JS, Stonebraker B, Lentz SS, et al. Intraperitoneal alpha-interferon in residual ovarian carcinoma: a phase II Gynecologic Oncology Group study, *Proc. Am. Soc. Clin. Oncol.,* **17** (1998) 358a.

12 Intraperitoneal Biologic Therapy for Ovarian Cancer

John C. Elkas, Oliver Dorigo, and Jonathan S. Berek

CONTENTS

1. INTRODUCTION

Epithelial ovarian carcinoma (EOC) is the leading cause of death from gynecologic malignancies in the United States, and is the fourth most common cause of cancer death in women. It is estimated that one in 70 women will develop ovarian cancer (OC) in her lifetime, and one in 100 will die of this disease. Although OC is sensitive to a variety of chemotherapeutic agents, the 5-yr survival for advanced disease remains only about 20%. Because of the poor long-term survival for advanced OC, investigators have sought to develop novel biologic therapies to combat this disease. Biologic therapies produce antitumor effects through the activation of the host's natural defense mechanisms. This may be particularly important in advanced OC, in which patients have been shown to be significantly immunocompromised *(1)*. Unfortunately, the initial trials of systemic biologic agents failed to elicit consistent responses in patients with OC.

The concept of the regional administration of drugs is appealing in patients whose tumors are confined to, and have not yet metastasized beyond, a definable body space, such as the peritoneal cavity. OC has been treated in a number of clinical trials with intraperitoneal (ip) cytotoxic chemotherapeutic agents, and has yielded a 20–30% complete response (CR) rate in patients with small-volume disease, after systemically administered chemotherapy *(2)*. Agents chosen for ip chemotherapy have a pharmacokinetic advantage when placed in the peritoneal cavity (i.e., a high peritoneal-plasma ratio, based on their mol wt and lipid solubility) and a steep dose–response curve, making them ideal agents for regional administration. Although the rationale for ip cytotoxic chemotherapy is based on the belief that a higher concentration of a drug

From: *Current Clinical Oncology: Regional Chemotherapy: Clinical Research and Practice*
Edited by: M. Markman © Humana Press Inc., Totowa, NJ

Table 1
Biological Response Modifiers

Group	Example
1. Microorganism	Bacille Calmette-Guérin, *Corynebacterium parvum,* attenuated *Streptococcus* (OK-432)
2. Chemically identified compounds from natural resources	Keyhole limpet hemocyanin, liposome-encapsulated muramyl tripeptide, Group B *Streptococcus* toxin, Diphtheria toxin fusion protein, Retinoic acid, β-carotene, Vitamin C
3. Polypeptides	Granulocyte-macrophage colony-stimulating factors (GM-CSF) and cytokines (interleukin-2 [IL-2], interferon-α [IFN-α], IFN-γ, tumor necrosis factor [TNF])
4. Synthetic compounds	Dexamethasone, monoclonal antibodies
5. Vaccines/gene therapy	IL-2 gene-modified tumor cell vaccines, herpes simplex virus-thymidine kinase (HSV-TK)/Gancyclovir suicide gene therapy, *p53* tumor suppressor gene therapy

Adapted with permission from *ref. 3.*

can be brought into direct contact with tumor cells, with subsequent increased concentration of agents in tumors, it is postulated that ip biologic therapy can activate regional mechanisms in the peritoneal cavity, leading to tumor lysis, with minimal systemic sequelae. Thus, regional biologic therapy could prove efficacious, even when previous intravenous (iv) treatment has been ineffective.

Recent advances in molecular biology, immunology, and cytokine biology have led to the availability of many new, promising regional biologic agents for the treatment of OC. Biologic response modifiers, including microorganisms, cytokines, monoclonal antibodies (MAbs), and activated lymphocytes, have been used to exert either direct antitumor responses or to activate components of the immune system to elicit tumoricidal activity (Table 1). In addition, advances in gene therapy using various vectors to deliver cytokines or tumor suppressor genes to malignant cells in the peritoneal cavity have led to the development of novel therapeutic approaches.

2. GENERAL CONCEPTS OF IMMUNOTHERAPY

2.1. Immunologic Mechanisms Involved in Control of Tumor Growth

Cellular and humoral immune mechanisms that are involved in control of tumor growth include cytotoxic T-cells, natural killer (NK) cells, macrophages, or lymphokine-activated killer (LAK) cells, and antibody-dependent cellular cytotoxicity (ADCC) mediated by complement activation *(4,5).* The interactions between the different components of the immune system are complex and not fully understood. However, a number of immune-mediated antitumor mechanisms have been well characterized, and are being applied to the development of biologic therapies for cancer.

2.2. T-Cells

T-lymphocytes have an integral role in the generation of immune responses, by acting as helper cells in both humoral and cellular immune systems. T-cell precursors originate in bone marrow and migrate to the thymus, where they mature into functional

T-cells. During this thymic maturation. T-cells learn to recognize antigen in the context of the major histocompatibility type of the individual.

T-cells can be distinguished from other types of lymphocytes by their cell-surface phenotype, as well as by differences in their biologic functions. Mature T-cells express the CD3 molecule and the T-cell antigen receptor, which is found in close association with the CD3 complex *(6,7)*. T-cells recognize antigen via the T-cell antigen receptor *(8)*. Its structure and molecular organization is similar to antibody molecules, which are the B-cell receptors for antigen.

There are two major subsets of mature T-cells, which are phenotypically and functionally distinct: T-helper/inducer cells, which express the CD4 cell-surface marker, and T-suppressor/cytotoxic cells, which express the CD8 marker *(9)*. The expression of these markers is acquired during the passage of T-cells through the thymus. CD8+ T-cells include cells that are cytotoxic and possess the ability to kill target cells bearing appropriate antigens. The CD8 T-cell subset also contains suppressor T-cells. Suppressor T-cells are cells are able to inhibit the biologic functions of B-cells or other T-cells.

Cytotoxic T-cells can be involved in antitumor responses *(10)*. These cells are able to recognize antigens on tumor cells via their antigen-specific T-cell receptor, stimulating a cascade of events that ultimately results in the lysis of the tumor cell. The ability of cytotoxic T-cells to kill tumor cells in vitro is most commonly measured by the release of ^{51}Cr from isotope-labeled target cells.

2.3. Natural Killer Cells

NK cells represent a subset of lymphocytes that share common cell-surface markers (CD56) with T-cells. NK cells characteristically have a large granular lymphocyte morphology *(11)*. NK cells can recognize and lyse tumor cells in vitro. NK activity is an innate form of immunity that does not require an adaptive memory response for optimal biologic function. NK antitumor activity can be augmented by exposure to several agents, especially cytokines like interleukin-2 (IL-2). Furthermore, ADCC can be elicited by NK-like cells, resulting in the lysis of tumor cells. The mechanisms of tumor cell killing in ADCC are not clearly understood, although close cellular contact between the ADCC effector cell and the target cell appears to be required.

2.4. Macrophages

Monocytes and macrophages are myeloid cells that play an important role in both innate and adaptive immune responses. As professional antigen-presenting cells, macrophages take up foreign antigen, process the antigen, and present it, in conjunction with major histocompatibility complex (MHC) molecules, to T-cells *(12,13)*. Helper/inducer (CD4) T-cells, bearing a T-cell receptor of appropriate antigen and self-specificity, are activated by antigen-presenting macrophages, and stimulated to produce certain cytokines like IL-2. In addition to their role as antigen-presenting cells, macrophages can play an important role in innate responses, by ingesting and killing microorganisms, or by becoming activated against tumor cells.

2.5. Adoptive Immunotherapy:
LAK Cells and Tumor-Infiltrating Lymphocytes

Exposure of peripheral blood monoclonal cells to IL-2 or other cytokines in vitro leads to the generation of cytotoxic effector cells called LAK cells *(14)*. These cells are effective cytotoxic cells for a variety of tumor cells, including tumor cells resistant to NK-cell or T-cell-mediated lysis. Tumor-infiltrating lymphocytes (TIL) can be isolated from tumors, and expanded in vitro by exposure to IL-2, to obtain tumor-specific cytotoxic cells.

2.6. Antitumor and Biologic Effects of Cytokines

Various cytokines appear to have antitumor effects in vitro and in vivo. However, in many instances, it has been difficult to discern whether these effects are the direct result of a cytokine-mediated antitumor effect or an indirect effect induced in some manner by cytokine exposure, such as activation of immune effector cells, or the induction of the secretion of other cytokines. Clearly, some cytokines, such as tumor necrosis factor (TNF), can have potent direct antitumor cytotoxic effects. Other cytokines, including some interferons (IFNs), may inhibit tumor growth by cytostatic and cytotoxic effects (Table 2).

3. NONSPECIFIC IMMUNOMODULATORS

3.1. Microorganisms

Early experimental biologic therapy for advanced-stage OC involved the use of microorganisms. *Corynebacterium parvum* was one of the original agents used for ip biologic therapy in OC. *C. parvum* is a heat-killed, Gram-negative anaerobic bacillus that induces a variety of immune responses. *C. parvum* can modulate biological mechanisms, and influence cellular responses to different stimuli. Exposure to *C. parvum* can also elicit various nonspecific immune responses, including an acute inflammatory response, predominantly through the induction and infiltration of neutrophils, attraction, activation, and cytotoxicity of macrophages, and enhanced cytotoxicity of NK cells and T-lymphocytes *(15,16)*.

Although iv treatment of OC patients with *C. parvum* failed to demonstrate antitumor responses, ip administration was efficacious. Studies by Berek et al. *(17)* and Bast et al. *(18)* reported a total of 21 patients treated with ip *C. parvum*. All patients had been treated with combination cytotoxic chemotherapy prior to biologic therapy. Of the 19 evaluable patients, there were six responders, including two CRs; all responding patients had macroscopic disease of less than 5 mm at the initiation of therapy. The most common initial side effect was abdominal pain (91%).

IP *C. parvum* has also been used for the palliation of ascites in OC patients. In a trial by Montovani et al. *(19)*, administration of ip *C. parvum* resulted in complete resolution of ascites in 3 of 8 patients, and a marked reduction in two others *(19)*. The palliative effect was sustained for 6–13 mo. Lichtenstein et al. *(20)* characterized the peritoneal exudates of OC patients treated intraperitoneally with *C. parvum*, and noted a predominance of neutrophils at 48 hr, and lymphocytes and macrophages at 7 and 14 d after injection. Peritoneal NK cytotoxicity increased during treatment in 6 of 9 patients tested. In addition, the increase of cytotoxic effectors, such as ADCC, in the peritoneal cavity correlated with the clinical response to the agent.

Although active in the treatment of OC, *C. parvum* did lead to significant morbidity through the induction of a profound local inflammatory reaction, including marked peritoneal fibrosis. This toxicity precluded more widespread testing, but the intense local inflammatory reaction may have been responsible for the killing and rejection of tumor cells by the intense, nonspecific activation of peritoneal immune cells.

Table 2
Cytokines

Cytokine	Biological activities
IL-1α, IL-β	↑ Stimulation of T-cells (cofactor), ↑ IL-2 production, ↑ IL-2 receptor expression, ↑ activity of macrophages and endothelial cells, ↑ acute-phase responses, ↑ catabolic processes, ↑ inflammation
IL-2	↑ Stimulation T-cells, ↑ cytotoxic T-lymphocyte (CTL) responses, ↑ growth and differentiation of B-cells, ↑ monocyte/macrophage activity
IL-3	↑ Early progenitor cell growth, ↑ growth of mature inducer cells, ↑ mast cell growth
IL-4	↑ CTL differentiation, ↑ growth of TILs, ↑ IL-2-induced LAK activity, ↑ colony growth with other factors, ↑ proliferation of activated B-cells
IL-5	↑ CTL differentiation, ↑ IL-2 receptor expression on T- and B-cells, ↑ IL-2-mediated LAK activity, ↑ proliferation and differentiation of eosinophilic precursors, ↑ immunoglobulin A (IgA) and IgM secretion by B-cells
IL-6	↑ Stimulation of T-cells, ↑ IL-2 production, ↑ CTL differentiation, ↑ NK and LAK cytotoxicity, ↑ MHC class I expression, ↑ carcinoembryonic antigen (CEA) expression, Ig secretion by B-cells, ↓ apoptosis of OC cells
IL-7	↑ Stimulation of T-cells in presence of co-stimulatory factors, ↑ LAK activity, ↑ generation and expansion of CTLs, ↑ cytokine secretion and antitumor activity of human monocytes
IL-8	Chemotactic factor for neutrophils, T- and B-cells, monocytes
IL-9	↑ Antigen specific T-helper cell clone stimulation, ↑ mast cell growth, ↑ IL-4-induced IgE synthesis by B-cells
IL-10	↓ Cytokine synthesis of T-helper cells, ↓ macrophage activity, ↓ monocyte-dependent stimulation of NK cell production of IFN-γ, ↑ T-cell precursors, ↑ CTL activity, ↑ MHC class II expression on B-cells
IL-11	↑ T-cell-dependent development of B-cells, ↑ megakaryocyte colony formation with IL-3
IL-12	↑ Stimulation of T-helper and T-killer cells independent of IL-2, ↑ induction of CTLs with IL-2, ↑ NK activity, ↑ IFN-γ production by resting B-cells
IL-13	↑ Stimulation, proliferation, and differentiation of human B-cells, ↑ IgE synthesis, ↑ MHC II expression on B-cells
IL-14	↑ B-cell proliferation, inhibits Ig secretion by B-cells
IL-15	↑ Stimulation of activated T-cells, ↑ generation of cytolytic cells and LAK cells
IL-16	Produced by mast cells, activates CD4+ T-cells
IL-17	↑ Secretion of cytokines (IL-6, IL-8, GM-CSF) from epithelial, endothelial, and fibroblastic cells; sustained proliferation of CD34+ cells
IL-18	Induces IFN-γ production from anti-CD3 activated T-helper cells (Th1) cells, ↑ Fas ligand expression, ↑ NK cell activity in vivo
G-CSF	↑ Growth of granulocyte colonies, ↑ activation mature granulocytes, ↑ proliferation of leukemic cells
GM-CSF	↑ Growth of granulocytes, monocytes, early erythrocyte progenitors, ↑ ADCC, ↑ activation of mature granulocytes and monocytes, ↑ chemotaxis for monocytes, ↑ production of M-CSF and TNF by monocytes
M-CSF	↑ Growth of monocyte colonies, ↑ survival of macrophages, ↑ ADCC by monocytes, ↑ production of cytokines, plasminogen activator oxygen reduction products, ↑ expression of Fc receptors, and MHC class II expression on macrophages
IFN-α	↓ Proliferation of certain tumor cells, ↓ viral proliferation, ↑ expression of Fc receptors, tumor-associated antigen, and MHC class I expression, ↑ NK activity, ↓ suppressor T-cell activity

(continued)

Table 2
(continued)

Cytokine	Biological activities
IFN-γ	↓ Viral proliferation, ↑ NK activity, ↑ expression of MHC class I and II, ↑ activation of macrophages, ↑ IL-2 receptor expression, ↑ Ig production by B-cells, ↑ CTL activation, ↑ expression of tumor-associated antigen
TNF	↑ T-cell proliferation, ↑ NK activity, ↑ macrophage activity, directly cytotoxic to tumor cells, ↑ acute-phase responses, ↑ expression of MHC I and II, ↑ production of other cytokines, cytokine receptor expression, mediates catabolic processes, septic shock, and inflammation

Another microorganism that has been used intraperitoneally as an nonspecific immunomodulator in the treatment of OC is the bacille Calmette-Guérin vaccine (BCG). BCG has been used in combination with attenuated *Streptococcus* (OK-432) for advanced OC by Ohkawa et al. *(21)*. OK-432 is an immunomodulator derived from a nonvirulent strain of type 3, group A *Streptococcus pyogenes*. These agents were administered intraperitoneally for 4 consecutive days, with weekly ip injections of doxorubicin, 5-fluorouracil, Endoxan, bleomycin, and mitomycin C. Although this was an uncontrolled study, the 60 evaluable patients treated had a 5-yr survival of 40%.

OK-432 has also been used singly in the treatment of OC. Kawagoe et al. *(22)* treated 12 patients, who had advanced OC with ascites, with ip OK-432, and noted complete resolution of ascites within 17 d after ip administration of OK-432. In addition, OK-432 prevented the reappearance of ascites for the study duration. The investigators postulated that regional administration of OK-432, unlike systemic therapy, promotes tumor cell lysis by local stimulation of T-cells and macrophages, and augmentation of NK cell activity in the peritoneal cavity. Koelbl et al. *(23)* also used ip OK-432 in 10 patients with advanced chemotherapy resistant OC. A CR was achieved in four patients for 14 mo (± 8.9 mo), and a partial response (PR) was seen in three patients for 2 mo (± 0.3 mo).

3.2. Cytokines

3.2.1. INTERFERON-a

IFN-α is capable of augmenting the cytotoxicity of autologous peripheral blood mononuclear cells to cancer cells *(24,25)*. The mechanism of action of IFN-α was thought to result from augmentation of NK cytotoxicity, which has been shown to be associated with tumor rejection. However, in clinical trials, augmentation of NK activity was not invariably associated with response to therapy. In vitro data suggests that the dominant mechanism for tumor cell lysis in the peritoneal cavity involves the direct effect of IFN on cancer cells, as is seen with cytotoxic chemotherapeutic agents *(26)*.

Recombinant human interferon-α (rhIFN-α) has been used in multiple clinical trials for OC. In phase II trials, systemic rhIFN-α has produced responses in only 10% in patients with advanced OC, and with significant systemic sequelae *(27)*. In contrast, ip rhIFN-α has produced higher response rates, and demonstrated only dose-dependent toxicity. Berek et al. *(28)* found that administration of ip rhIFN-α (25–50 million U), 3×/wk, was not tolerated, because of persistent general malaise, fever, and gastrointestinal toxicity. However, treatment with the same dose once a week was tolerated for 8–16 consecutive wk. Moore et al. *(29)*, in a Gynecologic Oncology Group (GOG) study, also noted a dose-dependent toxicity of ip IFN-α, with the maximum tolerated dose of 20×10^6 U on d 1 and 8 of a 21-d cisplatin-based chemotherapy cycle. In these studies, there was a paucity of significant neurotoxicity and renal toxicity. Most of the side effects of single-agent rhIFN-α appear to be complementary with cisplatin, but the general malaise and gastrointestinal toxicity produced by both may be additive when these agents are combined.

IP rhIFN-α has been most effective in OC patients with small-volume residual disease, i.e., microscopic disease or tumor nodules less than 5 mm, which persists after first-line chemotherapy. In the above-described study by Berek et al. *(28),* 14 patients with persistent EOC were treated with ip IFN-α at doses between 5×10^6 and 5×10^7 U over 4 wk, and then continued weekly for a total of 16 wk *(28).* Eleven patients underwent surgical reevaluation after therapy, which confirmed four pathological CRs (36%), one PR (9%), and disease progression in six patients (55%). Five of seven patients (71%) with residual tumor less than 5 mm had a surgically documented response; there was no response in the four patients whose tumors were greater than, or equal to, 5 mm.

Willemse et al. *(30)* reported a trial of ip rhIFN-α in 20 patients with advanced OC. Of 17 who had a reassessment laparotomy, five (29%) had CRs and four (24%) had PRs. Responses in both studies were confined to patients with minimal residual disease. The toxicity encountered in this trial was similar to that seen by Berek et al. *(28).* Overall, 28 surgically evaluated patients were treated in these two trials, with 14 (50%) PRs and nine (32%) CRs. All of the responding patients had microscopic or small-volume (less than 5 mm) residual disease. Therefore, the combined surgically defined CR rate in patients with minimal residual disease was 50% (9 of 18 patients). This data suggests that administration of ip rhIFN-α can result in regional control of small-volume disease confined to the peritoneal cavity. However, survival data are not available for these patients, so it is unclear whether ip rhIFN-α treatment can produce prolonged progression-free intervals.

There has been substantial in vitro evidence to suggest a synergy between IFN-α and standard cytotoxic agents (anthracyclines, actinomycin-D, vinca alkaloids, 5-fluorouracil, mitomycin, and cisplatin) *(31).* This synergy is seen only when tumor cells are exposed to IFN-α before the cytotoxic agent. Recent clinical trials have tested the synergy between cisplatin and ip IFN-α. In a multicenter phase I study, Berek et al. *(32)* showed that combined ip therapy with cisplatin and rhIFN-α can be administered safely to patients with residual OC after systemic chemotherapy. The maximum tolerated doses of the combination were 25×10^6 IU of rhIFN-α and 60 mg/m^2 of cisplatin. The therapy was best tolerated when given as one cycle every 3 wk. Of the eight patients who were treated with this dose, the median number of treatment cycles was six courses. Two CRs were noted after five and six treatment cycles, respectively, and PRs were seen in patients treated with four and eight cycles, respectively.

Nardi et al. *(33)* reported treatment with alternating weekly doses of 50 million U of ip rhIFN-α and 90 mg/m^2 cisplatin. In this trial, the surgically documented CR rate was 50% (7 of 14 patients); these responses were again confined to patients who started their treatment with microscopic or minimal residual disease (<5 mm). The toxicity was similar to that seen in the phase I and II trials of IFN-α alone. Therefore, the combination of ip cisplatin and IFN-α appeared to be tolerated in these patients, and resulted in a favorable response rate. The survival time of patients who had a CR was longer than that of patients who were nonresponsive. However, response rates were similar to those reported in other series of single-agent ip cisplatin administration, so that it was unclear whether the addition of IFN-α had any additive effect on the response rate.

Stuart et al. *(34)* used ip IFN-α alone in an effort to relieve symptoms of ascites in OC patients. Five of 10 patients reported symptomatic improvement of 2–7 wk duration, and toxicity was minimal at a dose of 10×10^6 U/m². Maenpaa et al. *(35)* combined ip IFN-α (20–50 million U) with mitoxantrone (20–50 mg) in patients with recurrent OC with ascites. Of 19 patients, one had a CR and seven had a PR, with a mean duration of response of 5 mo. With those results, Bezwoda et al. *(36)* treated patients for malignant ascites, with advanced OC, with ip rhIFN-α, some in combination with cisplatin. Seven responses were seen among 19 patients (36%) treated, and the combination of IFN-α and cisplatin produced a higher response rate than IFN-α alone: 5 of 7 patients (77%) who were treated with the combination responded, and 2 of 9 (22%), who were treated with cisplatin only, responded. Those authors concluded that the antitumor effect of cisplatin can be augmented by concomitant exposure to IFN-α. Furthermore, the clinical responses correlated with synergy between these two agents in vitro; thus, the antitumor effect of IFN-α is probably related to the direct inhibitory effect of the molecule, and not to immune modulation.

Frasci et al. *(37)* reported a trial of 41 patients with advanced OC, who were treated with an ip regimen of four cycles of cisplatin (75 mg/m²), mitoxantrone (20 mg/m²), and rhIFN-α (30 million U/m²). All patients had less than 2 cm residual disease after systemic cisplatin-based chemotherapy. Pathological CR was achieved in 23 of 37 (62%) evaluable patients. The 4-yr disease-free survival was 50%, and no relapse occurred after 32 mo. These observations again suggest that the combination of cytotoxic chemotherapy and ip IFN-α may be beneficial in advanced OC cancer, especially in patients with small-volume residual disease localized to the peritoneal cavity.

Contrastingly, when combined ip rhIFN-α and cisplatin treatment was tested by the GOG, a low response rate (7%) was seen *(38)*. This poor outcome is in contradiction to other phase I and II trials of cisplatin and ip IFN-α therapy in patients with persistent small-volume residual OC, in which response rates of 20–50% have been noted. However, similar findings were noted by the Italian North West Oncology Group *(39)*, who randomized patients to receive either three courses of ip carboplatinum or ip carboplatinum and IFN-α. They did not note any benefit with the addition of IFN-α therapy. These differences can probably be accounted for by the fact that, in these series, most evaluable patients had cisplatin-resistant disease, with maximum tumor sizes often larger than 5 mm. Further studies are currently ongoing, to assess the role of IFN-α in the treatment of OC.

3.2.2. INTERFERON-γ

Recombinant human interferon-γ (rhIFN-γ), like IFN-α, has been shown to have direct antitumor effects in vitro *(40)*. Because of its ability to activate the immune system, and its direct antitumor effects, IFN-γ has been evaluated in the treatment of OC. In a phase I trial, D'Acquisto et al. *(41)* treated 27 patients who had refractory OC with ip rhIFN-γ. IFN-γ was well tolerated when given weekly, and was associated with a 150–200-fold higher ip concentration, compared with systemic delivery. The major toxicity was fatigue and flu-like symptoms, with limited local toxicity at the highest dose level tested (8 million IU/m²). Similarly, Marth et al. *(42)* also conducted a phase I trial of ip IFN-γ and found a flu-like syndrome and fatigue to be the dose-limiting side effects. IFN-γ was also found to induce local macrophage activity, and to increase serum, urine, and ascites neopterin levels.

In a cooperative European trial, 40 patients, who had residual OC after initial cisplatin-based chemotherapy, were treated with ip rhIFN-γ at a dose of 20 million IU/m², twice weekly for a maximum of 4 mo *(43)*. Of the 30 evaluable patients, nine (30%) achieved a surgically defined CR. Ten of 23 patients (43%), whose largest residual tumor mass measured less than 2 cm, responded to IFN-γ therapy. Toxicity included fever, leukopenia, elevated transaminase levels, abdominal discomfort, and fatigue.

Recently, the same group reported the results of ip rhIFN-γ in 108 patients with residual disease at second-look laparotomy *(44)*. Patients were treated with 20×10^6 IU/m^2 twice a week for 3–4 mo. Of 98 assessable patients, 31 (32%) achieved a surgically documented response, including 23 patients (23%) with a CR. The median duration of response was 20 mo, and the 3-yr survival rate in responders was 62%. Side effects again included fever, flu-like syndrome, neutropenia, and liver enzyme disturbances, no significant peritoneal fibrosis was noted at reassessment laparotomy. These results have initiated plans for prospective trials of ip IFN-γ in the treatment of advanced OC.

3.2.3. TUMOR NECROSIS FACTOR-a

Recombinant human tumor necrosis factor-α (rhTNF-α) has shown significant anti-neoplastic activity in vitro and in vivo in animal models *(45)*. However, in phase I trials of systemic TNF-α, there was limited clinical activity, with considerable systemic toxicity, especially fevers, rigors, and significant hypotension *(46,47)*. As with other biologic response modifiers, it was postulated that the ip rhTNF-α would produce an increased antitumor effect and fewer systemic sequelae. In a phase I trial by Markman et al. *(48)*, rhTNF-α was administered safely when given intraperitoneally, with a marked pharmacokinetic advantage for ip administration, compared with systemic delivery. After the ip administration of 50 μg/m^2 rhTNF-α, peak TNF-α levels within the peritoneal cavity ranged from 15,000 to 59,000 pg/mL, compared with unmeasurable amounts in the systemic compartment (less than 50 pg/mL). TNF-α levels between 14,000 and 33,000 pg/mL persisted within the peritoneal cavity for as long as 6 h. Although the TNF was not detectable in plasma, patients experienced mild emesis, temperature elevations, and chills, even with ip TNF-α doses as low as 10 μg/m^2. Only one patient had a hypotensive episode, but abdominal discomfort was common. No clinical responses were observed in this trial.

TNF-α has been frequently used to control the formation of malignant ascites in OC. Kaufmann et al. *(49)* successfully treated 20 of 23 patients (87%) who had refractory recurrent malignant ascites from OC. All patients received three ip injections of 0.08–0.14 mg TNF-α/m^2. Side effects included flu-like symptoms combined with general malaise. Similarly, Raeth et al. *(50)* treated 32 patients who had symptomatic malignant ascites with a weekly infusion of rhTNF-α (80 mg/m^2). Twenty patients had OC, and 12 had several nonovarian malignancies. Patients received an average of 2.6 infusions of rhTNF-α. Of the 31 evaluable patients, 17 (55%) experienced complete resolution of ascites 30 d after the initiation of therapy, and 14 patients exhibited partial control of malignant ascites. Only one patient had a relapse during the follow-up period of approx 8 mo. The most significant side effects were fever, chills, abdominal pain, and emesis.

A randomized trial was recently concluded, based on the mounting evidence supporting the efficacy of TNF-α in reducing or eliminating malignant ascites from OC *(51)*. Thirty-nine patients with refractory malignant ascites from OC received either 0.06 mg/m^2 rhTNF-α intraperitoneally per week after paracentesis or paracentesis alone. None of the 18 evaluable patients who received rhTNF-α in conjunction with paracentesis had either a CR or PR. Side effects were consistent with those seen in previous studies.

Table 3
Clinical Trials Using IP Injection of IL-2 in OC Patients

Ref.	Treatment	Clinical response	Side effects
Beller et al. (57)	IL-2	1/8 PR	Flu-like Sx, neuropathy, anemia
Chapman et al. (58)	IL-2	3/7 NC	Hypovolemia, fever, chills, azotemia
Panici et al. (59)	IL-2	1/11 CR	Hypotension, CNS toxicity, oliguria
Edwards et al. (53)	IL-2	6/35 CR	Local-regional toxicity
		3/35 PR	
Steis et al. (55)	IL-2 + LAK	2/10 PR	Flu-like Sx, edema, ip fibrosis, anemia
Freedman et al. (56)	IL-2 + TIL	4/8 PR	Flu-like Sx, hypotension, anemia
Stewart et al. (60)	IL-2 + LAK	1/10 PR	Flu-like Sx, anemia abdominal pain
Urba et al. (54)	IL-2 + LAK	2/7 PR	IP fibrosis

NC = no change; Sx = symptoms.

This report, unlike the others cited, utilized paracentesis prior to the administration of TNF-α, and this may account for the discrepancy in results. Further studies are needed to evaluate the efficacy of this treatment for patients with malignant ascites, when alternative therapies have been ineffective. In addition, the potential of TNF to augment the antitumor effect of a cytotoxic chemotherapeutic agent offers another potential immunotherapeutic strategy. Even low doses of TNF-α can significantly augment the antitumor properties of drugs such as cisplatin, mitoxantrone, doxorubicin, and cyclophosphamide in vitro (52). Therefore, the use of ip TNF-α, administered in conjunction with cytotoxic chemotherapy, could offer a therapeutic advantage, and minimize the systemic toxicity of TNF-α immunotherapy.

3.2.4. IL-2/ADOPTIVE IMMUNOTHERAPY

IP IL-2 has been used in a number of clinical trials in OC, either alone or in conjunction with cellular immunotherapy (Table 3). Although IL-2 therapy has not resulted in prolongation of survival, a number of favorable clinical responses have been observed, including CRs. One of the most convincing studies demonstrating the antitumor effect of IL-2 is by Edwards et al. (53): Treatment of 45 patients with ip IL-2 at doses ranged from 6×10^4 to 3×10^7 IU/m^2/d. IL-2 was given with either continuous 7-d infusions, followed by 7-d intervals, or by weekly infusions over 24 h. Significant regional dose-limiting toxicity was seen with the 7-d infusions, determining the maximum tolerated dose at 600,000 IU/m^2. Weekly administration of IL-2 was tolerated significantly better. Among 35 evaluable patients, six CRs and three PRs (26% total response rate) were confirmed at reassessment laparotomy.

As noted, IL-2 has also been used in conjunction with cellular immunotherapy in the treatment of OC. Urba et al. (54) treated 12 patients, who had persistent OC or colon cancer confined to the peritoneal cavity, with ip IL-2 and autologous LAK cells. Two of six evaluable OC patients had PRs, and three of eight colon cancer patients had PRs. No CRs were documented. Similarly, Steis et al. (55) treated 22 patients who had tumors confined to the peritoneal cavity with ip IL-2 and LAK therapy, and six responses were noted. In this series, sepsis, hypotension, and peritoneal fibrosis was encountered. The LAK + IL-2-induced peritoneal fibrosis, like that seen with *C. parvum*, probably resulted from the induction of cells that promote the deposition of collagen.

More recently, Freedman et al. (56) treated eight patients with IL-2-expanded TILs + IL-2, followed by several cycles of IL-2 alone (56). Four of eight patients (50%)

had PRs to include ascites or solid tumor regression. Toxicity included one case of peritonitis and four episodes of grade 3 anemia. Although adoptive immunotherapy remains in the developmental stages, early preliminary data supports further investigation into this realm of therapy for OC.

4. SPECIFIC IMMUNOSTIMULATION

4.1. Monoclonal Antibodies

4.1.1. BISPECIFIC AND CHIMERIC ANTIBODIES

Bispecific antibodies possess two antigen recognition sites, which are usually directed against a tumor-associated antigen and an antigen on immune effector cells. The antibody links the tumor cell via the tumor-associated antigen recognition site directly to an immune effector cell. Furthermore, binding of the antibody to the immune effector cell initiates tumor lysis. MDX-210, for example, is a bispecific antibody that recognizes Fc-receptor on monocytes and macrophages, as well as the cell-surface product of the *HER-2-neu* oncogene. It has been used in a number of clinical trials as systemic, but not yet ip treatment, and found to be well tolerated and immunologically and clinically active *(61)*. Optimization of the dose and schedule of MDX-210, and development of combination treatments with cytokines, which modulate immune effector cells, are currently underway, and may enhance the efficacy of this novel therapeutic approach in, for example, *HER-2/neu*-overexpressing OC.

Several investigators have shown that TIL, isolated from the ascites of OC patients, can be expanded in culture, and show lytic activity against autologous and allogeneic tumor cells in vitro *(62)*. However, clinical responses have been limited because of lack of specificity and/or activity of injected TILs. A number of investigators are currently attempting to overcome these obstacles by redirecting TILs against OC cells through specific ligands *(63)*. Hwu et al. *(64)* have developed a chimeric single-chain antibody–T-cell receptor construct, which combines antigen specificity via the variable portion of an antibody recognition site with the signaling components of a T-cell receptor. TILs expressing the chimeric protein on the cell surface are subsequently able to recognize tumor-associated antigen on OC cells. Upon linking to the appropriate ligand, the TILs are activated via the signaling pathways of the attached T-cell receptor component. The feasibility of this approach was demonstrated in vitro, as well as in vivo, by targeting a folate-binding protein on the human OC cell line IGROV1 *(65)*. Expression of the chimeric protein on TILs isolated from human melanoma led to significantly increased in vitro cytotoxicity of TILs against the IGROV1 cell line, compared to that of unmodified TILs. Furthermore, treatment of animals with established IGROV1 tumors resulted in significantly increased survival, compared to control groups.

4.1.2. RADIOCONJUGATES

MAbs can be utilized to deliver therapeutic doses of irradiation to OC cells through the use of radionuclides. As with other biologic response modifiers discussed, in vivo evidence suggests that the route of administration plays an integral role in determining the clinical performance of radiolabeled MAbs, because more lesions are detected and can be treated with ip administration than with systemic. The radionuclides available for therapeutic use include copper-67, bromine-77, bromine-82, yttrium-90, technetium-99m, indium-111, iodine-125, iodine-131, lutetium-177, rhenium-186, and astatine-211. Of those listed, ^{186}Re and ^{90}Y may be the most suited for radioimmunotherapy, because they have long half-lives, an ability to produce stable daughter products, emit little or no γ-radiation, have intermediate β-energy, and form relatively stable chelates with antibodies. A number of small phase I and II clinical studies, with the use of ip radiolabeled MAbs, have been reported to date.

An early study by Epenetos et al. *(66)* administered ^{131}I-labeled HMFG1, HMFG2, AUA1, or H17E2 intraperitoneally to a cohort of 24 patients: Eight with large-volume disease showed no response; 9 patients with less than 2 cm disease displayed a PR. Toxicity included mild abdominal pain, fever, diarrhea, and moderate pancytopenia. Similarly, Stewart et al. *(67)* used ^{131}I-labeled HMFG1, HMFG2, AUA1, and H17E2 intraperitoneally: In 31 evaluable patients, a CR was noted in 3 of 6 patients with microscopic disease, and PRs in 2 of 15 patients with less than 2 cm disease. No responses were noted in their eight patients with greater than 2 cm disease. Ward et al. *(68)* also used an ip [13]I-labeled antibody in a series of seven patients with small-volume disease. They noted a temporary control in ascites in several patients, but 6 of 7 patients had disease progression within 3 mo.

Finkler et al. *(69)* and Hnatowich et al. *(70)* used a radiolabeled OC125 MAb. Only one transient response in 12 patients was noted by Hnatowich; three responses were reported by Finkler in his cohort of four patients who had less than 2 cm disease at initiation of treatment. No responses were seen by Finkler in his 16 patients with greater than 2 cm residual disease. Muto et al. *(71)* did not report a response in their study of 28 patients treated with a radiolabeled OC125 antibody. Although response rates in these studies varied, patients with minimal disease at time of therapy appeared to have the best chance for an objective disease response.

Recently, Alvarez et al. *(72)* treated 27 persistent/recurrent OC patients after platinum-based chemotherapy with ip [117]Lu-CC49. One of 13 patients with gross disease had greater than 50% reduction in tumor volume after therapy. Two of nine patients with less than 1 cm disease were disease-free at 5 mo after therapy, and four of five patients with microscopic disease were without evidence of disease at a minimum of 6 mo. Marrow suppression was the dose-limiting toxicity encountered in this phase I/II study. Like previous studies using various radiolabeled MAbs, the key to prolonged disease-free survival was small-volume disease at initiation of therapy. Residual disease greater than 1–2 cm requires radiation doses of at least 50–60 Gy, which is higher than safely attainable in the peritoneal cavity; however, small-volume disease should be treatable in this manner. Further studies are underway, evaluating a number of ip radiolabeled MAbs, to include the addition of paclitaxel as a radiation sensitizer to enhance antitumor activity.

4.1.3. ANTI-IDIOTYPES

Anti-idiotypic antibodies present the mirror image of an antigen expressed on the surface of the tumor, and can generate humoral and cellular antitumor immune responses. Activation of the idiotypic network has been attempted in several clinical trials in OC, using different antibodies as systemic treatment. However, the efficacy of ip administration of anti-idiotypes has yet to be studied.

A radiolabeled antibody against the tumor antigen, CA-125, was used for diagnostic purposes in 62 patients with OC *(73)*. A significant anti-idiotypic antibody (Ab2) level was found in 28 patients, which increased with repetitive applications. Twenty patients with Ab2 concentrations >10,000 U/mL had a significantly higher survival rate than the patients with lower levels of Ab2. In another study, 26 of 50 OC patients, receiving anti-CA-125 murine MAb B43.13., were found to have elevated anti-idiotypic antibodies *(74)*.

Human anti-mouse antibodies are observed frequently after immunoscintigraphy with MAbs directed against CA-125. In 58 patients with advanced OCs, who had received MAb (OC125) against the cancer-associated antigen, CA-125, for diagnostic purposes, induction of anti-idiotypic antibodies led to a prolongation of survival, and induction of antitumoral immunity *(75)*. It is possible that anti-idiotypic immune responses may trigger an antitumor effect, either by suppressing the growth of CA-125-expressing cancer cells directly, or by activating the patient's immune response via induction of Ab3.

The concept of stimulating anti-idiotypic network responses is still being explored, and has not been evaluated as ip treatment. The efficacy of this approach will depend on the tumor specificity of the antigenic determinant of the therapeutic anti-idiotype. It will therefore be necessary to generate or identify more OC-specific antigens. Furthermore, the efficacy of the ip application of this approach might be limited by the lack of insufficient numbers of immune cells in the peritoneal cavity, which are able to recognize these antibodies and stimulate antitumor immune responses.

5. GENE THERAPY

Advances in molecular biology have allowed the modification of genetic material with the ability to transfer genes into cells, either to replace a missing or malfunctioning gene, or to provide a new function to a cell *(76)*. Various novel therapeutic strategies have been developed in recent years to inhibit tumor growth directly, or to stimulate a systemic immune response against the cancer.

Several methods are currently used to transfer genes into mammalian cells *(77)*. These methods differ in accuracy, efficiency, and stability of gene expression. Physical methods include electroporation, gene gun, and chemical methods, such as calcium–phosphate or diethylaminoethyl-dextran transfection *(78)*. The DNA transferred by these techniques is usually in the form of plasmid DNA. In general, physical methods yield low gene transfer efficiencies.

Liposomes consist of positively charged lipid molecules that possess the ability to bind negatively charged DNA *(79)*. This lipid–DNA complex subsequently fuses with the membrane of the host cell, to release the DNA into the cytoplasm, or is taken up by the cell via endocytosis. Some of the DNA molecules relocate into the nucleus, and use the host cell's transcription machinery to express the foreign gene *(80)*.

Viral gene transfer systems, such as retroviruses and adenoviruses (Ads), are the most commonly used vectors in vitro and in vivo *(81,82)*. Retroviral vectors bind to most human cells via a receptor, but only infect replicating cell lines. Fusion between the viral envelope and the target cell membrane releases the viral core particle into the cytoplasm. The viral RNA is reverse transcribed into proviral DNA, which subsequently translocates into the cell nucleus. Integration of proviral DNA into the cell's genome is only possible if the host cell undergoes a cell division shortly after the infection. Such integration yields stable transfectants that can be selected in vitro via drug resistance genes, and that maintain transgene expression over an extended period of time. The efficiency of retroviral gene transfer and subsequent transgene expression in vivo is low, chiefly because of inactivation by complement *(83)*.

Ads are able to infect most cells, including nondividing cells, via receptors on the cell surface. In contrast to retroviruses, Ads are not subject to complement inactivation, and have been used in vivo with better transfection efficiency than other vector systems

(84). However, immune responses against viral proteins can interfere with the effectiveness of subsequent injections of Ads in vivo.

5.1. Immunogene Therapy

In order to avoid frequently encountered severe toxicities associated with high doses of cytokines, several investigators have used the transfer of cytokine genes into tumor cells to co-present tumor-associated antigen and the immunostimulatory cytokine *(85)*. The injection of cytokine gene-modified tumor cells has resulted in significant antitumor immune responses in several animal tumor models. In these studies, the transfer of cytokine genes into tumor cells has reduced or abrogated the tumorigenicity of the cells after implantation into syngeneic hosts. Furthermore, treated animals developed systemic antitumor immunity, and were protected against subsequent tumor challenges with the unmodified parental tumor *(86,87)*.

Based on the biological rationale of increasing the immunogenicity of OC cells by transfer of an immunostimulatory cytokine gene, Santin et al. *(88)* have developed an IL-4-secreting human OC cell line, using retroviral-mediated gene transduction. The cell line, termed UC1107E, was shown to express IL-4 between 900 and 1300 pg/mL/ 10^5 cells/48 h. Characterization of this cell line revealed expression of MHC I and HER-2/neu surface antigens. Similarly, the investigators generated a cell line transduced with the gene for granulocyte-macrophage colony-stimulating factor *(89)*. Mixed with autologous tumor cells, these cell lines could be used as a tumor cell vaccine in OC patients. The presence of alloantigens and IL-4 at the local injection site may provide two potent signals for recognition of the autologous tumor cells by the immune system. Besides providing strong stimuli to the immune system, the allogeneic vaccine concept would also permit better standardization and higher practicability for clinical use.

Although the transfer of cytokine genes into OC cells has stimulated potent antitumor effects in some preclinical models, the immunostimulatory effects in patients might be influenced by factors in the tumor microenvironment. One reason for the failure of the immune system to develop an effective antitumor response is the production of immunosuppressive factors, such as TGF-β, by tumor cells *(90)*. The biological importance of TGF-β as an immunosuppressive factor in, for example, OC was shown by Hirte et al. *(91,92)*. These studies demonstrated that ascites from patients with OC inhibited the generation of LAK cells in vitro via the effect of TGF-β.

Stimulation of antitumor immune responses against gynecologic malignancies with, for example, genetically modified tumor cell vaccines is a promising gene therapy approach *(93)*. The stimulation of systemic antitumor immunity has the potential to eradicate metastases at distant sites. Preliminary data from ongoing clinical immunogene therapy trials in a variety of cancers indicate that the injection of genetically modified tumor cell vaccines in patients is tolerated without significant toxicity. However, the most effective approaches have yet to be identified.

5.2. Tumor-Suppressor Gene Therapy

The *p53* tumor suppressor gene plays an important role in the maintenance of normal cell growth and differentiation *(94)*. Inactivation of the *p53* gene by mutation is still the most commonly detected genetic lesion in human cancer. The protein encoded by the *p53* gene induces expression of several growth-inhibitory genes, such as *WAF1*. The *WAF1*-encoded protein p21 inhibits cyclin-dependent kinases that are necessary for the cell to proceed through the cell cycle. Cells with genetic damage are arrested in the G1 phase of the cell cycle to allow DNA repair. If DNA repair is unsuccessful, *p53* can trigger apoptosis (programmed cell death). Mutations of the *p53* gene may result in a biologically altered gene product with loss of antiproliferative activity, and possibly a dominant-negative effect via complex formation with the wild-type protein. Mutation and overexpression occur in 15% of stage I/II and 50% of stage III/IV EOC, suggesting a major role in the development and maintenance of the malignant phenotype *(95–98)*.

Restoration of normal *p53* function in cancer cell lines with mutated or missing p53 protein has resulted in growth inhibition in vitro and decreased tumorigenicity in vivo in a variety of cancer cell lines. For example, Santoso et al. *(99)* used a recombinant Ad to transfect the human OC cell line 2774, which contains an Arg273His *p53* mutation, with the wild-type *p53* gene. Transfected cells showed significant (>90%) growth inhibition, compared to untransfected controls.

A number of clinical trials are currently investigating the feasibility of Ad-mediated *p53* transfer intraperitoneally into OC. Patients with advanced OCs that bear *p53* mutations, are treated with ip infusion of 1000-cc wild-type *p53*-Ad-containing solutions. These treatments are given repetitively in 1–3 wk intervals, to maximize transfection efficiency and antitumor effects. Preliminary results have shown that this therapy is well tolerated by the patient. Antitumor effects have been reported in single cases, but the efficacy of this approach needs to be determined in further clinical trials. Inflammatory responses have been observed in some patients, which might be attributed either to an immune response against adenoviral proteins or to secondary responses to the tumor caused by presentation of different antigens after expression of wild-type *p53* in tumor cells, with subsequent cell death. It is therefore possible that the *p53* tumor suppressor strategy as ip treatment of OC not only induces apoptosis, but generates antitumor immune responses, that are clinically significant.

REFERENCES

1. Khoo SK and Mackay EV. Immunologic reactivity of female patients with genital cancer: status in preinvasive, locally invasive and disseminated disease, *Am. J. Obstet. Gynecol.*, **119** (1974) 1018–1025.
2. Markman M and Howell SB. Intraperitoneal chemotherapy for ovarian cancer, In Alberts DS, Surwit EA (eds), *Ovarian Cancer.* Martinus Nijhoff, Boston, 1985, pp. 179–212.
3. Clark JW. Biological response modifiers. *Cancer Chemother. Biol. Response Modif.* **17** (1997) 287–315.
4. Benjamini E, Rennick DM, and Sell S. Tumor immunology, In Stites DP, et al. (eds), *Basic and Clinical Immunology,* Lange, Los Altos, CA, 1984, 223.
5. Boyer P, Berek JS, and Zigelboim J. Lymphocyte activation by recombinant interleukin-2 in ovarian cancer patients, *Obstet. Gynecol.*, **73** (1989) 793–797.
6. Marx JL. T-cell receptor—the genes and beyond, *Science,* **227** (1985) 733–755.
7. Hedrick SM, Cohen DI, Nielsen EA, and Davis MM. Isolation of cDNA clones encoding T-cell-specific membrane-associated proteins, *Nature,* **308** (1984) 149–153.
8. Williams AF. T-lymphocyte receptor—elusive no more, *Nature,* **308** (1984) 108–109.
9. Kotzin BL, Benike CJ, and Engleman EG. Induction of immunoglobulin secreting cells in the allogenic mixed leukocyte reaction: regulation by helper and suppressor lymphocyte subsets in man, *J. Immunol.*, **127** (1981) 931–935.
10. Berke G. Functions and mechanisms of lysis induced by cytotoxic lymphocytes and natural killer cells, In *Paul's Fundamental Immunology,* Raven, New York, 1989, pp. 735–764.
11. Herberman RB. *Natural Cell-Mediated Immunity Against Tumors,* Academic, New York, 1980, 973.
12. Lanzavecchia A. Antigen-specific interaction between T and B cells, *Nature,* **314** (1985) 537–539.
13. Unanue ER and Allen PM. Basis for the immunoregulatory role of macrophages and other accessory cells, *Science,* **236** (1987) 551–557.

14. Grimm EA, Mazumder A, Zhang HZ, and Rosenberg SA. Lymphokine activated killer cell phenomenon: lysis of NK resistant fresh solid tumor cells by IL-2 activated autologous human peripheral blood lymphocytes, *J. Exp. Med.,* **155** (1982) 1823–1841.

15. Halpern B. *Corynebacterium parvum: application in experimental and clinical oncology,* Plenum, New York, 1975.

16. Chen MF, Suzuki H, and Yano S. Induction of murine lymphokine-activated killer-like cells by *Corynebacterium parvum (C. parvum)* in vitro: Lysis of tumor cells and macrophages by *C. parvum*-induced killer cells. *Anticancer Res.,* **12** (1992) 451–456.

17. Berek JS, Knapp RC, Hacker NF, et al. Intraperitoneal immunotherapy of epithelial ovarian cancer with *Corynebacterium parvum, Am. J. Obstet. Gynecol.,* **152** (1985) 1003–1010.

18. Bast RC, Berek JS, Obrist R, et al. Intraperitoneal immunotherapy of human ovarian carcinoma with *Cornyebacterium parvum, Cancer Res.,* **43** (1983) 1395–1401.

19. Mantovani A. Intraperitoneal administration of *Corynebacterium parvum* by chemical fractionation, *Int. J. Immunopharmacol.,* **2** (1981) 437–446.

20. Lichtenstein A, Berek JS, Bast RC, et al. Activation of peritoneal lymphocyte cytotoxicity in patients with ovarian cancer by intraperitoneal treatment with *Corynebacterium parvum, J. Biol. Response Mod.,* **3** (1984) 371–378.

21. Ohkawa K and Ohkawa R. Locoregional immunotherapy and chemotherapy in advanced ovarian cancer cytotoxicity, *Asian Oceania Fed. Obstet. Gynecol.,* (October 1981) 352.

22. Kawagoe K and Masuda J. Advanced ovarian cancer treated by intraperitoneal immunotherapy with OK-432, *Jpn. J. Clin. Oncol.,* **16** (1986) 137–142.

23. Koelbl H, Micksche M, Gitsch G, Hanzal E, and Nowotny C. Treatment with biologic response modifiers in patients with ovarian cancer, *Eur. J. Obstet. Gynecol. Reprod. Biol.,* **41** (1991) 64–69.

24. Zighelboim J, Niio Y, Berek JS, and Bonavida B. Immunologic control of ovarian cancer, *Nar. Immunol. Cell Growth Regul.,* **7** (1988) 216–225.

25. Philip R. Cytolysis of tumor necrosis factor (TNF)-resistant tumor targets. Differential cytotoxicity of monocytes activated by the interferons, IL-2, and TNF. *J. Immunol.* **140** (1988) 1345–1349.

26. Berek JS, Cantrell JL, Lichtenstein AK, et al. Immunotherapy with biochemically dissociated fractions of proprionebacterium acnes in a murine ovarian cancer model, *Cancer Res.,* **44** (1984) 1871–1875.

27. Niloff TM, Knapp RC, Jones G, et al. Recombinant leukocyte alpha interferon in advanced ovarian carcinoma, *Cancer Treat. Rep.,* **69** (1985) 895–896.

28. Berek JS, Hacker NF, Lichtenstein AK, et al. Intraperitoneal recombinant alpha-interferon for salvage immunotherapy in stage III epithelial ovarian cancer: a Gynecologic Oncology Study group, *Cancer Res.,* **45** (1985) 4447–4453.

29. Moore DH, Valea F, Walton LA, Soper J, Clarke-Pearson D, and Fowler WC Jr. Phase I study of intraperitoneal interferon-alpha 2b and intravenous cis-platinum plus cyclophospamide chemotherapy in patients with untreated stage III epithelial ovarian cancer: a gynecologic Ongolocy Group pilot study, *Gynecol. Oncol.,* **59** (1995) 267–272.

30. Willemse PH, DeBries EGE, Aalers JG, et al. Intraperitoneal human recombinant interferon alpha-2b in minimal residual ovarian cancer, *Eur. J. Cancer,* **26** (1990) 353–358.

31. Aapro MS, Alberts DS, and Salmon SE. Interaction of human leukocyte interferon with vinca alkaloids and other chemotherapeutic agents against human tumors in clonogenic assay, *Cancer Chemother. Pharmacol.,* **10** (1983) 161–166.

32. Berek JS, Welander C, Schink JC, Grossberg H, Montz FJ, and Zigelboim J. Phase I–II trial of intraperitoneal cisplatin and alpha-interferon in patients with persistent epithelial ovarian cancer, *Gynecol. Oncol.,* **40** (1991) 237–243.

33. Nardi M, Cognetti F, Pollera CF, et al. Intraperitoneal recombinant alpha-2-interferon alternating with cisplatin as salvage therapy for minimal residual disease ovarian cancer. A phase II study, *J. Clin. Oncol.,* **8** (1990) 1036–1041.

34. Stuart GC, Nation JG, Snider DD, and Thunberg P. Intraperitoneal interferon in the management of malignant ascites, *Cancer,* **27** (1993) 1423–1429.

35. Meanpaa J, Kivinen S, Raisanen I, Sipiila P, Vayrynen M, and Grohn P. Combined intraperitoneal interferon alpha-2b and mitoxantrone in refractory ovarian cancer, *Ann. Chir. Gynaecol.,* **208(suppl)** (1994) 25–27.

36. Bezwoda WR, Golombick T, Dansey R, and Keeping J. Treatment of malignant ascites due to recurrent/refractory ovarian cancer: the use of interferon-alpha or interferon-alpha plus chemotherapy in vivo and in vitro, *Eur. J. Cancer,* **27** (1991) 1423–1429.

37. Frasci G, Tortoriello A, Facchini G, et al. Carboplatin and alpha-2b interferon intraperitoneal combination as first-line treatment of minimal residual ovarian cancer. A pilot study, *Curr. J. Cancer,* **30A** (1994) 946–950.

38. Moore DH, Valea F, Walton LA, Soper J, Clarke-Pearson D, and Fowler WC Jr. Phase I study of intraperitoneal interferon-alpha 2b and intravenous cis-platinum plus cyclophospamide chemotherapy in patients with untreated stage III epithelial ovarian cancer: a gynecologic Oncology Group pilot study, *Gynecol. Oncol.,* **59** (Nov. 1995) 267–272.

39. Bruzzone M, Rubagotti A, Gadducci A, et al. Intraperitoneal carboplatin with or without interferon-alpha in advanced ovarian cancer patients with minimal residual disease at second look: a prospective randomized trial of 111 patients, Gruppo Oncologic Nord Ovest, *Gynecol. Oncol.,* **65** (1997) 499–505.

40. Golub SH. Immunological and therapeutic effects of interferon treatment of cancer patients, *Clin. Immunol. Allergy,* **4** (1984) 377.

41. D'Acquisto R, Markman M, Hakes, et al. Phase I trial of intraperitoneal recombinant gamma-interferon in advanced ovarian carcinoma, *J. Clin. Oncol.,* **6** (1988) 689–695.

42. Marth C, Mull R, Gastl G, et al. Intraperitoneal installation of gamma interferon for the treatment of refractory ovarian carcinoma, *Geburtshilfe Frauenheilkd* **49** (1989) 987–991.

43. Pujade-Lauraine E, Colombo N, Maner N, et al. Intraperitoneal human r-interferon gamma in patients with residual ovarian carcinoma at second look laparotomy, *Proc. Am. Soc. Clin. Oncol.,* **9** (1990) 156.

44. Pujade-Lauraine E, Guastalla JP, Colombo N. et al. Intraperitoneal recombinant interferon gamma in ovarian cancer patients with residual disease at second-look laparotomy, *J. Clin. Oncol.,* **14** (1996) 343–350.

45. Old LJ. Tumor necrosis factor, *Science,* **230** (1985) 630–632.

46. Chapman PB, Lester TS, Casper ES, et al. Clinical pharmacology of recombinant human tumor necrosis factor in patients with advanced cancer, *J. Clin. Oncol.,* **5** (1987) 1942–1951.

47. Spriggs DR, Sherman ML, and Michie H. Recombinant human tumor necrosis factor administered as a 24-hr intravenous infusion. A phase I and pharmacologic study, *J. Natl. Cancer Inst.,* **80** (1988) 1039–1044.

48. Markman M, Ianotti N, Hakes T, et al. Phase I trial of intraperitoneal recombinant tumor necrosis factor, *Proc. Am. Soc. Clin. Oncol.,* **8** (1989) 64.

49. Kaufmann M, Schmid H, Raeth U, et al. Therapy of ascites with tumor necrosis factor in ovarian cancer, *Geburtshilfe Frauenheilkd,* **9** (1990) 678–682.

50. Rath U, Kaufmann M, Schmid H, et al. Effect of intraperitoneal recombinant human tumour necrosis factor alpha on malignant ascites, *Eur. J. Cancer,* **27** (1991) 121–125.

51. Hirte HW, Miller D, Tonkin K, et al. Randomized trial of paracentesis plus intraperitoneal tumor necrosis factor-alpha paracentesis alone in patients with symptomatic ascites from recurrent ovarian carcinoma, *Gynecol. Oncol.,* **64** (1997) 80–87.

52. Bonavida B, Tsuchitani T, Zighelboim J, and Berek JS. Synergy is documented in vitro with low dose tumor necrosis factor, cisplatin, and doxorubicin in ovarian cells, *Gynecol. Oncol.,* **38** (1990) 333–339.

53. Edwards RP, Gooding W, Lembersky BC, et al. Recombinant interleukin-2 continuous infusion in ovarian cancer patients with minimal residual disease at second-look, *Cancer Treat. Rev.,* **16** (1989) 123–127.

54. Urba WJ, Clark JW, Steis RG, et al. Intraperitoneal lymphokine-activated killer cell/interleukin-2 therapy in patients with intra-abdominal cancer: immunologic considerations, *J. Natl. Cancer Inst.,* **19** (1989) 602–611.

55. Steis RG, Urba WJ, VanderMolen LA, et al. Intraperitoneal lymphokine-activated killer-cell and interleukin-2 therapy for malignancies limited to the peritoneal cavity, *J. Clin. Oncol.,* **10** (1990) 1618–1629.

56. Edwards RP, Gooding W, Lembersky BC, Colonello K, Hammond R, Paradise C, et al. Comparison of toxicity and survival following intraperitoneal recombinant interleukin-2 for persistent ovarian cancer after platinum: twenty-four-hour versus 7-day infusion, *J. Clin. Oncol.,* **15** (1997) 3399–3407.

57. Beller U, Abraham C, James L, et al. Phase IB study of low-dose intraperitoneal recombinant interleukin-2 in patients with refractory advanced ovarian cancer: rational and preliminary report, *Gynecol. Oncol.,* **34** (1989) 407–412.

58. Chapman PB, Kolitz JE, Hakes TB, et al. Phase I trial of intraperitoneal recombinant interleukin-2 in patients with ovarian carcinoma, *Invest. New Drugs,* **3** (1988) 179–188.

59. Panici PB, Scambia G, Greggi S, et al. Recombinant interleukin-2 continuous infusion in ovarian cancer patients with minimal residual disease at second-look, *Cancer Treat. Rev.,* **16** (1989) 123–127.

60. Stewart JA, Belinson JL, Moore AL, et al. Phase I trial of intraperitoneal recombinant interleukin-2/lymphokine-activated killer cells in patients with ovarian cancer, *Cancer Res.*, **50** (1990) 6302–6310.

61. Valone FH, Kaufman PA, Guyre PM, et al. Clinical trials of bispecific antibody MDX-210 in women with advanced breast or ovarian cancer that overexpresses HER-2/neu, *J. Hematother.*, **4** (1995) 471–475.

62. Lucci JA, Manetta A, Cappuccini F, et al. Immunotherapy of ovarian cancer. II. In vitro generation and characterization of lymphokine-activated killer T cells from the peripheral blood of recurrent ovarian cancer patients, *Gynecol. Oncol.*, **45** (1992) 129–135.

63. Hwu P and Rosenberg SA. Genetic modification of T cells for cancer therapy: an overview of laboratory and clinical trials, *Cancer Detect. Prev.*, **18** (1994) 43–50.

64. Hwu P, Yang JC, Cowherd R, et al. In vivo antitumor activity of T cells redirected with chimeric antibody/T-cell receptor genes, *Cancer Res.*, **55** (1995) 3369–3373.

65. Hwu P, Shafer GE, Treisman J, et al. Lysis of ovarian cancer cells by human lymphocytes redirected with a chimeric gene composed of an antibody variable region and the Fc receptor g chain, *J. Exp. Med.*, **178** (1993) 361–366.

66. Epenetos AA, Hooker G, and Krausz T. Antibody-guided irradiation of malignant ascites ovarian cancer: a new therapeutic method possessing specificity against cancer cells, *Obstet. Gynecol.*, **68** (1986) 71s–74s.

67. Stewart JS, Hird V, Snook D, et al. Intraperitoneal radioimmunotherapy for ovarian cancer: pharmacokinetics, toxicity and efficacy of 131 I labelled monoclonal antibodies, *Int. J. Radiat. Oncol. Biol. Phys.*, **16** (1989) 405–413.

68. Ward B, Mather S, Shepaherd J, et al. Treatment of intraperitoneal malignant disease with monoclonal antibody guided 131I radiotherapy, *Br. J. Cancer*, **58** (1988) 658–662.

69. Finkler NJ, Muto MG, Kassis AI, et al. Intraperitoneal radiolabelled OC125 in patients with advanced ovarian cancer, *Gynecol. Oncol.*, **34** (1989) 339–344.

70. Hnatowich DJ, Mardirossian G, and Rose PG. Intraperitoneal therapy of ovarian cancer with Yttrium-90-labelled monoclonal antibodies: preliminary observations, *Antibiot. Immunoconjug. Radiopharmacol.*, **4** (1991) 359–371.

71. Muto MG, Finkler NJ, Kassis AI, et al. Intraperitoneal radioimmunotherapy of refractory ovarian carcinoma utilizing iodine-131-labelled monoclonal antibody OC125, *Gynecol. Oncol.*, **45** (1992) 265–272.

72. Alvarez RD, Partridge EE, Khazeli MB, et al. Intraperitoneal radioimmunotherapy of ovarian cancer with 177-Lu-CC49: a phase I/II study, *Gynecol. Oncol.*, **65** (1997) 94–101.

73. Schmolling J, Wagner U, Reinsberg J, Biersack HJ, and Krebs D. Immune reactions and survival of patients with ovarian carcinomas after administration of 131I-F(Ab)2 fragments of the OC 125 monoclonal antibody, *Geburtshilfe Frauenheilkd.*, **55** (1995) 200–203.

74. Madiyalakan R, Sykes TR, Dharampaul S, et al. Antiidiotype induction therapy: evidence for the induction of immune response through the idiotype network in patients with ovarian cancer after administration of anti-CA125 murine monoclonal antibody B43.13, *Hybridoma*, **14** (1995) 199–203.

75. Wagner U, Reinsberg J, Schmidt S, et al. Monoclonal antibodies and idiotypic network activation for ovarian carcinoma, *Cell Biophys.*, **24/25** (1994) 237–242.

76. Sobol RE, Shawler DL, Dorigo O, Gold D, Royston I, and Fakhrai H. Immunogene therapy of cancer, In Sobol RE, Scanlon KJ (eds), *Internet Book of Gene Therapy*, Appleton and Lange, Norwalk, 1995, pp. 175–180.

77. Vile R and Russell SJ. Gene transfer technologies for the gene therapy of cancer, *Gene Ther.*, **1** (1995) 88–89.

78. Kriegler M. *Gene Transfer and Expression. A Laboratory Manual.* New York, Stockton, 1990.

79. Puyal C, Milhaud P, Bienvenue A, and Philippot JR. New cationic liposome encapsulating genetic material. A potential delivery system for polynucleotides, *Eur. J. Biochem.*, **228** (1995) 697–703.

80. Hofland H and Huang L. Inhibition of human ovarian carcinoma cell proliferation by liposome-plasmid DNA complex, *Biochem. Biophys. Res. Commun.*, **207** (1995) 492–496.

81. Jolly D. Viral vectors systems for gene therapy, *Cancer Gene Ther.*, **1** (1994) 51–64.

82. Miller AD. Retroviral vectors, *Curr. Top. Microbiol. Immunol.*, **3** (1993) 102–109.

83. Welsh RM, Cooper NR, Jensen FC, and Oldstone MBA. Human serum lyses RNA tumour viruses, *Nature*, **257** (1975) 612–614.

84. Addison CL, Braciak T, Ralston R, et al. Intratumoral injection of an adenovirus expressing interleukin

2 induces regression and immunity in a murine breast cancer model, *Proc. Natl. Acad. Sci. USA*, **92** (1995) 8522–8526.

85. Miller AR, McBride WH, Hunt K, and Economou JS. Cytokine-mediated gene therapy for cancer, *Ann. Surg. Oncol.*, **1** (1994) 436–450.

86. Dorigo O, Shawler DL, Royston I, Sobol RE, Berek JS, and Fakhrai H. Combination of transforming growth factor beta antisense and interleukin-2 gene therapy in the murine ovarian teratoma model *Gynecol. Oncol.*, **71** (1998) 204–210.

87. Shawler DL, Dorigo O, Gjerset RA, Royston I, Sobol RE, and Fakhrai H. Comparison of gene therapy with interleukin-2 (IL-2) gene modified fibroblasts and tumor cells in the murine CT-26 model of colorectal carcinoma, *J. Immunother.*, **17** (1995) 201–208.

88. Santin AD, Ioli GR, Hiserodt JC, et al. Development and characterization of an IL-4-secreting human ovarian carcinoma cell line, *Gynecol. Oncol.*, **58** (1995) 230–239.

89. Santin AD, Ioli GR, Hiserodt JC, et al. Development and in vitro characterization of a GM-CSF secreting human ovarian carcinoma tumor vaccine, *Int. J. Gynecol. Cancer*, **5** (1995) 401–410.

90. Sulitzenau D. Immunosuppressive factors in human cancer, *Adv. Cancer Res.*, **60** (1993) 247–267.

91. Hirte W, Clark DA, O'Connell G, Rusthoven J, and Mazurka J. Reversal of suppression of lymphokine-activated killer cells by transforming growth factor-beta in ovarian carcinoma ascitic fluid requires interleukin-2 combined with anti-CD3 antibody, *Cell Immunol.*, **142** (1992) 207–216.

92. Hirte H and Clark DA. Generation of lymphokine-activated killer cells in human ovarian carcinoma ascitic fluid: identification of transforming growth factor-beta as a suppressive factor, *Cancer Immunol. Immunother.*, **32** (1991) 296–302.

93. Dorigo O and Berek JS. Gene therapy for ovarian cancer: development of novel treatment strategies, *Internat. J. Gynecol. Cancer*, **7** (1997) 1–13.

94. Vogelstein B and Kinzler KW. p53 function and dysfunction, *Cell*, **70** (1992) 523–526.

95. Hartmann LC, Podratz KC, Keeney GL, et al. Prognostic significance of p53 immunostaining in epithelial ovarian cancer, *J. Clin. Oncol.*, **12** (1994) 64–69.

96. Kupryjanczyk J, Thor AD, Beauchamp R, et al. p53 gene mutations and protein accumulation in human ovarian cancer, *Proc. Natl. Acad. Sci. USA*, **90** (1993) 4961–4965.

97. Runnebaum IB, Tong XW, Moebus V, et al. Multiplex PCR screening detects small p53 deletions and insertions in human ovarian cancer cell lines, *Hum. Genet.*, **93** (1994) 620–624.

98. Berchuck A, Kohler MF, Marks JR, et al. p53 tumor suppressor gene frequently is altered in gynecologic cancers, *Am. J. Obstet. Gynecol.*, **170** (1994) 246–252.

99. Santoso JT, Tang DC, Lane SB, et al. Adenovirus-based p53 gene therapy in ovarian cancer, *Gynecol. Oncol.*, **59** (1995) 171–178.

13 Intraperitoneal Therapy with Fluoropyrimidines in the Treatment of Ovarian and Gastrointestinal Cancers

Franco M. Muggia, Tamar Safra, Susan Jeffers, Agustin Garcia, and Susan Groshen

CONTENTS

1. INTRODUCTION AND GENERAL PRINCIPLES

Dose–effect relationships are the underlying rationale for exploring local-regional administration of drugs *(1)*. The role of dose-intensity (or, more specifically, dose-density) in improving results from chemotherapy of solid tumors has been a subject of frequent debate. Unfortunately, systemic administration of most drugs are subject to a relatively narrow range of dose escalation, even with the use of myelopoietic growth factors to ameliorate the dose-limiting toxicities of many of the most common anticancer drugs. Moreover, accumulating clinical experience suggests that dose–effect relationships beyond the usual tolerance range do not lead to tangible evidence of greater benefit with increasing doses. For example, ovarian cancer (OC) trials testing platinum dose-intensity have been almost uniformly disappointing *(2,3)*. When the disease is predominantly confined to the peritoneal cavity, however, the dose-intensification (as defined by the pharmacologic advantage expressed as intraperitoneal (ip) area under the curve (AUC)/plasma AUC) achieved through ip administration varies from severalfold to several log-fold among various drugs tested *(4)*. This degree of dose-intensification would be expected to show enhanced effects, even for drugs in

From: *Current Clinical Oncology: Regional Chemotherapy: Clinical Research and Practice*
Edited by: M. Markman © Humana Press Inc., Totowa, NJ

which such dose–effect relationships are considered to be almost flat beyond the usually employed dose per cycle, such as has been described for carboplatin *(5)*.

Another key principle of ip therapy is that the drugs to be used demonstrate activity against the cancer being treated. Because most of the tumor is beyond the surface, and penetration through several cell layers is needed in order to fulfill the pharmacologic advantage underlying ip drug administration, the intrinsic sensitivity of the tumor to the ip drug being used is particularly important. Howell et al. *(6)* has stressed a third principle: ip drugs show local tolerance at doses that regularly achieve therapeutic systemic levels. If these conditions are fulfilled, tumor exposure to drug levels via capillary flow will be at least equivalent to those of the drug given systemically. Accordingly, this has been verified with cisplatin in animal models *(7)*, and is also supported by clinical data from the same authors: Peritoneal tumor nodules have the same platinum content by either the ip or intravenous (iv) drug administration in the central areas, but the outer layers contain more platinum when the drug is given ip *(8)*.

Fluoropyrimidines are of great interest because of their activity against gastrointestinal (GI) cancers. However, special pharmacologic considerations described below preclude fulfilling this last principle regularly with these drugs. Cytocidal concentrations in the ip cavity are accompanied by several logs lower systemic concentrations *(9–19)*. However, rather than considering the failure to fulfill Howell's principle a problem for ip-administered fluoropyrimidines, such a feature may actually lead to a useful therapeutic strategy through combinations of ip and systemic drug administration, thus maximizing the antitumor effects of these drugs against peritoneal, as well as juxtaperitoneal, metastases.

2. PHARMACOLOGIC ASPECTS OF IP FLUOROPYRIMIDINES

The pharmacology of fluoropyrimidines, introduced clinically in the 1950s by Heidelberger, focused early on the role of the liver in its catabolism. The nucleoside, floxuridine (5-fluoro-2′–deoxyuridine [FUDR]) is more completely metabolized than is the base, 5-fluorouracil (5-FU). Comparative studies by Ensminger et al. *(20)* established the high first-pass extraction of FUDR following intra-arterial administration. It was this striking pharmacologic property that led the authors of this chapter to study the ip administration of this drug, following the suggestion by the Gastrointestinal Tumor Study Group *(21)*. The 3-d schedule chosen for study represented a compromise of a schedule emphasizing its time-dependent antitumor activity and practical considerations excluding even longer schedules. Pharmacologic study of its daily administration for 3 d established pharmacokinetic parameters for this drug *(13)*, which have been confirmed in two subsequently published studies *(15,16)*, and one published only in abstract form *(17)*. Table 1 indicates parameters from these studies, usually obtained during the first cycle. Serial studies obtained in several patients, however, indicate that the clearance increases on repeated cycles (an observation also made with 5-FU, when comparing d 1 to d 5 administration) *(12)*.

Studies with ip 5-FU were among the first to be carried out by the group at the National Cancer Institute that pioneered the systematic pharmacologically based administration of ip drugs *(9,10)*. These studies included documentation of hepatic extraction, and the fact that levels of 5-FU in the hepatic veins were barely above those of systemic administration *(10)*. Consequently, the very high concentration at peritoneal surfaces did not necessarily indicate high levels in the liver, as had initially been hoped. IP

Table 1
Pharmacokinetics of IP FUDR and IP LV

Parameter	3g FUDR n = 18	160 mg (RS)–LV n = 6	160 mg (S)–LV n = 11
$t^{1/2}$(h)	3.0	3.74	5.3
range	1.9–5.0	.81–4.08	2.6–13.1
AUC_{PF}			
(μg/h/mL)	4451	831	711
SD	2405	1036	318
CL_{PL}			
(mL/min)	14.9	10.1	4.6
SD	9.2	4.7	2.7
AUC ratio			
IP/PL	997	9.7	44.5
SD	999	7.0	25.0

n, patient number; Pf = peritoneal fluid; PL = plasma.
Data used with permission from refs. *15* and *16*.

drug administration was therefore unlikely to prove more effective than systemic administration for the treatment of liver metastases.

However, both FUDR and 5-FU achieved millimolar concentration in the peritoneum, with only occasional hematologic and mucosal intolerance. Moreover, FUDR had excellent local tolerance, and substantial ip levels of 5-FU were achieved from the ip FUDR. The effect of ip 5-FU on the peritoneum and patient tolerance was quite variable in the initial study utilizing every-4-h ip dwells. In fact, the toxicity of a daily × 5 ip administration was less than following iv administration. More recently, reports of sclerosing peritonitis raise a concern of their relationship to 5-FU *(22)*.

The systemic levels of both drugs after ip administration are quite variable. It would be expected, from the pharmacologic findings indicative of saturable kinetics, that ip dose escalations within the same patient, in order to achieve systemic dose-limiting toxicities, may result in a disproportionate increase in systemic drug levels, and may unpredictably lead to prohibitive toxicities. More reasonably, one may consider systemic administration of the fluoropyrimidine to supplement ip dosing: the 2–3-log pharmacologic advantage for either of the fluoropyrimidines, given ip, would then also be accompanied by adequate systemic levels attainable in all patients. Such ip–systemic combinations have had only limited study, with continuous-infusion 5-FU given with ip cisplatin *(23)*. However, the mild toxicity spectrum in the FUDR studies, described in the next subheading, provide some impetus to explore this total-fluoropyrimidine therapy. In fact, two patients have been treated by the authors with ip FUDR, followed by 14 d iv 5-FU. The logistics of providing such continuous therapy may prove impractical. With the availability of oral fluoropyrimidine prodrugs (capecitabine, tegafur, and uracil; oral 5-FU with the dihydropyrimidine dehydrogenase inhibitor, 776C85), such ip–systemic approaches may become easier to explore in the treatment of patients with ip cancers of GI origin.

Gemcitabine (2′,2′-difluorodeoxycytidine), with its superior activity against pancreatic cancer, compared to 5-FU, is the latest fluoropyrimidine to join the therapeutic armamentarium. Its ip administration is being studied in combination with ip cisplatin. In keeping with the experience of other antimetabolites, and its inactivation by cytidine deaminase, ip gemcitabine results in substantial pharmacologic advantage at reasonable local tolerance, and dose-limiting thrombocytopenia (47).

Another aspect of ip drug delivery is lymphatic uptake. In animal studies with thoracic duct cannulation, 5-FU had superior uptake, compared to etoposide (24). Such studies indicate whether a drug achieves sufficient uptake in lymphatic channels, and may have implications for their therapeutic potential against retroperitoneal spread of cancer. There are no human studies on this pharmacologic determinant, but the importance of tissue penetration is emphasized by the recent review by Dedrick and Flessner (25). Moreover, they stress that maneuvers designed to increase peritoneal × area product have been mostly unexplored. One such method may be utilizing a glucose polymer, icodextrin, which permits long-term continuous ambulatory ip treatments, maintaining a fluid volume within the peritoneal cavity. The pharmacokinetics and tolerance of prolonged ip 5-FU by this method have been reported in 17 patients (26).

The authors have chosen to pursue further studies with ip FUDR, because several aspects render it attractive for ip administration, and superior to 5-FU: Concentrations achieved in the peritoneal cavity are more than 6 logs above what is needed to demonstrate cytotoxicity of epithelial cancer cell lines; the pharmacokinetics of FUDR indicate very efficient clearance by the liver, contributing to the safe attainment of high ip levels, with minimal systemic toxicities in most subjects; tumoricidal levels of both 5-FU and FUDR are observed after ip FUDR; FUDR has considerably greater solubility than 5-FU, and the risk of any drug precipitation at an acid pH is totally obviated; and biochemical modulation, based on enhancing ternary complex formation between the fluoropyrimidine, the folate cofactor, and thymidylate synthase (e.g., using leucovorin [IV] or hydroxyurea), is more relevant to FUDR than to 5-FU (27).

3. PHASE I STUDIES OF IP FUDR

3.1. Dose-Escalation Study of Single-Agent IP FUDR

The first study of ip FUDR was initiated simultaneously in 1986 at New York University (NYU) and the University of Southern California (USC) (13). The starting dose was 500 mg (total dose, and not per m^2) in 2 L normal saline for 2 d. Dose escalations proceeded to 3 d, and then escalated doses, given first to three patients for 2 d, and subsequently for 3 d. Dose-limiting toxicities, such as stomatitis, diarrhea, or myelosuppression, were not frequent, even at 3000 mg for 3 d, and individual patients who began at 3000 mg were escalated to 7000 mg × 3 d without dose-limiting toxicities, with treatments being repeated every 3 wk. However, based on the pharmacokinetics that were determined and the millimolar concentrations achieved, the 3000 mg × 3 d was selected as the recommended dose for phase II study. The Southwest Oncology Group (SWOG) launched such a phase II study in patients with OC in 1988, and the toxicities observed indicated that the selected dose schedule was quite satisfactory, although grade 3 and 4 neutropenia and thrombocytopenia were observed in 15% of patients. Dose escalation to 4500 mg × 3 d was carried out in some patients; two received the dose on a per-m^2 basis, and experienced myelosuppression. During the conduct of this study, HT3 inhibitors were introduced as antiemetics, and the sometimes-troublesome same-day nausea and vomiting were drastically reduced with either iv or oral ondansetron or granisetron. Because of ease of administration and accumulating favorable clinical experience, a number of additional studies with ip FUDR were carried out at USC.

3.2. Dose-Escalation Study of IP (R,S)-Leucovorin Given with IP FUDR

This study assessed the tolerance and the pharmacokinetics of FUDR at the 3000 mg × 3 d dose schedule, given with ip LV starting at 5 mg × 3 d and eventually by doubling the dose in cohorts of three patients, escalating to 640 mg × 3 d. LV had no obvious effect on the toxic events that were recorded *(15)*. At Memorial Sloan-Kettering Cancer Center (MSKCC), a similar study was carried out, and a dose was recommended of 2000 mg/m^2 × 3 d with ip LV (a dose-schedule quite analogous to the authors) *(28)*. In unpublished experience, they have also tested lower doses in an every-12-h × -6 schedule, attempting to provide more continued exposure to higher levels of FUDR.

3.3. Pharmacologic Study of IP FUDR with Three Fixed Doses of IP (S)-Leucovorin

The results of this study were comparable to the previous one, and again suggested no obvious toxicity from the concomitant administration (S)-LV tested at doses of 160, 320, or 640 mg *(16)*. In subsequent experience in combination with cisplatin *(29)*, however, the author observed a greater incidence of mucosal toxicities (even in cycles given without cisplatin) than had been observed in the phase II study by the SWOG in a similar population *(30)*, and have concluded that ip LV might add to the GI toxicity of ip FUDR. In more recent studies, therefore, the authors have dropped LV.

3.4. Dose-Escalation Study of Continuous-Infusion IV Hydroxyurea with IP FUDR and (R,S)-Leucovorin

This study, published only in abstract form *(17)*, again utilized FUDR at a dose of 3000 mg × 3 d + 640 mg LV; the infusion of hydroxyurea was ongoing. Grade 3 thrombocytopenia and grade 4 neutropenia occurred in three instances each, out of five patients entered at the highest dose of iv hydroxyurea of 3.6 g/m^2/d. The recommended dose for phase II study of iv hydroxyurea is 3.0 g/m^2/d, to be given with ip FUDR and LV. Antitumor effects were noted, but not at extraperitoneal sites in patients with GI cancers and liver metastases entered to assess whether this type of modulation would enhance the activity of fluoropyrimidines at sites other than in the peritoneum. For this reason, the authors have considered the combination of ip FUDR with systemic fluoropyrimidines as potentially more promising for future development.

3.5. Phase I/II Study of IP FUDR and LV Combined with Cis- or Carboplatin

Patients were treated with the usual dose of ip 3000 mg FUDR, and ip 320 mg LV × 3 d, to be followed by ip 60 mg/m^2 cisplatin on the third day, repeated every 3 wk. In patients with OC and minimal residual disease, treatment tolerance was to be assessed for six courses. Eighteen patients were entered, with 11 having minimal residual disease OC. Partial or full substitution of cisplatin with carboplatin was effected for patients with preexisting neuropathy. The results indicated excellent hematologic tolerance of the combination with cisplatin alone, and with 30 mg/m^2 cisplatin + carboplatin at an AUC of 3; however, myelosuppression delaying treatment courses was occasionally seen with carboplatin at an AUC of 5 in patients with moderate neuropathy. Because of mucositis, the LV has been dropped in 10 additional patients who have been treated since publication of this study. Also, because toxicity has been minimal, an increase of the cisplatin dose to 75 mg/m^2, in those patients experiencing no toxicity to the first cycle, has been proposed in a recent study to be conducted by the Eastern Cooperative Oncology Group (ECOG).

In all these phase I trials, the usual complications secondary to the presence of an ip catheter have been seen. These have been detailed in prior publications. However, in the randomized phase II study by the SWOG (*see* next subheading) these complications were fewer in the FUDR arm *(30)*. Nevertheless, one should be cognizant not only of the common outflow obstruction, but also inflow problems (which are probably catheter-related), and problems with perforations and infections that occur in less than 10% of patients.

4. CLINICAL EXPERIENCE OF IP FUDR IN OC

In the phase I studies at USC, exclusive of the combinations with platinums or with hydroxyurea, 10 patients, all pretreated with a number of prior platinum-containing regimens, received 2–5 cycles of therapy (median three). Three patients showed signs of progression, two discontinued for logistical reasons (one with 20-mo follow-up prior to detection of progressive disease), and five were interrupted because of new availability of paclitaxel: Three of these had demonstrated a decrease in CA-125. A six-year follow-up is available in one of these patients, who had received ip FUDR with (S)-LV for three cycles for small-volume residual disease in the peritoneal cavity, detected at second-look laparotomy. She also had a small right pleural effusion, and, with persistently elevated CA-125, it was elected to treat her with paclitaxel. One yr later, while still receiving paclitaxel, she had a laparotomy for volvulus, and no malignant disease was noted at exploration. She has had no abdominal manifestations while requiring prolonged systemic therapy for extraabdominal (axilla, pleura) metastases.

The randomized phase II study in OC patients with minimal residual disease at second-look laparotomy by the SWOG indicated that ip FUDR was the likely choice, instead of ip mitoxantrone, in a pick-the-winner design. The completion rate of six courses for FUDR was 67% (vs 42% for mitoxantrone). The median relapse-free survival in the FUDR arm was 37 mo, and seven of the 28 evaluable patients remained in a disease-free state from 3.5 to 7+ yr *(30,* and unpublished update). Analogous results have been reported with consolidation treatments, such as whole abdominal radiation *(31)*, or interleukin-2 *(32)*, and slightly inferior results with ip consolidation from one institution utilizing a combination of cytarabine, cisplatin, and bleomycin, but this series included up to 2 cm residual disease *(33)*. In the absence of concurrent controls, it is difficult to extrapolate from these results regarding antitumor efficacy. In the SWOG study, the presence of a mitoxantrone arm, showing inferior results, suggests that FUDR had antitumor effects resulting in delay of relapses and some long-term benefit. Normalization of CA-125 in those patients with abnormal findings at the outset further point to such antitumor effects *(30)*.

IP 5-FU has been studied in combination, and as a single agent, for minimal residual disease OC. The largest study is by the Gynecologic Oncology Group, and reports many adverse effects *(34)*. The combination studies included frontline administration with cisplatin *(35)*, as randomized consolidation *(36)* in an inconclusive trial because of size, and as part of phase I and pharmacologic study with cisplatin *(37)*.

The authors have been accumulating experience with FUDR and platinums in patients receiving this therapy as consolidation for minimal residual disease at reassessment. At USC, 18 such patients have been treated since the 11 included in prior publication

(29). Four patients continue disease-free, exceeding 3 yr from onset of treatment. The authors have opened additional studies at NYU in 1997, and through the ECOG in 1998.

5. CLINICAL EXPERIENCE OF IP FUDR IN GI CANCERS

A subset of patients with colorectal cancer (CRC) recur predominantly in the peritoneum, and have been excellent candidates for treatment in phase I ip studies. Nine patients were entered in FUDR + LV studies, and received 2–14 cycles of treatment (median, 5). One patient, failing 5-FU with measurable disease on CT scan, manifested a partial response, and another patient a decrease in carcinoembryonic antigen for 8 mo. Thirteen patients with CRC were entered in the ip FUDR + LV + iv hydroxyurea protocol: Seven of these completed six cycles of treatment, and showed no progression from 4 to 12 mo *(17).* Sugarbaker et al. *(38)* had already explored the possibility that ip fluoropyrimidines could decrease peritoneal metastases in high-risk CRC patients as an adjuvant following resection. Their trial, which utilized ip 5 FU × 5 d for six courses, and compared it to ip, did not demonstrate any differences in recurrences or survival, but fewer peritoneal recurrences were documented in the ip group. a pilot study recently carried out in a similar high-risk population by the MSKCC group, with ip FUDR, has yielded encouraging results *(18).*

An occasional patient with gastric cancer (GC) has been treated in the phase I studies. One patient sustained a remarkable decrease in ascites, but progressed in extraperitoneal sites, and one of two patients with GC in the hydroxyurea protocol had stable disease for 4 mo. A large 5-FU + cisplatin neoadjuvant study was launched at USC in patients with potentially resectable GC: Two cycles of ip FUDR + cisplatin were given as consolidation postsurgical resection *(39).* The results have recently been published as a final report by Crookes et al. *(40)* and, with a median followup of 45 mo, show a median survival exceeding 4 yr. Their conclusions state: "This program of preoperative and postoperative ip chemotherapy has been found to be safe and appears to decrease gastric carcinoma recurrence rates and increase survival compared with historical control." IP consolidation with FUDR has also been adopted by the group at MSKCC.

In other GI cancers, such as small bowel and pancreas origin, some antitumor effects have been noted in the phase I studies. One patient, with ascites from an ileal carcinoma complicating Crohn's disease, experienced a brief 2-mo remission before developing intestinal obstruction. One patient diagnosed as an unknown primary cancer, probably of pancreatic origin, had a 9-mo remission in ascites and markers.

6. CLINICAL EXPERIENCE OF IP FUDR IN PSEUDOMYXOMA PERITONEII OR APPENDICEAL PRIMARIES

In the initial phase I study, one man with advanced pseudomyxoma peritoneii and multiple masses after two resections, was treated with FUDR for over 1 yr, and experienced some relief in ascites formation and decreased CEA. In the ip FUDR + LV studies, five patients with appendiceal primaries were treated and received 2, 3, 6, 6, and 11 cycles of ip FUDR. The two patients receiving this as first chemotherapy were reassessed after two and 11 cycles: the first had microscopic residual, and, after adding cisplain, had no evidence of disease at 31 mo; the other one had a negative reassessment, but had progressive disease 14 mo later. In the ip FUDR + LV + iv hydroxyurea, four patients with appendiceal primaries were entered. All of them were previously untreated: Two patients with minimal disease have shown no recurrence more than 1 yr after completing their treatment; one patient with bulky disease was stable for 4 mo. Two patients (one man with unknown primary and a woman, at a few months postresection of a rectosigmoid carcinoma and adjuvant 5-FU) had manifestations best characterized as a bulky pseudomyxoma peritoneii with large mucinous omental caking, peritoneal and pelvic mucinous deposits leading to abdominal distention, and no liver metastases. Both entered the protocol, and showed minor decreases in their markers, and were subsequently subjected to near-total palliative resection and drainage of their mucinous masses. The man was consolidated with additional ip FUDR, and is alive with disease 3+ yr later.

Others have also considered a role for ip therapy in this disease. Sugarbaker et al. have published their experience with aggressive surgical and perioperative ip approaches *(41–43)*. Favorable results from ip therapy have also been published from other groups *(44)*.

7. CONCLUSIONS AND FUTURE DIRECTIONS

In the extensive clinical experience with ip FUDR, principally originating in three centers (NYU, USC, and MSKCC), the drug has been demonstrated to possess ideal features for ip administration: excellent local and subjective tolerance at readily achievable cytotoxic concentrations. The feasibility of administering repeated cycles of treatment with little morbidity has been proven in a multi-institutional setting, and in the various pilot studies. The drug has also been shown to be suitable for combinations with platinum compounds, drugs that have shown a superiority over iv treatment in randomized trials of OC *(45,46)*, and promising results in GC described above.

The authors have documented antitumor activity against GI and OC in phase I studies, including patients with various degrees of assessibility and exposure to prior therapies. The purpose of this chapter was to build a rationale for the integration of ip drug administration in current therapeutic strategies. This is an important step to consider, because the track record in eliminating peritoneal spread of disease by systemic drug therapy in GI cancers is quite dismal, and, in OC, only the initial platinum-based regimens have curative potential by the systemic route.

A most important future direction, therefore, should be the integration of ip drugs in phase III studies. In OC, the authors have proposed a trial comparing reassessment to no reassessment, following complete responses to initial platinum-based chemotherapy of suboptimally debulked disease. The patients randomized to reassessment would undergo debulking (if appropriate), and then be consolidated with ip cisplatin, if negative, or with ip cisplatin + FUDR, if positive for residual disease. Introducing a new drug, such as FUDR, to which no patient has been previously exposed, is an obvious rationale for its selection over other candidate ip drugs. Statistical considerations have been performed, taking into account 33% with negative assessment (with an anticipated median survival of 4 yr), 50% with <0.5 cm (with an anticipated median survival of 3 yr), and 17% with 0.5–1 cm residual (with an anticipated median survival of 2 yr). A 50% improvement in median survival with ip therapy in the reassessed population would require 330 patients for a one-sided 0.05 level, and a power of 0.80.

In GI cancer, the neoadjuvant strategy has been widely adopted. A randomization, including ip FUDR (and cisplatin) after resection, vs only continued systemic therapy, could indicate the efficacy and morbidity of such ip consolidation. Similarly, in CRC patients at high risk of ip dissemination (e.g., ovarian or omental spread, T3 tumors with adherences, multiple positive regional nodes) should be assessed for trials, including ip or systemic consolidation. Such trials, however, would require that surgical teams be ready to place ip catheters at the time of their intervention, and such a step would require much greater awareness than there has been to date of the limitations of the various approaches to control peritoneal spread of disease. Similarly, experience with pseudomyxoma peritoneii indicates that ip FUDR should be considered further as a therapeutic modality: Randomized phase II clinical trials might prove informative in this relatively rare entity.

Exploration of ip FUDR in combinations other than platinums is particularly relevant for the treatment of GI cancers. For example, an ip FUDR oral fluoropyrimidine combination could prove to have promising efficacy in colon cancer with peritoneal spread. Other combinations of interest are with topoisomerase I inhibitors, and the authors are beginning studies with ip administration of these agents. At present, no other therapeutic leads appear more promising in control of small-volume GI cancer spread throughout the peritoneal than ip administration of FUDR alone, or in combination.

REFERENCES

1. Los G and McVie JG. Experimental and clinical stages of intraperitoneal chemotherapy, *Eur. J. Cancer*, **26** (1990) 755–762.
2. Hoskins WJ, McGuire WP, Brady MF, et al. Effect of diameter of largest residual disease on survival after primary cytoreductive surgery in patients with suboptimal residual epithelial ovarian carcinoma, *Am. J. Obstet. Gynecol.*, **170** (1994) 974–980.
3. McGuire WP, Hoskins WJ, Brady MF, et al. Assessment of dose-intensive therapy in suboptimally debulked ovarian cancer: a Gynecologic Oncology Group study, *J. Clin. Oncol.*, **13** (1995) 1589–1599.
4. Markman M. Intraperitoneal antineoplastic agents for tumors principally confined to the peritoneal cavity, *Cancer Treat. Rev.*, **13** (1986) 219–242.
5. Jodrell DI, Egorin MJ, Canetta R, et al. Relationships between carboplatin exposure and tumor response and toxicity in patients with ovarian cancer, *J. Clin. Oncol.*, **110** (1992) 520–528.
6. Howell SB, Pfeifle CL, Wung WE, et al. Intraperitoneal cisplatin with systemic thiosulfate protection, *Ann. Intern. Med.*, **97** (1982) 845–851.
7. Los G, Mutsaers PHA, van der Vijgh, Baldew GS, de Graaf PW, and McVie JG. Direct diffusion of cis-diamminedichloroplatinum (II) in intraperitoneal rat tumors after intraperitoneal chemotherapy: a comparison with systemic chemotherapy, *Cancer Res.*, **49** (1989) 3380–3384.
8. Los G, Mutsaers PHA, Lenglet WJM, Baldew JS, and McVie JG. Platinum distribution in intraperitoneal tumors after intraperitoneal cisplatin treatment, *Cancer Chemother. Pharmacol.*, **25** (1990) 389–394.
9. Speyer JL, Collins JM, Dedrick RL, et al. Phase I and pharmacological studies of 5-fluorouracil administered intraperitoneally, *Cancer Res.*, **40** (1980) 567–572.
10. Speyer JL, Sugarbaker PH, Collins JM, Dedrick RL, Klecker RW Jr, and Myers CE. Portal levels and hepatic clearance of 5-fluorouracil after intraperitoneal administration in humans, *Cancer Res.*, **41** (1981) 1916–1922.
11. Archer SG, McCullock RK, and Gray BN. Comparative study of the pharmacokinetics of continuous portal vein infusion versus intraperitoneal infusion of 5-fluorouracil, *Reg. Cancer Treat.*, **2** (1989) 105–111.
12. Sugarbaker PH, Graves T, DeBruijn EA, et al. Early postoperative intraperitoneal chemotherapy as an adjuvant to surgery for peritoneal carcinomatosis from gastrointestinal cancer: pharmacological studies, *Cancer Res.*, **50** (1990) 5790–5794.
13. Muggia FM, Chan KK, Russell C., et al. Phase I and pharmacologic evaluation of intraperitoneal 5-fluoro-2′-deoxyuridine, *Cancer Chemother Pharmacol.*, **28** (1991) 241–250.
14. Muggia F, Chan K, Tulpule A, and Retzios A. Importance of pharmacokinetics for developing new therapies, In Kimura K, Carter SK, Ogawa M, Eds. *Cancer Chemotherapy: Challenges for the Future*, Vol. 7, Exerpta Medica, Tokyo, 1992, pp. 305–313.
15. Muggia FM, Tulpule A, Retzioa A, et al. Intraperitoneal 5-fluoro-2′-deoxyuridine with escalating doses of leucovorin: pharmacology and clinical tolerance, *Invest. New Drugs*, **12** (1994) 197–206.

16. Israel VK, Jiang C, Muggia FM, et al. Intraperitoneal 5-fluoro-2'-deoxyuridine (FUDR) and (s)-leucovorin for disease predominantly confined to the peritoneal cavity: a pharmacokinetic and toxicity study, *Cancer Chemother. Pharmacol.*, **37** (1995) 32–38.

17. Garcia A, Spears CP, Kutsch K, et al. Phase I and pharmacologic study of intravenous hydroxyurea infusion given with intraperitoneal 5-fluoro-2'-deoxyuridine (FUDR) and leucovorin, *Cancer Chemother. Pharmacol.*, submitted.

18. Kelsen DP, Saltz L, Cohen AM, et al. Phase I trial of immediate postoperative intraperitoneal floxuridine and leucovorin plus systemic 5-fluorouracil and levamisole after resection of high risk colon cancer, *Cancer*, **74** (1994) 2224–2233.

19. Gyves J, Ensminger W, Stetson P, et al. Constant intraperitoneal 5-fluorouracil infusion through a totally implanted system, *Clin. Pharmacol. Ther.*, **35** (1984) 83–89.

20. Ensminger W, Rosowsky A, and Raso V. Clinical pharmacologic evaluation of hepatic arterial infusion of 5-fluoro-2'-deoxyuridine and 5-fluorouracil, *Cancer Res.*, **38** (1978) 3784–3792.

21. Gastrointestinal Tumor Study Group. Workshop on intraperitoneal chemotherapy, *Semin. Oncol.*, **12 (Suppl. 4)** (1985) 1–123.

22. Atiq OT, Kelsen DP, and Shiu MH. Phase II trial of postoperative adjuvant intraperitoneal cisplatin and fluorouracil and systemic fluorouracil chemotherapy in patients with resected gastric cancer, *J. Clin. Oncol.*, **11** (1993) 425–433.

23. Reichman B, Markman M, Hakes T, et al. Phase I trial of concurrent intraperitoneal and continuous infusion of 5-fluorouracil plus intraperitoneal cisplatin in patients with refractory cancer, *Reg. Cancer Ther.*, **1** (1989) 223–228.

24. Lindner P, Heath DD, Shalinsky DR, Howell SB, Naredi P, and Hafstrom L. Regional lymphatic exposure following ip administration of 5-fluorouracil, carboplatin, and etoposide, *Surg. Oncol.*, **2** (1993) 105–112.

25. Dedrick RL and Flessner MF. Pharmacokinetic problems in peritoneal drug administration: tissue penetration and surface exposure, *J. Natl. Cancer Inst.*, **89** (1997) 480–487.

26. Cafier CS, Kerr DJ, Young AM, Neoptolemos JP, et al. Prolonged intraperitoneal infusion of 5-fluorouracil using a novel solution, *Br. J. Cancer*, **74** (1996) 2032–2035.

27. Keyomarsi K and Moran RK. Folinic acid augmentation of the effects of fluoropyrimidines on murine and human leukemic cells, *Cancer Res.*, **46** (1986) 4229–4335.

28. Smith JA, Morris A, Duafala ME, Bertino JR, Markman M, and Kleinberg M. Stability of flosuridine and leucovorin calcium admixtures for intraperitoneal administration, *Am. J. Hosp. Pharm.*, **45** (1989) 985–989.

29. Muggia FM, Jeffers S, Muderspach L, et al. Phase I/II study of intraperitoneal floxuridine and platinums (cisplatin and/or carboplatin), *Gynecol. Oncol.*, **66** (1997) 290–294.

30. Muggia FM, Liu PY, Alberts DS, et al. Intraperitoneal mitoxantrone or floxuridine: effects on time-to-failure and survival of patients with minimal residual ovarian cancer after second-look laparotomy: a randomized phase II study by the Southwest Oncology Group, *Gynecol. Oncol.*, **61** (1996) 395–402.

31. Sedlacek TV, Spyropoulos P, Cifaldi R, Glassburn J, and Fisher S. Salvage therapy for ovarian carcinoma using whole abdomen radiation therapy, *Proc. Am. Soc. Clin. Oncol.*, **16** (1997) 353a (Abstract).

32. Edwards RP, Gooding W, Lembersky BC, et al. Comparison of toxicity and survival following intraperitoneal recombinant interleukin-2 persistent ovarian cancer after platinum twenty-four hour versus 7-day infusion, *J. Clin. Oncol.*, **15** (1997) 3399–3407.

33. Piver MS, Recio FO, Baker TR, and Driscoll D. Evaluation of survival after second-line intraperitoneal cisplatin-based chemotherapy for advanced ovarian cancer, *Cancer*, **73** (1994) 1693–1698.

34. Walton LA, Blessing JA, and Homesley HD. Adverse effect of intraperitoneal fluorouracil in patients with optimal residual ovarian cancer after second-look laparotomy: a Gynecologic Oncology Group study, *J. Clin. Oncol.*, **7** (1989) 466–470.

35. Doroshow J, Braly P, Hoff S, et al. Intraperitoneal (ip) chemotherapy with cisplatin (p) and 5-fluorouracil (FU): an active regimen for refractory ovarian cancer (oc), *Proc. Am. Soc. Clin. Onc.*, **5** (1986) 117 (Abstract).

36. Louie KG, Ozols RF, Myers CE, et al. Long-term results of a cisplatin-containing combination chemotherapy regimen for the treatment of advanced ovarian carcinoma, *J. Clin. Oncol.*, **4** (1986) 579–85.

37. Schilsky RL, Choi KE, Grayhack J, et al. Phase I clinical and pharmacologic study of intraperitoneal cisplatin and fluorouracil in patients with advanced intraabdominal cancer, *J. Clin. Oncol.*, **8** (1990) 2054–2061.

38. Sugarbaker PH, Gianola FJ, Speyer JL, Wesley R, Barofsky I, and Myers CE. Prospective randomized trial of intravenous versus intraperitoneal 5-fluorouracil in patients with advanced primary colon or rectal cancer, *Surgery,* **98** (1985) 414–421.

39. Leichman L, Silberman H, Leichman CG, et al. Preoperative systemic chemotherapy followed by adjuvant postoperative intraperitoneal therapy for gastric cancer: a University of Southern California pilot program, *J. Clin. Oncol.,* **10** (1992) 1933–1942.

40. Crookes P, Leichman CG, Leichman L, et al. Systemic chemotherapy for gastric carcinoma followed by postoperative intraperitoneal therapy: a final report, *Cancer,* **79** (1997) 1767–1775.

41. Sugarbaker PH, Kern K, and Lack E. Malignant pseudomyxoma peritonei of colonic origin: natural history and presentation of a curative approach to treatment, *Dis. Colon Rectum,* **30** (1987) 772–779.

42. Sugarbaker PH, Zhu BW, Sese GB, et al. Peritoneal carcinomatosis from appendiceal cancer: results of 69 patients treated by cytoreductive surgery and intraperitoneal chemotherapy, *Dis. Colon Rectum,* **36** (1993) 323–329.

43. Sugarbaker PH, Cunliffe W, Belliveau JF, et al. Rationale for perioperative intraperitoneal chemotherapy as a surgical adjuvant for gastrointestinal malignancy, *Reg. Cancer Treat.,* **1** (1988) 66–79.

44. Gough DB, Donohue JH, Schutt AJ, et al. Pseudomyxoma peritonei. Long-term survival with an aggressive regional, *Ann. Surg.,* **219** (1994) 112–119.

45. Alberts DS, Liu PY, Hannigans EV, et al. Intraperitoneal cisplatin plus intravenous cyclophosphamide versus intravenous cisplatin plus intravenous cyclophosphamide for stage III ovarian cancer, *N. Engl. J. Med.,* **335** (1996) 1950–1955.

46. Markman M, Bundy B, Benda J, et al. Randomized phase 3 study of intravenous (iv) cisplatin (cis)/paclitaxel (PAC) versus moderately high dose iv carboplatin (carb) followed by iv PAC and intraperitoneal (ip) cis in optimal residual ovarian cancer: an intergroup trial (GOG, SWOG, ECOG), *Proc. Am. Soc. Clin. Oncol.,* **17** (1998) 361a (Abstract).

47. Aghajanian C, Sabbatini P, Hensley M, et al. A phase I trial of intraperitoneal (IP) cisplatin with IP gemcitabine in patients (PTs) with epithelial ovarian cancer. *Proc. Am. Soc. Clin. Oncol.* **18** (1999) 370a (Abst. #1428).

14 Cytoreductive Surgery and Intraperitoneal Chemotherapy for Peritoneal Surface Malignancies

Paul H. Sugarbaker

CONTENTS

1. INTRODUCTION

Changes in the use of chemotherapy in patients with peritoneal carcinomatosis, peritoneal sarcomatosis, and peritoneal mesothelioma have shown favorable results of treatment. A change in route of drug administration has occurred: Chemotherapy is given intraperitoneally, or by combined intraperitoneal (ip) and intravenous (iv) routes. In this new strategy, iv chemotherapy alone is rarely indicated. Also, a change in timing has occurred: Chemotherapy begins in the operating room, and may be continued for the first 5 d postoperative (PO). A change in selection criteria of treatment of cancer has also occurred. The lesion size (LS) of peritoneal implants is of crucial importance. Only patients with small-sized ip tumor nodules, with limited distribution within the abdomen and pelvis, are likely to show prolonged benefit. Meticulous cytoreductive surgery is necessary prior to the ip chemotherapy instillation. Aggressive treatment strategies for large-volume invasive ip cancer will not produce long-term benefits, and are often the cause of excessive morbidity or mortality. The initiation of treatments for peritoneal surface malignancy (PSM) must occur as early as possible in the natural history of these diseases, in order to achieve the greatest benefits. The greatest change that now needs to occur with PSM is a change in oncologists' attitudes toward these diseases. They may be cured if treated early with aggressive local-regional treatment strategies.

2. BACKGROUND

Most cancers that occur within the abdomen or pelvis will disseminate by three different routes: hematogenous metastases, lymphatic metastases, and through peritoneal

From: *Current Clinical Oncology: Regional Chemotherapy: Clinical Research and Practice*
Edited by: M. Markman © Humana Press Inc., Totowa, NJ

spaces to surfaces within the abdomen and pelvis. In a substantial number of patients with abdominal or pelvic malignancy, surgical treatment failure is isolated to the resection site or to peritoneal surfaces. This leads to a hypothesis that suggests that the elimination of peritoneal surface spread may have an impact on the survival of these cancer patients, and that a leading cause of death and suffering in patients with these malignancies is progression of peritoneal surface disease. Prior to the use of cytoreductive surgery and ip chemotherapy, these conditions were uniformly fatal, eventually resulting in intestinal obstruction over the course of months or years. Occasionally, patients with low-grade malignancies, such as pseudomyxoma peritonei, survived for several years, but all end-result reporting have shown fatal outcomes.

Current technology for the administration of ip chemotherapy demands that it be used as an integral part of the surgical procedure. Surgically directed chemotherapy involves several conceptual changes in chemotherapy administration. First, an ip, rather than an iv, route for chemotherapy is used. The ip route, when properly utilized, will allow uniform distribution of a high concentration of anticancer therapy at the site of the malignancy. This is achieved by the surgeon intraoperatively manipulating the intestinal contents to uniformly distribute the chemotherapy. In the early PO period, the patient's position if repeatedly changed, to assist gravity in maintaining an optimal chemotherapy distribution. Second, chemotherapy administration is timed so that all of the malignancy, except for microscopic residual disease, will have been removed prior to chemotherapy treatments, which means that the limited penetration of chemotherapy into tissues (approx 1 mm) will be adequate to eradicate all tumor cells. Also, the chemotherapy will be used prior to the construction of any anastomosis, so that suture line recurrences should also be eliminated. Finally, patient selection must occur, so that these aggressive management strategies, cytoreductive surgery, and ip chemotherapy are used as early in the natural history of the cancer as possible. No longer can the clinician wait for the patient to become symptomatic to begin treatments. Even protocols to prevent peritoneal surface spread, which may occur after the resection of a primary gastrointestinal (GI) or gynecologic malignancy, must be considered. Treatment of patients with an invasive malignancy that has a wide distribution of large-volume cancer will not produce long-term benefits. As soon as oncologists believe that PSM can be cured, they will initiate aggressive treatments in a timely fashion. This chapter is designed to acquaint physicians with methods for treatment and prevention developed for peritoneal carcinomatosis, sarcomatosis, and mesothelioma.

2.1. Peritoneal–Plasma Barrier

IP chemotherapy gives high response rates within the abdomen, because the peritoneal plasma barrier provides dose-intensive therapy *(1)*. Figure 1 shows that large-mol-wt substances, such as mitomycin C (MMC), are confined to the abdominal cavity for long time periods *(2)*, which means that the exposure of peritoneal surfaces to pharmacologically active molecules can be increased considerably by giving the drugs via the ip route, rather than by the iv route.

For chemotherapy agents used to treat peritoneal carcinomatosis or peritoneal sarcomatosis, the area under the curve (AUC) ratios of ip to iv exposure are favorable. Table 1 presents the AUC (ip/iv) for the drugs in routine clinical use in patients with peritoneal seeding *(3–5)*. In the author's studies, these include 5-fluorouracil (5-FU), MMC, doxorubicin, cisplatin, paclitaxel, and gemcitabine.

One should not assume that the ip administration of chemotherapy eliminates their systemic toxicities. Although the drugs are sequestered within the peritoneal space,

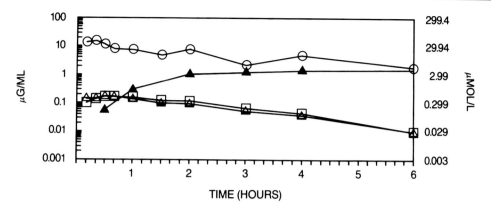

Fig. 1. Large mol wt compounds, when instilled into the peritoneal cavity, are sequestered at that site for long time periods. The physiologic barrier to the release of ip drugs is called "the peritoneal plasma barrier." In this experiment, 15 mg MMC was infused into the cavity as rapidly as possible. IP, iv portal venous and urine MMC concentrations were determined by high pressure liquid chromatography assay. . = peritoneal fluid, ▲ = urine, ∪ = plasma, ∨ = portal plasma. Adapted with permission from ref. 2.

Table 1
Area Under Curve Ratios of Peritoneal
Surface Exposure to Systemic Exposure
for Drugs Used to Treat Intra-abdominal Cancer

Drug	Mol wt	AUC
5-fluorouracil	130	250
Mitomycin C	334	75
Doxorubicin	544	500
Cisplatin	300	20
Paclitaxel	808	1000
Gemcitabine	263	50

they eventually are cleared into the systemic circulation. For this reason, the safe dose of most drugs instilled into the peritoneal cavity are identical to the iv dose. The exceptions are drugs with hepatic degradation, such as 5-FU and gemcitabine. An increased dose of approx 50% is usually possible with 5-FU. The dose for a 5-d course of iv 5-FU is approx 500 mg/m²/d; for ip 5-FU, the dose if 750 mg/m²/d. This considerable (50%) increase in dose of 5-FU is of great advantage in eliminating peritoneal carcinomatosis.

2.2. Tumor Cell Entrapment

The author has advanced the tumor cell entrapment hypothesis to explain the rapid progression of PSM in patients who undergo treatment using surgery alone. This theory relates the high incidence and rapid progression of peritoneal surface implantation to free ip tumor emboli, as a result of serosal penetration by cancer; leakage of malignant cells from transected lymphatics; dissemination of malignant cells directly from the cancer specimen, as a result of surgical trauma and backflow of venous blood; fibrin entrapment of intra-abdominal tumor emboli on traumatized peritoneal surfaces; and promotion of these entrapped tumor cells through growth factors involved in the wound healing process. This phenomenon may cause a high incidence of surgical treatment failure in patients treated for primary GI cancer. Also, the reimplantation of malignant cells into peritonectomized surfaces in a reoperative setting must be expected.

Chemotherapy used in the perioperative period not only directly destroys tumor cells, but it also eliminates viable platelets, while blood cells, and monocytes form the peritoneal cavity, which diminishes the promotion of tumor growth associated with the wound healing process. Consequently, the results of ip chemotherapy show a reduction in local recurrence, and peritoneal surface recurrence in patients with intra-abdominal cancer. Removal of the leukocytes and monocytes also decreases the ability of the abdomen to resist an infectious process; therefore, strict aseptic technique is imperative when administering the chemotherapy, or when handing abdominal tubes and drains.

In order to interrupt this widespread implantation of tumor cells on abdominal and pelvic surfaces, the abdominal cavity is flooded with chemotherapy in a large volume of fluid during the operation (heated intraoperative ip chemotherapy) and in the PO period (early PO ip chemotherapy). Some patients with a guarded prognosis may receive adjuvant ip and systemic chemotherapy *(6)*. Therefore, the strategy for treatment and prevention of peritoneal carcinomatosis and sarcomatosis involves not only a change in the route (from iv to ip), but also a change in the timing (PO to perioperative) of chemotherapy administration.

This new approach to surgical treatment of abdominal and pelvic malignancy begins in the operating room after a complete resection of a primary cancer, or after the complete cytoreduction of peritoneal carcinomatosis, peritoneal sarcomatosis, or peritoneal mesothelioma. The proper placement of tubes and drains and temperature probes is needed prior to initiation of ip chemotherapy. Suture lines or repair of seromuscular tears occurs after the ip chemotherapy is completed. Before abdominal closure, the temperature probes are removed, but the tubes and drains are left in place for early PO ip lavage and chemotherapy.

2.3. Prior Limited Benefits with IP Chemotherapy

The use of ip chemotherapy in the past has met with limited success and acceptance by oncologists. There have been three major impediments to greater success. First, intracavitary instillation allows limited penetration of drug into tumor nodules: Only the outermost layer (approx 1 mm) of a cancer nodule is penetrated by the chemotherapy, which means that only minute tumor nodules can be definitely treated. In most trials, oncologists have attempted to treat established disease, and this selection of patients has caused disappointment with ip drug use. Microscopic residual disease is the ideal target for ip chemotherapy protocols.

A second cause for limited success with ip chemotherapy is a nonuniform drug distribution. Patients treated by drug instillation into the abdomen or pelvis uniformly have had prior surgery, which invariably causes scarring within the abdomen and pelvis. The adhesions create multiple barriers to the free access of fluid. Although the instillation of a large volume of fluid will partially overcome the problems created by adhesions, frequently, large surface areas will have no access to chemotherapy. In addition, limited access from adhesions is impossible to predict, and may increase with repeated instillations of chemotherapy.

Also, surgery results in fibrin deposits on surfaces that have been traumatized by cancer resection. Free ip cancer cells become trapped within the fibrin. The fibrin is infiltrated by platelets, neutrophils, and monocytes, as part of the wound healing process. As collagen is laid down, the tumor cells are then entrapped by scar tissue, which is dense and poorly penetrated by ip chemotherapy.

Poor drug distribution is also caused by gravity. IP fluid does not uniformly contact all parietal and visceral peritoneal surfaces. Gravity pulls the fluid to dependent portions of the abdomen and pelvis, especially the pelvis, abdominal gutters, and the right retrohepatic space. Unless the patient frequently changes position, the surfaces between bowel loops and the anterior abdominal wall will remain relatively untreated.

The third and final obstacle to success with the administration of ip chemotherapy is the difficulty and dangers of long-term peritoneal access. There has been no technical solution to the requirement for reliable repeated access to the peritoneal space. Access in the operating theater is now completely safe, and temporary access in the early PO period is safe for the patient. However, repeated instillations of large volumes of chemotherapy solution causes great inconvenience, and can result in a large number of serious complications. Whether the oncologist chooses repeated paracentesis or an indwelling catheter, complications, such as pain upon instillation, bowel perforation, instillation into soft tissues, or inability to infuse or drain, occur repeatedly. Prolonged peritoneal access is a technical challenge without a known solution.

The problems with prolonged peritoneal access have led numerous surgical oncologists to adopt what has been referred to as the "big bang" approach. All visible abdominal or pelvic cancer should be completely extirpated by surgery; then, in the operating room, a high dose of heated chemotherapy is delivered to eradicate the remaining tiny tumor nodules and microscopic cancer cells that remain. This means that all abdominal and pelvic components of the cancer, including persistent PSM, are eliminated. Systemic components of the disease now become the responsibility of the medical oncologist.

2.4. Proper Patient Selection for IP Chemotherapy

Perhaps the greatest impediment to lasting benefits from ip chemotherapy should be attributed to improper patient selection. In most ip chemotherapy protocols, the patients, from a theoretical perspective, would not benefit much, if at all. A great number of patients with gross intra-abdominal disease have been treated, but, even with extensive prior cytoreductive surgery, the patient is not likely to have lasting benefit. Rapid recurrence of ip cancer, combined with progression of lymph nodal or systemic disease, are likely to interfere with any long-term benefits in these patients. Patients who benefit will have minimal disease isolated to peritoneal surfaces that have access to chemotherapy, so that complete eradication of disease can occur. Partial responses are not of great benefit in PSMs. Complete and durable responses are the reasonable goal. Of course, where the patient starts at the time of initiation of treatment will have great bearing on the response achieved. Early and asymptomatic patients must be selected for ip chemotherapy protocols.

2.5. Clinical Assessments of PSM

In the past, peritoneal carcinomatosis was considered to be a fatal disease process. The only assessment used was either carcinomatosis present with a presumed fatal outcome or carcinomatosis absent with curative treatment options available. Currently, there are four important clinical assessments of PSM that need to be used to select patients who will benefit from treatment protocols: the invasive character of the malignancy, the preoperative computed tomography (CT) scan of abdomen and pelvis, the Peritoneal Cancer Index (PCI), and the completeness of cytoreduction (CC) score.

The invasive character of a PSM will have profound influence on its treatment options. Noninvasive tumors may have extensive spread on peritoneal surfaces, and yet be completely resectable by peritonectomy procedures. Also, these noninvasive malignancies are unlikely to metastasize by lymphatics to lymph nodes or by the blood to liver and other systemic sites. Therefore, protocols for cytoreductive surgery and ip chemotherapy may have a curative intent in patients with pseudomyxoma peritonei and peritoneal mesothelioma. Also, some low-grade sarcomas may be aggressively treated, with cure as a goal for cytoreductive surgery and ip chemotherapy. Pathology review and an assessment of the aggressive or nonaggressive nature of a malignancy must occur.

The preoperative CT scan of chest, abdomen, and pelvis is of great value in planning treatments for peritoneal surface disease: Systemic metastases can be clinically excluded and pleural surface spread ruled out. Unfortunately, the CT scan should be regarded as an inaccurate test by which to quantitate peritoneal carcinomatosis from adenocarcinoma (ACA) or mesothelioma. The malignant tissue progresses on the peritoneal surfaces, and its shape conforms to the normal contours of the abdominopelvic structures. This is quite different from the metastatic process in the liver or lung, which progresses as three-dimensional tumor nodules, and can be accurately assessed by CT.

However, the CT scan has been of great help in locating and quantitating mucinous ACA within the peritoneal cavity (7). These tumors produce copious colloid material that is readily distinguished by shape and density from normal structures. Using two new but distinctive radiologic criteria, those patients with resectable mucinous peritoneal carcinomatosis can be selected from those with nonresectable malignancy. This keeps patients who are unlikely to benefit from reoperative surgery from undergoing cytoreductive surgical procedures.

The two radiologic criteria found to be most useful are segmental obstruction of small bowel, and presence of tumor greater than 5 cm in greatest dimension on small bowel surfaces or directly adjacent to small bowel mesentery. These criteria reflect radiologically the biology of the mucinous ACA. The obstructed segments of bowel signal an invasive character of malignancy that would be unlikely to be completely cytoreduced. The mucinous cancer on small bowel and small bowel mesentery indicates that the mucinous cancer is no longer redistributed. This means that small bowel surfaces or small bowel mesentery will have residual disease after cytoreduction, because these surfaces are impossible to peritonectomize (Figs. 2 and 3).

The CT is also of great help in the identification of nodules of recurrent sarcoma and sarcomatosis. The recurrences on peritoneal surfaces are nodular, and the result of fibrin entrapment of traumatically disseminated sarcoma cells. In a CT scan with maximal filling of bowel by oral contrast, even small 1-cm nodular sarcoma recurrences are imaged.

The third assessment of peritoneal surface malignancy is the PCI. This is a clinical summary of both LS and distribution of PSM. It should be used in the decision-making process as the abdomen is explored. To arrive at a score, the size of ip nodules must be assessed. The LS score should be used. The number of nodules is not scored, only the size of the largest nodules. An LS-0 score means that no malignant deposits are visualized. A LS-1 score signifies that tumor nodules less than 0.5 cm are present. A LS-2 score signifies tumor nodules between 0.5 and 5.0 cm. LS-3 signifies tumor nodules greater than 5.0 cm in any dimension. If there is a confluence of tumor, the lesion size is scored as 3.

In order to assess the distribution of peritoneal surface disease, the abdominopelvic regions are utilized, (Fig. 4). For each of these 13 regions, a LS score is determined. The summation of the LS score in each of the 13 abdominopelvic regions is the PCI for that patient. A maximal score is 39 (13 × 3).

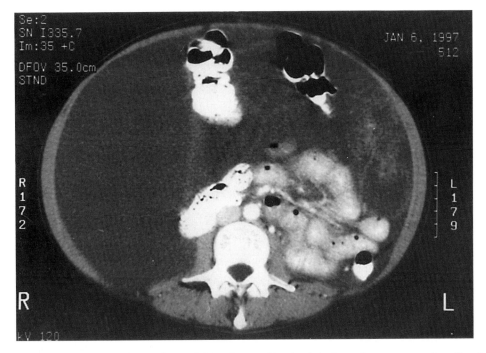

Fig. 2. Patient with grade 1 mucinous ACA of appendiceal origin (pseudomyxoma peritonei), who had a CC, and remains disease-free at 2 yr postoperatively. The mucinous tumor is very extensive, but the small bowel loops are of normal caliber, and are not distended by air. Also, the small bowel has become compartmentalized by the mucinous tumor. The small bowel surfaces and small bowel mesentery remain tumor free.

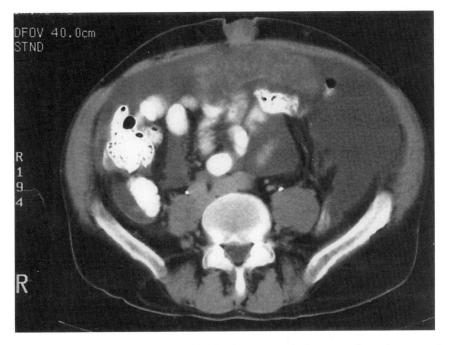

Fig. 3. Patient with grade 2 mucinous ACA who has recurred after extensive prior cytoreductive surgery. Small bowel loops are slightly distended, contain small volumes of air, and its mesenteric surface is coated by mucinous tumor nodules. This patient has less than 5% likelihood of a CC.

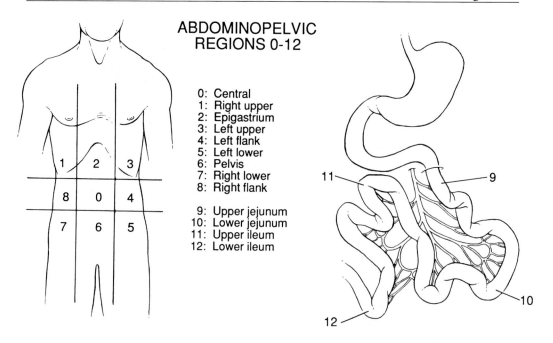

Fig. 4. Peritoneal Cancer Index is a composite score of LS 0 to 3 in abdominal-pelvic regions 0–12.

The PCI has been validated to date in three separate situations. First, Steller et al. *(8)* used it successfully to quantitate ip tumor in a murine peritoneal carcinomatosis model. Gomez et al. *(9)* showed that the PCI could be used to predict long-term survival in patients having a second cytoreduction for peritoneal carcinomatosis. Berthet et al. *(10)* showed that the PCI predicted benefits for treatment of peritoneal sarcomatosis from recurrent visceral or parietal sarcoma. The patients with a favorable prognosis had a score of less than 12.

There are some caveats in the use of the PCI. First, noninvasive malignancy on peritoneal surfaces may be completely cytoreduced. Diseases such as pseudomxyoma peritonei and peritoneal mesothelioma are in this category. In these situations, the status of the abdomen and pelvis after cytoreduction may have no relationship to the status at the time of abdominal exploration, i.e., even though the surgeons may find an abdomen with a PCI of 39, it can be converted to an index of 0 by cytoreduction. In these diseases, the prognosis will only be related to the condition of the abdomen after the cytoreduction (completeness of cytoreduction score).

A second caveat for the PCI is that cancers may invade anatomically crucial sites. For example, invasive cancer not cleanly resected on the common bile duct will cause a poor prognosis, despite a low PCI. Invasion of the base of the bladder, or unresectable disease on a pelvic side wall, may, by itself, result in residual invasive cancer after cytoreduction, and imply a poor prognosis. Also, unresectable cancer along the small bowel may by itself confer a poor prognosis. In other words, invasive cancer at crucial anatomic sites may function as systemic disease in assessing prognosis with invasive cancer. This poor prognosis information may override a favorable PCI score.

The final assessment to be used for prognosis of PSM is the CC score. This information is of less value to the surgeon in planning treatments than the PCI, because it is not available until after the cytoreduction is complete, not as the abdomen is being explored.

If, during exploration, it becomes obvious that cytoreduction will not be complete, the surgeon may decide that a palliative debulking rather than an aggressive cytoreduction with ip chemotherapy, will provide symptomatic relief. However, in both noninvasive and invasive PSM, the CC score is a major prognostic indicator. It has been shown to function with great accuracy in pseudomyxoma peritonei, peritoneal mesothelioma, colon cancer, peritoneal carcinomatosis, and sarcomatosis *(11)*.

2.6. Clinical Evidence that Cytoreductive Surgery and IP Chemotherapy Benefit Patients with PSM

Treatments for peritoneal carcinomatosis and sarcomatosis have been shown to provide prolonged survival, with a portion of patients alive at 5 yr and considered cured. The strategy for treating these patients has always involved three essential components: First is a complete cytoreduction, utilizing peritonectomy procedures, with an attempt to remove all visible tumor; assuming that microscopic residual disease will eventuate in recurrence in all these patients, the second essential component is perioperative ip chemotherapy; and it is becoming increasingly clear that proper patient selection is the third essential component of these treatment strategies. Although no one questions the essential nature of complete cytoreduction and accurate patient selection, many oncologists are not convinced that ip chemotherapy is of benefit to prevent recurrence of peritoneal surface disease. Data from prospective trials and from clinical observations suggest that ip chemotherapy can reduce or eliminate the recurrence of peritoneal carcinomatosis after surgery to remove large-volume disease.

The first data comes from prospective clinical trials. Sugarbaker et al. *(12)* conducted a trial in patients with poor-prognosis colon cancer. IV 5-FU was randomized against ip 5-FU. Each cycle of treatment was given for 5 d, and the treatments were repeated on a monthly basis for 1 yr. Patients who recurred were explored, and the status of their disease was assessed during the surgery. A statistically significant decrease in the incidence of peritoneal carcinomatosis occurred in patients who had received ip 5-FU ($P = 0.003$). In this small group of poor-prognosis patients, there was no improvement in survival. There was a great reduction in the incidence of recurrence of peritoneal carcinomatosis in the patients receiving ip 5-FU.

Several prospective randomized studies in peritoneal carcinomatosis from gastric cancer (GC) have been reported. The meta-analysis of eight trials is shown in Fig. 5. In all but one of these trials, the ip chemotherapy was given in the perioperative period. There was an improved survival in all seven trials utilizing perioperative ip chemotherapy *(13)*.

In the study by Yu et al. *(13)*, perioperative ip MMC and 5-FU were used for the first 5 d following gastrectomy. The risk of recurrence was nearly twice as great in patients who had surgery alone, compared to those patients who had surgery plus perioperative chemotherapy. In patients with stage III disease, the odds ratio was 4 in favor of the ip chemotherapy. In patients who had positive lymph nodes, the odds ratio was 8. These data strongly suggest that microscopic residual disease can be eliminated by perioperative ip chemotherapy.

Strong data from Mayo Clinic *(14)*, in patients with pseudomyxoma peritonei, shows that ip chemotherapy is effective in this patient population. In their report on 56 patients, the only long-term survivors were those who had both surgery and ip chemotherapy. Patients who had only repeated surgeries had a median survival of 3 yr, and only 5% of these patients were alive at the end of 5 yr.

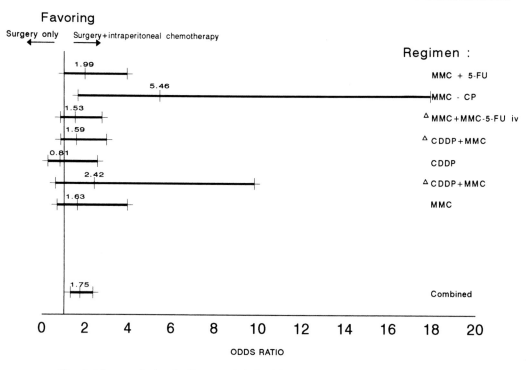

Fig. 5. Meta-analysis of adjuvant trials in GC using perioperative chemotherapy.

The patterns of recurrence in patients with and without ip chemotherapy show marked differences in the abdomen and at other anatomic sites. Zoetmulder and Sugarbaker *(15)* have shown that diaphragm perforation in patients with pseudomyxoma peritonei, which occurred at the time of cytoreduction, was associated with disease progression within the pleural space in 10 of 11 patients. Disease control within the abdomen where ip chemotherapy was used occurred in all of the patients, which strongly suggested that small-volume disease that entered the chest without ip chemotherapy resulted in progression. A much larger residual disease found in the abdomen was controlled with perioperative ip chemotherapy. Likewise, if drain tracts are used in patients with known peritoneal carcinomatosis, they will become involved by disease. Drain tracts in patients undergoing cytoreductive surgery with ip chemotherapy seldom, if ever, develop disease within the tract. Likewise, the abdominal incision is frequently involved if surgery only is used to remove peritoneal carcinomatosis or sarcomatosis. If the surgery is combined with ip chemotherapy, disease within the abdominal incision is not seen. This is also true in ovarian cancer (OC) patients with vaginal cuff recurrence. If the vaginal cuff is closed without ip chemotherapy, OC is inoculated into this anatomic site. If ip chemotherapy is used after an OC cytoreduction, no recurrence within the vaginal cuff has been observed.

A final site for disease occurrence is the laparoscopy ports after laparoscopy in patients with suspected peritoneal carcinomatosis. Almost invariably, the laparoscopy ports become involved by cancer, because disease is disseminated by the puncture sites through the abdominal wall *(16)*.

There is a definite correlation of the pattern of failure in patients receiving early PO ip chemotherapy with dye studies that show nonuniform distribution of chemotherapy in a closed abdomen (Fig. 6). Zoetmulder and Sugarbaker *(15)* found that recurrence

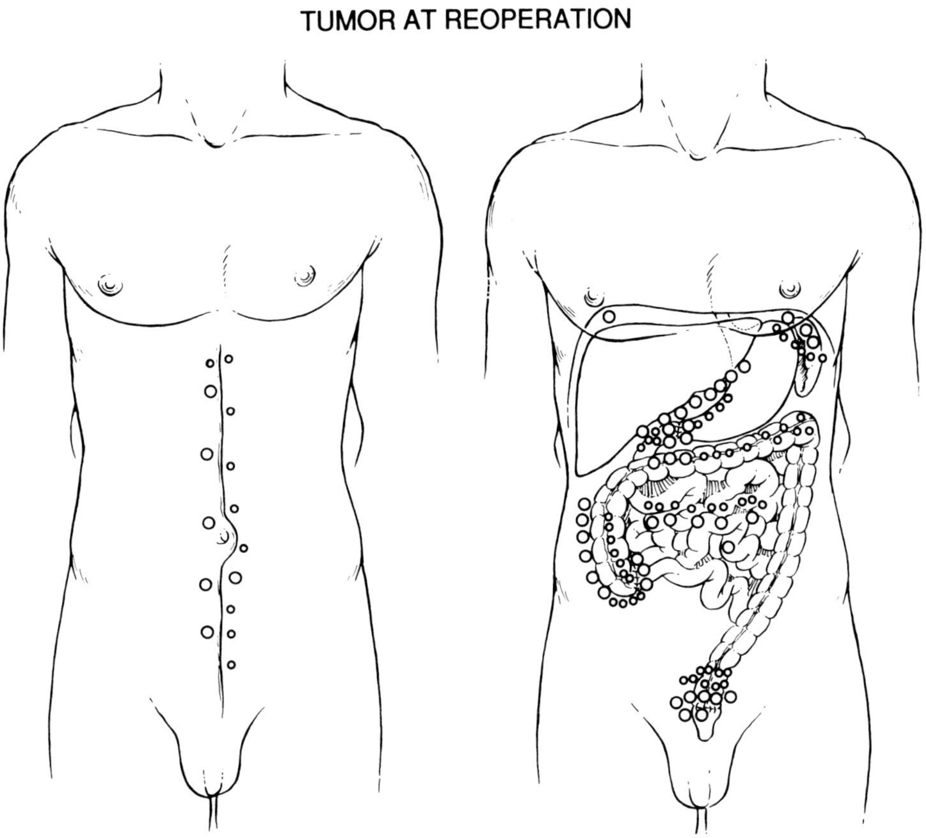

TUMOR AT REOPERATION

Fig. 6. Patterns of recurrence of a closed method for ip chemotherapy. Adapted with permission from ref. *15.*

in patients with pseudomyxoma peritonei was most likely to occur within the abdominal incision, with colorectal or gastrojejunal suture lines, and at the base of the small bowel mesentery. Of course, the closure of the abdominal incision and suture lines prevent adequate chemotherapy access at these sites. Another area for frequent recurrence was the anterior surface of the stomach. Dye studies have shown that the left lobe of the liver almost invariably becomes adherent to the anterior surface of the stomach in patients treated with a closed ip chemotherapy technique. Also, dye studies have demonstrated poor chemotherapy access to the base of the small bowel mesentery. This data strongly suggests that pseudomyxoma peritonei recurs where there is imperfect exposure to the ip chemotherapy. Other sites that have been noted to have a high incidence of recurrence after use of ip chemotherapy are the inverted appendiceal stump and umbilical fissure.

Elias et al. (personal communication) show an interesting pattern of recurrence in those patients who were treated using a peritoneal expander to deliver ip chemotherapy. They reported a high incidence of recurrent disease where the peritoneal expander contacted the peritoneal surface of the upper abdomen. Cancer cells were pressed into the peritoneal surface at this site, and were prevented from coming into contact with the chemotherapy drug.

The remarkably high response rate in patients with malignant ascites shows that ip chemotherapy is able to treat peritoneal surface disease. The marked effectiveness of ip chemotherapy on patients with malignant ascites attests to the reliable responses that occur with ip chemotherapy.

Surgery has been used for many decades in an attempt to treat patients with recurrent intra-abdominal cancer. The fact that surgery alone has been unsuccessful is well established. Patients with peritoneal seeding have never experienced long-term survival by surgery alone. Data presented in this chapter suggests that there is a high salvage rate in properly selected patients who are treated with cytoreductive surgery combined with adequate ip chemotherapy. These data together strongly suggest that ip chemotherapy is an essential component of treatment protocols for PSMs.

2.7. Proper Surgical Techniques for PSM

If a surgeon operates on a patient with PSM, certain requirements are necessary: One must know how to perform peritonectomy procedures, dissect using lasermode electrosurgery, and prevent cancer implantation into traumatized peritoneal surfaces, suture lines, all transabdominal puncture sites, and the abdominal wound closure.

Peritonectomy procedures are necessary if one is to successfully treat PSMs with curative intent, and are used in the areas of visible cancer progression, in an attempt to leave the patient with only microscopic residual disease. Small tumor nodules can be removed using electroevaporation. Involvement of the visceral peritoneum frequently requires resection of the structure. PSM tends to involve the viscera at three definite sites, where the bowel is anchored to the retroperitoneum, and a reduction in peristalsis causes less mobility of the visceral peritoneal surface. The rectosigmoid colon, as it comes up out of the pelvis, is a nonmobile portion of the bowel. Also, it is a dependent site, and, therefore, frequently requires resection. Usually, a complete pelvic peritonectomy involves stripping of the abdominal sidewalls, the peritoneum overlying the bladder, the cul-de-sac, and the rectosigmoid colon. The ileocecal valve is another area where there is limited mobility. Resection of the terminal ileum and a small portion of the right colon is often necessary. A final site often requiring resection is the antrum of the stomach, which is fixed to the rectoperitoneum at the pylorus. Tumor accumulates in the subpyloric space, and may cause intestinal obstruction as a result of gastric outlet obstruction. Occasionally, tumor in the lesser omentum will cause a confluence of disease on the lesser curvature. This may require a total gastrectomy, because of encasement of the vascular supply to the stomach. The other peritonectomy procedures have been presented (17).

In order to adequately perform cytoreductive surgery, the surgeon must use lasermode electrosurgery. Peritonectomies and visceral resections using the traditional scissor and knife dissection will unnecessarily disseminate a large number of tumor emboli within the abdomen. Also, clean peritoneal surfaces devoid of cancer cells are less likely to occur. Lasermode electrosurgery leaves a margin of heat necrosis that is less likely to contain persistent malignant cells. Electroevaporation of tumor and normal tissue at the margins of resection minimizes both the blood loss with peritoneal striping and the likelihood of persistent disease within a peritonectomy site.

Finally, extensive cytoreductions may actually harm patients in the long run, rather than help them. Extensive removal of peritoneal surfaces without ip chemotherapy will allow tumor cells to become implanted within a deeper layer of the abdomen and pelvis, which may lead to obstruction of vital structures, such as ureters. Also, deep involvement of the pelvic sidewall, or tissues along vascular structures, may occur. If a surgeon is to attempt to treat PSM, he must become thoroughly familiar with the techniques of intraoperative chemotherapy, early PO chemotherapy, and delayed ip

Table 2
Current Indications for IP Chemotherapy

Symptomatic malignant ascites
Pseudomyxoma peritonei after complete cytoreduction (CC)
Peritoneal mesothelioma after CC
Primary colon or rectal cancer:
    Small volume and limited distribution peritoneal seeding
    Perforated colon cancer
    Colon cancer with adjacent organ involvement
    Colon cancer with spread to ovaries
    Colon cancer with positive ip cytology
    Tumor spill with resection of primary colon or rectal cancer
Recurrent colon or rectal cancer:
    Small volume and limited-distribution of peritoneal seeding
    Colon cancer causing Krukenberg ovarian tumor
    Tumor spill with resection of recurrent cancer
    CC of recurrent disease at more than a single site
Recurrent OC with spread limited to peritoneal surfaces:
    Limited or absent iv chemotherapy options
    Long free interval between initial treatment and recurrence
Primary GC after complete resection with limited peritoneal seeding:
Primary of recurrent abdominopelvic sarcoma
    Sarcomatosis following CC
    Primary abdominopelvic sarcoma with equivocal margins of resection
    Primary abdominopelvic sarcoma with tumor spill during resection

chemotherapy. Complete cytoreduction, combined with aggressive perioperative ip chemotherapy and proper patient selection, are the three definite requirements of treatment strategies for PSM.

3. INDICATIONS FOR IP CHEMOTHERAPY

3.1. Large-Volume, Low-Grade ACA and Sarcoma

IP chemotherapy is a treatment option for PSM, and is currently used in clinical pathways in the Gastrointestinal Oncology Program at the Washington Cancer Institute. Table 2 presents the current indications for the use of ip chemotherapy. ACA of low malignant potential usually arises in the appendix, and seeds the abdominal and pelvic cavity extensively. These noninvasive malignancies can be eradicated from the abdomen by peritonectomy procedures. Cytoreductive surgery, followed by ip chemotherapy, should be considered the standard therapy for patients with peritoneal carcinomatosis from low-grade mucinous tumors. Also, treatments have demonstrated benefits for patients with peritoneal surface disease from grade I sarcoma and mesothelioma.

3.2. Moderate- to High-Grade ACA

Higher-grade ACAs of colonic or other GI cancer sites are selectively treated with cytoreductive surgery followed by ip chemotherapy *(18)*. It should be noted that, in patients with large-volume, high-grade cancer, only palliative treatments for peritoneal carcinomatosis should be considered. Approximately 10% of the total number of colon and rectal cancer patients have peritoneal seeding documented at the time of resection of the primary cancer. The clinical pathway shown in Fig. 7 presents treatment options as currently practiced for peritoneal carcinomatosis from primary colon cancer.

3.3. Importance of Tumor Volume and Distribution in Patients with Moderate- to High-Grade ACA

In the current approach to high-grade ACA, tumor volume and tumor distribution are the fundamental criteria for the selection of patients for treatment with ip chemotherapy. The treatment of bulk disease from moderate- to high-grade cancer in the abdominal cavity by ip chemotherapy is to be avoided. Only patients with low-volume, high-grade peritoneal surface cancer should be treated with ip chemotherapy. Small-lesion-size peritoneal seeding, with limited distribution on peritoneal surfaces, should be expected to respond, and constitutes an indication for treatment. If large-volume, low-grade disease is present, a complete surgical cytoreduction must precede ip chemotherapy administration.

3.4. Prevention of Peritoneal Carcinomatosis in High-Risk Patients

A major role for ip chemotherapy is the prevention of subsequent peritoneal carcinomatosis or sarcomatosis. Virtually every patient who has a free intra-abdominal perforation of GI cancer through the malignancy itself develops peritoneal carcinomatosis. The author recommends intraoperative and early PO ip chemotherapy treatments for all patients with perforated GI cancer.

Not infrequently, patients who are undergoing a resection of a large intra-abdominal tumor will have a tumor spill. This may be common with advanced primary or recurrent rectal malignancy and recurrent colonic cancer. It may occur almost routinely in the resection of advanced GC. If there is a tumor spill, then, in order to prevent subsequent development of peritoneal carcinomatosis or sarcomatosis, the author recommends the use of ip chemotherapy. Limited peritoneal seeding, perforation, and tumor spill are considered absolute indications for the use of perioperative ip chemotherapy.

3.5. Microscopic Residual Disease as Target of Adjuvant IP Chemotherapy

In patients with established peritoneal surface disease, maximal surgical efforts, combined with maximal tolerable ip chemotherapy, are needed to attempt a curative effort. All studies suggest, however, that the extent of disease present at the initiation of treatments has a profound effect on outcome. Minimal peritoneal spread of cancer requires minimal peritonectomy and less severe chemotherapy, to result in long-term survival. In primary cancer without clinical evidence of peritoneal seeding, adjuvant treatments may be designed to prevent peritoneal dissemination. The target of perioperative ip chemotherapy is microscopic residual disease. The surgery to remove the primary cancer is not changed. However, intraoperative chemotherapy with manual distribution of drug should be sufficient to eliminate small numbers of cancer cells that remain following surgery. It is possible that the greatest benefit from ip chemotherapy will come from its adjuvant use in cancers that have a high propensity for local-regional recurrence: GC, pancreatic cancer, retroperitoneal sarcoma, and OC.

4. METHODS

4.1. Heated Intraoperative IP Chemotherapy Administration

In the operating room, heated intraoperative chemotherapy is used (6). Heat is part of the optimizing process, and is used to bring as much dose intensity to the abdominal

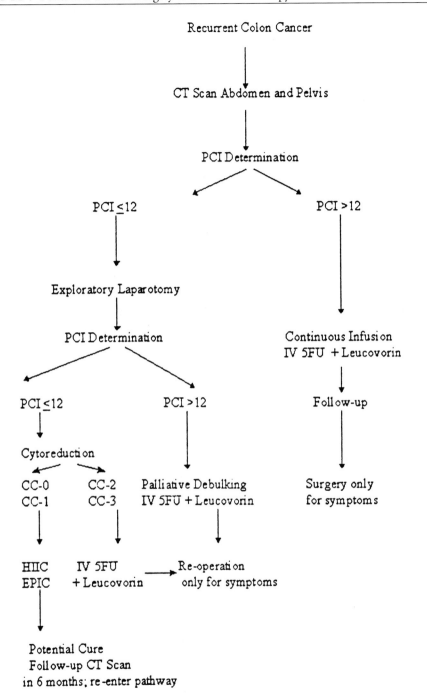

Fig. 7. Clinical pathway for peritoneal seeding from colon cancer. PCI = Peritoneal Cancer Index; CC = completeness of cytoreduction; IV 5-FU = intravenous 5-fluorouracil; HIIC = heated intraoperative ip chemotherapy; EPIC = early postoperative ip chemotherapy.

Table 3
Benefits of Using Heated Intraoperative IP Chemotherapy

Heat increases drug penetration into tissue.

Heat increases the cytotoxicity of selected chemotherapy agents.

Heat has an antitumor effect by itself.

Intraoperative chemotherapy allows manual distribution of drug and heat uniformly to all surfaces of abdomen and pelvis.

Renal toxicities of chemotherapy given in the operation room can be avoided by careful monitoring of urine output during chemotherapy perfusion.

Time that elapses during the heated perfusion allows a normalization of many parameters (temperature, blood clotting, hemodynamic, and so on).

and pelvic surfaces as possible. Hyperthermia with ip chemotherapy has several advantages. First, heat by itself has more toxicity for cancerous tissue than for normal tissue. This predominant effect on cancer increases as the vascularity of the malignancy decreases. Second, hyperthermia increases the penetration of chemotherapy into tissues. As tissues soften in response to heat, the elevated interstitial pressure of a tumor mass may decrease and allow improved drug penetration. Third, and probably most important, heat increases the cytotoxicity of selected chemotherapy agents. This synergism occurs only at the interface of heat and body tissue at the peritoneal surface. The rationale for using heated chemotherapy as a surgically directed modality in the operating room is listed in Table 3.

After cancer resection is complete, the Tenckhoff catheter and closed suction drains are placed through the abdominal wall, and made watertight with a purse-string suture at the skin. Temperature probes are secured to the skin edge. Using a running 2×0 monofilament suture, the skin edges are secured to the edge of the self-retaining retractor. A plastic sheet is incorporated into these sutures to create a covering for the cavity. A slit in the plastic cover is made to allow the surgeon's double-gloved hand access to the abdomen and pelvis (Fig. 8). During the 2 h perfusion, all the anatomic structures within the peritoneal cavity are uniformly exposed to heat and to chemotherapy. The surgeon gently but continuously abrades all viscera, to keep adherence of peritoneal surfaces to a minimum. A roller pump forces the chemotherapy solution into the abdomen through the Tenckhoff catheter, and pulls it out through the drains. A heat exchanger keeps the fluid being infused at 44–45°C, so that the ip fluid is maintained at 42–43°C. The circuit used for the administration of heated intraoperative ip chemotherapy is diagrammed in Fig. 9. The smoke evacuator is used to pull air from beneath the plastic cover through activated charcoal, preventing any possible contamination of air in the operating room by chemotherapy. Standardized orders for heated intraoperative ip chemotherapy are given in Table 4.

After the intraoperative perfusion is complete, the abdomen is suctioned dry of fluid. The abdomen is then reopened, and reconstructive surgery is performed. No anastomoses are constructed until after the chemotherapy perfusion is complete.

4.2. Immediate PO Abdominal Lavage

In order to keep the catheters for drug instillation and abdominal drainage clear of blood clots and tissue debris, an abdominal lavage is begun in the operating room. This requires tubes and drains to be positioned prior to closure of the abdomen. The author has utilized large volumes of fluid rapidly infused, and then drained from the

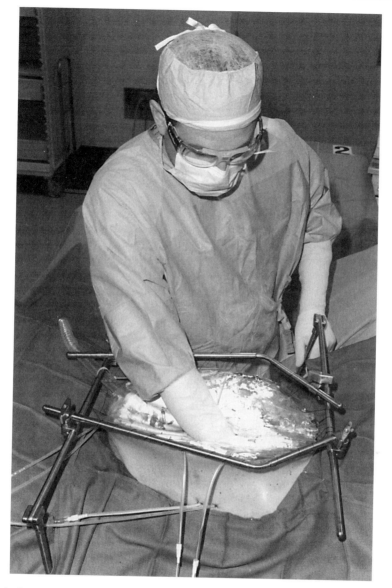

Fig. 8. Surgical manipulation of the abdominal contents after complete resection of cancer assures uniform distribution of heat and chemotherapy.

abdomen after a short dwell time. The standardization orders for immediate PO lavage are given in Table 5. All intra-abdominal catheters are withdrawn before the patient is discharged from the hospital.

4.3. Early PO IP Chemotherapy for ACA

IP chemotherapy, following complete cytoreduction in patients with appendiceal cancer, colonic cancer, rectal cancer, GC, or other GI ACAs, has utilized 5-FU. In pretreated OC, patients who have demonstrated neurologic toxicities from systemic cisplatin should never use it again. These patients are also treated with 5-FU. The standard orders for early PO administration of ip 5-FU are shown in Table 6.

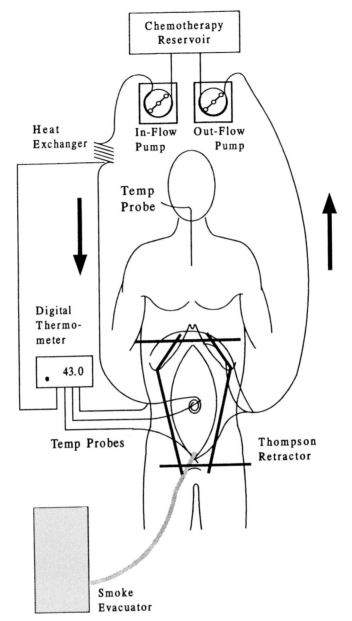

Fig. 9. Circuit for heated intraoperative ip chemotherapy perfusion. All plastic tubes are positioned in a standardized fashion except the Tenckhoff catheter for the heated intraoperative perfusion. It is placed at the anatomic site at which the surgeon thinks there is the greatest likelihood of recurrence. This allows for regional dose intensity of the heated chemotherapy.

4.4. Induction or Adjuvant IP Chemotherapy for ACA

Standard therapy, for all patients with peritoneal seeding from moderate- or high-grade cancer who are treated with ip chemotherapy, involves at least four cycles of treatment. The only patients who do not receive all four cycles of ip chemotherapy are those patients who have grade 1 tumor and a complete cytoreduction. All other patients have at least four cycles of chemotherapy directed at both systemic and ip sites. One

Table 4
Standardized Orders for Heated Intraoperative IP Chemotherapy

Mitomycin orders
1. For adenocarcinoma from appendiceal, colonic, rectal, gastric, and pancreatic cancer, add mitomycin ____ mg to 2 L 1.5% peritoneal dialysis solution.
2. Dose of mitomycin: for males 12.5 mg/m^2; for females 10 mg/m^2.
3. Use 33% dose reduction for heavy prior chemotherapy, marginal renal function, age greater than 60 yr, extensive intraoperative trauma to small bowel surfaces, or prior radiotherapy.
4. Send 1 L of 1.5% peritoneal dialysis solution to test the perfusion circuit.
5. Send 1 L of 1.5% peritoneal dialysis solution for immediate postoperative lavage.
6. Send the above to operating room ____ at ____ o'clock.

Cisplatin and doxorubicin orders
1. For sarcoma, ovarian cancer, and mesothelioma; add cisplatin ____ mg to 2 L 1.5% peritoneal dialysis solution. The dose of cisplatin is 50 mg/m^2.
2. Add doxorubicin ____ mg to the same 2 L 1.5% peritoneal dialysis solution. The dose of doxorubicin is 15 mg/m^2.
3. Use 33% dose reduction for heavy prior chemotherapy, marginal renal function, age greater than 60 yr, extensive intraoperative trauma to small bowel surfaces, or prior radiotherapy.
4. Send 1 L 1.5% peritoneal dialysis solution for test of the perfusion circuit.
5. Send 1 L 1.5% peritoneal dialysis solution for immediate postoperative lavage.
6. Send the above to operating room ____ at ____ o'clock.

Table 5
Standardized Orders for Immediate PO Abdominal Lavage

Day of operation:
1. Run in 1000 mL 1.5% dextrose peritoneal dialysis solution as rapidly as possible. Warm to body temperature prior to instillation. Clamp all abdominal drains during infusion.
2. No dwell time.
3. Drain as rapidly as possible through Tenckhoff catheter and abdominal drains.
4. Repeat irrigations every 1 h for 4 h, then every 4 h until returns are clear; then every 8 h until chemotherapy begins.
5. Change dressing at Tenckhoff catheter and abdominal drain skin sites using sterile technique once daily and as necessary.
6. Standardized precautions must be used for all body fluids from this patient.

of these cycles is the intraoperative and early PO ip treatment. The other three cycles are on a monthly basis. Each cycle consists of 5 consecutive days of therapy (Table 7).

The preferred method for peritoneal access for the first cycle of adjuvant chemotherapy is to have a catheter placed by paracentesis, and to assess the adequacy of chemotherapy distribution radiologically. A majority of patients treated for peritoneal carcinomatosis have extensive peritoneal adhesions. To maximize distribution, chemotherapy is administered through a temporary catheter, which is placed under radiologic control by paracentesis (8.3 French All Purpose Drain Catheter, Meditech, Watertown, MA). Routinely, the author has used a CT scan with ip contrast to demonstrate uniform distribution of fluid within the abdomen.

Standardized orders for induction ip and systemic chemotherapy for ACAs are the same as for adjuvant ip chemotherapy. IP chemotherapy is only given to patients with

Table 6
Standardized Orders for Early PO IP Chemotherapy with 5-FU

Postoperative Days 1–5
1. Add to ____ mL 1.5% dextrose peritoneal dialysis solution:
   (a) ____ mg 5-fluorouracil (650 mg/m², maximal dose 1300 mg)
   (b) 50 mEq sodium bicarbonate
2. Intraperitoneal fluid volume: 1 L for patients <2.0 m², 1.5 L for >2.0 m².
3. Drain all fluid from the abdominal cavity prior to instillation, then clamp abdominal drains.
4. Run the chemotherapy solution into abdominal cavity through Tenckhoff catheter as rapidly as possible. Dwell for 23 h and rain for 1 h prior to next instillation.
5. Continue to drain abdominal cavity after final dwell until Tenckhoff catheter is removed.
6. Use 33% dose reduction for heavy prior chemotherapy, age greater than 60 yr, or prior radiotherapy.
7. Gravity distribution.

Table 7
Standardized Orders for Adjuvant IP 5-FU and IV Mitomycin Chemotherapy

Cycle no. _____
1. CBC, platelets, profile A, and appropriate tumor marker prior to treatment; and CBC, platelets 10 d after initiation of treatments.
2. 5-fluorouracil ____ mg 750 mg/m² (maximum dose 1600 mg) and 50 mEq sodium bicarbonate in 1000 cc 1.5% dextrose peritoneal dialysis solution via intraperitoneal catheter q day × 5 d. Last dose ____. Dwell for 23 h, drain for 1 h. Continue with next administration, even if no drainage obtained.
3. On d 3 (Date _____): 500 cc lactated Ringer's solution intravenously over 2 h prior to mitomycin infusion. Mitomycin ____ mg (10 mg/m²) (Maximum dose 20 mg) in 200 cc 5% dextrose and water intravenously over 2 h.
4. Follow routine procedure for peripheral extravasation of a vesicant if extravasation should occur.
5. Compazine 25 mg per rectum q 4 h prn for nausea. OUTPATIENT ONLY: May dose × 4 for use at home.
6. Percocet 1 tablet PO q 3 h prn for pain. OUTPATIENT ONLY: May dose × 4 for use at home.
7. Routine vital signs.
8. Out of bed ad lib.
9. Diet: Regular as tolerated.
10. Daily dressing change to intraperitoneal catheter skin exit site.
11. Use 33% dose reduction for age greater than 60 yr or prior radiotherapy.

low-volume disease that is not confluent in the abdomen. After delivering the three cycles of combined ip and systemic chemotherapy in patients who receive ip chemotherapy prior to surgery, all treatments are discontinued for at least 2 mo. If surgery follows ip chemotherapy too quickly, an increased complication rate will occur (19–21). After the patient has recovered full activity, a complete exploratory laparotomy, with meticulous cytoreduction of all residual cancer, is performed. A final cycle of intraoperative and early PO ip chemotherapy is utilized.

4.5. Clinical Results of Treatment

Patients are frequently encountered who have large volumes of ascites, which may be caused by breast cancer, GC, mucinous malignancies of the colon or appendix, or OC. IP chemotherapy is uniformly successful in eliminating debilitating ascites. This usually requires two or three instillations of a systemic dose of appropriate chemotherapy into the abdomen. The treatment regimen, outlined in this chapter as induction or adjuvant ip chemotherapy, is often used. Also, Link et al. *(22)* used mitoxantrone in this clinical situation. In a few patients, persistent ascites will require a moderate cytoreduction, in order to separate bowel loops, remove bulk disease, and allow the use of a single cycle of heated intraoperative ip chemotherapy. During the cytoreduction, large masses of tumor are removed. This generally includes the greater and lesser omentum and penduculated tumor masses. No attempt at a complete cytoreduction is made. The patient is treated for 90 min with heat and the appropriate chemotherapy. Also, early PO ip chemotherapy is suggested. The responses achieved in patients who are debulked, and then given chemotherapy, are more lasting than in patients given chemotherapy only.

4.6. Appendix Cancer and Pseudomyxoma Peritonei Syndrome

The paradigm for treatment of peritoneal carcinomatosis is the same as for appendiceal malignancy. Experience with approx 350 patients has been reported *(23,24)*. Strategies used included peritonectomy procedures, combined with perioperative ip chemotherapy with MMC and 5-FU. Survival was statistically significant for both the invasive character of the mucinous tumor and the completeness of cytoreduction. Patients with pathology of adenomucinosis and a complete cytoreduction showed an 85% 5-yr survival. In patients with the pseudomyxoma/carcinoma hybrid pathology, complete cytoreduction resulted in a 56% 5-yr survival. Patients with mucinous ACA had a 33% 5-yr survival.

4.7. Primary Peritoneal Surface Malignancy

A confusing and poorly understood group of tumors that has been successfully treated with peritonectomy and perioperative ip chemotherapy are the primary PSMs, including mesothelioma, papillary serous ACA, and primary peritoneal ACA. As with appendiceal ACA, survival is heavily dependent on the invasive character of the tumor and the completeness of cytoreduction. The 3-yr survival in a group of 39 patients with primary peritoneal tumors was 44%. Further experience with this group of patients is necessary. Currently, all patients are being treated with heated intraoperative cisplatin and doxorubicin. A second-look procedure with initiation of these same treatments is performed in 9 mo *(25)*.

4.8. Peritoneal Carcinomatosis from Colon Cancer

To date, 150 patients have been treated who have peritoneal carcinomatosis from colon cancer. Gomez Portilla et al. *(9)* and Sugarbaker et al. *(18)* reviewed their treatment with this disease process: Preoperative PCI score and distribution of abdominopelvic regions together determined the prognosis. The PCI provided a combined score found to be valuable in selecting patients for treatment. In 45 patients who had a complete cytoreduction, there was a 53% 5-yr survival. If the PCI was less than 10, there was a 63% 5-yr survival. If less than three abdominal regions were involved, the

5-yr survival was 48%. An aggressive approach was suggested to peritoneal surface spread of ACA of the colon in selected patients.

4.9. Sarcomatosis

Berthet et al. *(10)* have reviewed their experience with cytoreductive surgery and ip chemotherapy for treatment of selected patients with sarcomatosis. If the PCI at the time of abdominal exploration was less than 13, there was a 75% 5-yr survival. In those who had a PCI of 13 or more, the 5-yr survival was only 13%. The completeness of cytoreduction was also statistically significant for an improved prognosis: Twenty-seven patients with a complete cytoreduction had a 5-yr survival of 39%; sixteen patients with a CC-2 or CC-3 resection had a survival of 14%.

4.10. Peritoneal Seeding from GC

Extensive studies *(26,27)* with peritoneal seeding from GC have been conducted in Japan, but reports from Western series are not available. Survival rates for patients treated with heated intraoperative ip chemotherapy at the time of gastrectomy vary from 10–43%. Further work in this field is necessary; however, a strong recommendation for the treatment of Western patients with peritoneal seeding from GC by experienced oncologists can be made from current available data.

4.11. Recurrent and Obstructing GI Cancer

Averbach and Sugarbaker *(28)* looked at their experience with an problematic group of patients, who developed intestinal obstruction after prior treatment for a GI malignancy. With aggressive treatments using a second-look surgery, peritonectomy procedures, and ip chemotherapy, an R-O resection resulted in a 5-yr survival in 60% of the patients, and an R-2 or R-3 resection resulted in a zero 5-yr survival. The patients with appendiceal malignancy had a greatly improved survival, compared to those with colon cancer or other diagnoses. A free interval of greater than 2 yr between primary malignancy and the onset of obstruction also correlated favorably with prolonged survival. Only patients with ip chemotherapy used in conjunction with cytoreductive surgery were shown to have prolonged survival.

4.12. Morbidity and Mortality

The morbidity and mortality of 181 consecutive patients, who had cytoreductive surgery and four cycles of combined regional and systemic chemotherapy for peritoneal carcinomatosis, has been reported *(29)*. In these 181 patients, there were three treatment-related deaths (2%). Fistula formation was a great problem in those patients who had intestinal obstruction, prior radiation therapy, or prior ip chemotherapy. Nineteen of those 72 patients (26%) developed a bowel perforation postoperatively. Only 2 of 109 patients (2%) with more normal bowel developed a fistula. Anastomotic leakage occurred in 10 of 181 patients (6%).

4.13. Alternative Approaches

Peritoneal carcinomatosis has been treated in the past with systemic chemotherapy. No long-term survivors have been described in the literature. Palliative surgery can give temporary relief of intestinal obstruction. These efforts have always been categorized as low-value surgery, because long-term survival was rarely achieved. Other therapies, including ip immunotherapy, ip isotopes, and ip labeled monoclonal antibody, have not shown reproducible beneficial treatments. Alternative approaches to cytoreductive surgery and ip chemotherapy for peritoneal carcinomatosis have not been reported.

4.14. Patient Care Considerations

The major detrimental side effect of combined cytoreductive surgery and ip chemotherapy is prolonged ileus. Patients may have a nasogastric tube in place, with large volumes of secretions being aspirated for 2–4 wk postoperatively. The length of time required for nasogastric suctioning seems related to the extent of the peritonectomy procedure and the extent of prior abdominal adhesions that required lysis.

The most life-threatening problem is the fistula, which is a sidewall perforation of the small bowel. Patients need to be made aware of the possibility of a fistula, before cytoreductive surgery and ip chemotherapy are contemplated. As mentioned above, the anastomotic leak rate of 6% is low.

Following these treatments, the patient is maintained on parenteral feeding for 2–4 wk. Approximately 20% of patients, especially those who have had extensive prior procedures, will need parenteral feeding when they leave the hospital.

REFERENCES

1. Jacquet P, Vidal-Jove J, Zhu BW, and Sugarbaker PH. Peritoneal carcinomatosis from intraabdominal malignancy: natural history and new prospects for management, *Acta Belg. Chir.*, **94** (1994) 191–197.
2. Sugarbaker PH, Graves T, DeBruijn EA, et al. Rationale for early postoperative intraperitoneal chemotherapy (EPIC) in patients with advanced gastrointestinal cancer, *Cancer Res.*, **50** (1990) 5790–5794.
3. Sugarbaker PH, Cunliffe W, Israel M, and Sweatman TW. Early postoperative intraperitoneal adriamycin: pharmacologic studies and a preliminary clinical report, *Reg. Cancer Treat.*, **4** (1991) 127–131.
4. Markman M. Intraperitoneal taxol, In Sugarbaker PH (ed), *Peritoneal Carcinomatosis: Drugs and Diseases*, Kluwer, Boston, 1996, pp. 1–5.
5. Pestieau SR, Stuart OA, Chang D, Jacquet P, and Sugarbaker PH. Pharmacokinetics of intraperitoneal gemcitabine in a rat model. submitted
6. Sugarbaker PH. *Cytoreductive Surgery and Intraperitoneal Chemotherapy: A Manual for Physicians and Nurses*, Ludann, Grand Rapids, 1995.
7. Jacquet P, Jelinek J, and Sugarbaker PH. Abdominal computer tomographic scan in the selection of patients with mucinous peritoneal carcinomatosis for cytoreductive surgery, *J. Am. Coll. Surg.*, **181** (1995) 530–538.
8. Steller EPH. Comparison of four scoring methods for an intraperitoneal immunotherapy model, In *Enhancement and Abrogation: Modifications of Host Immune Status Influence IL-2 and LAK Cell Immunotherapy*, Erasmus Universitait, Rotterdam, 1988, pp. 56–63.
9. Gomez Portilla A, Sugarbaker PH, and Chang D. Second-look surgery after cytoreduction and intraperitoneal chemotherapy for peritoneal carcinomatosis from colorectal cancer: analysis of prognostic features, *World J. Surg.*, in press.
10. Berthet B, Sugarbaker TA, and Chang D. Quantitative methodologies for selection of patients with recurrent abdominopelvic sarcoma for treatment, *European J. Cancer,* **35** (1999) 413–419.
11. Jacquet P and Sugarbaker PH. Clinical research methodologies in diagnoses and staging of patient with peritoneal carcinomatosis, In Sugarbaker PH (ed), *Peritoneal Carcinomatosis: Principles of Management*, Kluwer, Boston, 1996, pp. 359–374.
12. Sugarbaker PH, Gianola FJ, Speyer JL, Wesley R, Barofsky I, and Meyers CE. Prospective randomized trial of intravenous versus intraperitoneal 5-fluorouracil in patients with advanced primary colon or rectal cancer, *Surgery*, **98** (1985) 414–421.
13. Yu W, Whang I, Suh I, Averbach A, Chang D, and Sugarbaker PH. Prospective randomized controlled trial of adjuvant early postoperative intraperitoneal chemotherapy as an adjuvant to resectable gastric cancer, *Ann. Surg.*, **228** (1998) 347–354.
14. Gough DB, Donahue JH, Schutt AJ, et al. Pseudomyxoma peritonei: long-term survival with an aggressive regional approach, *Ann. Surg.*, **219** (1994) 112–119.

15. Zoetmulder FAN and Sugarbaker PH. Patterns of failure after complete cytoreduction and early postoperative intraperitoneal chemotherapy, *Eur. J. Cancer*, **32A** (1996) 1727–1733.
16. Jacquet P and Sugarbaker PH. Wound recurrence after laparoscopic colectomy for cancer: new rationale for intraoperative intraperitoneal chemotherapy, *Surg. Endosc.*, **10** (1996) 295–296.
17. Sugarbaker PH. Peritonectomy procedures, *Ann. Surg.*, **221** (1995) 29–42.
18. Sugarbaker PH, Schellinx MET, Chang D, Koslowe P, and von Meyerfeldt M. Peritoneal carcinomatosis from adenocarcinoma of the colon, *World J. Surg.*, **20** (1996) 585–592.
19. Esquivel J, Vidal-Jove J, Steves MA, and Sugarbaker PH. Morbidity and mortality of cytoreductive surgery and intraperitoneal chemotherapy, *Surgery*, **113** (1993) 631–636.
20. Murio EJ and Sugarbaker PH. Gastrointestinal fistula following cytoreductive procedures for peritoneal carcinomatosis: incidence and outcome, *J. Exp. Clin. Cancer Res.*, **12** (1993) 153–158.
21. Fernandez-Trio V and Sugarbaker PH. Diagnosis and management of postoperative gastrointestinal fistulas: a kinetic analysis, *J. Exp. Clin. Cancer Res.*, **13** (1994) 233–241.
22. Link K, Hepp G, Staib L, Butzer U, Bohm W, and Beger HG. Intraperitoneal regional chemotherapy (IPRC) with mitoxantrone, In Sugarbaker PH (ed), *Peritoneal Carcinomatosis: Drugs and Diseases,* Kluwer, Boston, 1996, pp. 31–40.
23. Sugarbaker PH. Peritoneal carcinomatosis from appendiceal cancer: a paradigm for treatment of abdomino-pelvic dissemination of gastrointestinal malignancy, *Acta Chir. Austriaca*, **28** (1996) 4–8.
24. Sugarbaker PH, Ronnett B, Archer A, et al. Management of pseudomyxoma peritonei of appendiceal original, *Adv. Surg.*, **30** (1997) 233–280.
25. Sugarbaker PH. Primary peritoneal surface tumors: mesothelioma, adenocarcinoma and papillary serous, in progress.
26. Yonemura Y, Fujimura T, Nishimura G, et al. Effects of intraoperative chemohyperthermia in patients with gastric cancer with peritoneal dissemination, *Surgery*, **119** (1996) 437–444.
27. Fujimoto S, Shrestha RD, Kokubin M, et al. Intraperitoneal hyperthermic perfusion combined with surgery effective for gastric cancer patients with peritoneal seeding, *Ann. Surg.*, **208** (1988) 36–41.
28. Averbach AM and Sugarbaker PH. Recurrent intraabdominal cancer with intestinal obstruction: management of 42 patients by surgery and intraperitoneal chemotherapy, *Int. Surg.*, **80** (1995) 141–146.
29. Sugarbaker PH and Jablonski KA. Prognostic features of 51 colorectal and 130 appendiceal cancer patients with peritoneal carcinomatosis treated by cytoreductive surgery and intraperitoneal chemotherapy, *Ann. Surg.*, **132** (1995) 124–132.

15 Memorial Sloan-Kettering Cancer Center Experience with Intraperitoneal Chemotherapy for Gastric Cancer

Eileen M. O'Reilly and David P. Kelsen

CONTENTS

INTRODUCTION

Worldwide, gastric cancer (GC) remains a major cause of cancer mortality. Although its incidence has declined over the last few decades, it remains a major public health problem, now ranking eighth globally in terms of annual cancer-related deaths. In addition, the number of patients with newly diagnosed proximal gastric and gastroesophageal junction adenocarcinomas continues to rise *(1–3)*.

Approximately 22,600 new cases of GC are diagnosed per year in the United States *(4)*, where the survival rate for resectable GC is generally poor, with an overall 5-yr survival rate of 15–30%. This contrasts with the survival rates of GC in other ethnic populations, e.g., the Japanese, in whom 5-yr survival rates may approach 50% *(5)*. Survival in patients with GC is dependent on the stage of the disease at the time of presentation. In the United States, two-thirds of patients traditionally present with

From: *Current Clinical Oncology: Regional Chemotherapy: Clinical Research and Practice*
Edited by: M. Markman © Humana Press Inc., Totowa, NJ

advanced-stage III or IV disease *(6,7)*, which are associated with 5-yr survival rates of 20 and 5%, respectively.

Despite optimum surgery, i.e., an R0 resection (negative margins), a majority of patients with transmural or node-positive GCs, relapse *(8)*. After surgery, approx 60% of patients recur, most commonly in the peritoneal cavity and/or the liver *(9–11)*. Metastatic disease outside the abdomen occurs in 20–40%, but is less frequent than intra-abdominal relapse, and is rarely the first site of recurrence. Peritoneal carcinomatosis from GC has a very poor prognosis, and is associated with high morbidity, such as progressive abdominal distention and recurrent bowel obstruction *(12,13)*. Thus, effective therapy to the peritoneal cavity at the time of surgery, for patients with high-risk stage II or III GC, might improve overall long-term survival, change the failure pattern, and decrease morbidity from recurrent GC.

Postoperative (PO) adjuvant chemotherapy *(14,15)* has been extensively investigated, in an attempt to improve overall survival for surgically resectable GC patients, but this approach has not conclusively shown an impact on overall long-term survival for this disease in Western populations. Thus, new approaches are mandated. Two novel approaches, neoadjuvant chemotherapy *(16–18)* and intraperitoneal (ip) chemotherapy, have shown promise, and are actively being studied in many clinical trials of this disease conducted by both U.S. and Eastern investigators.

This chapter reviews the Memorial Sloan-Kettering Cancer Center (MSKCC) experience with ip chemotherapy administered in the adjuvant phase II setting of surgically resected high-risk GC, and reviews international adjuvant random-assignment ip chemotherapy phase III trials. Combined neoadjuvant and adjuvant phase II studies, both completed and ongoing, at MSKCC and at other U.S. centers, will also be discussed.

2. INTRAPERITONEAL CHEMOTHERAPY

IP chemotherapy involves the administration of chemotherapy directly into the abdominal cavity. The major advantage of ip chemotherapy in stomach cancer relates to the early administration of high doses of chemotherapy drugs to the sites with the highest risk of recurrence. Additionally, high levels of drugs are also achieved in the portal vein, which feeds the liver, also a very common site of relapse in GC *(19)*. Markman et al. *(20)*, have shown that peritoneal metastases (PMs) from ovarian cancer refractory to iv cisplatin, have a 42% response to cisplatin when given intraperitoneally. Similar data is available for intrahepatic perfusion in refractory colon cancer using floxuridine (FUDR) *(21)*, a drug which is now used extensively for ip therapy of GC. The pharmacokinetic advantages of ip chemotherapy have been well reviewed elsewhere *(22,23)*.

Supporting preclinical data for a regional-based approach includes work by Archer and Grey *(19)*. In a rat model, ip chemotherapy treated both hepatic and PMs. In a clinical trial in patients with colon cancer, Sugarbaker et al. *(24)* have demonstrated a change in the failure patterns of the disease with ip therapy, namely, a decrease in the occurrence of PMs, but with no overall survival advantage.

The rationale for the use of this approach in stomach cancer is based on the failure patterns of the disease. As noted above, even in the setting of optimally resected GC, local-regional failure remains common, and generally is the initial site of relapse. The failure patterns of GC have been established by both second-look surgical procedures and autopsy series *(8–10)*.

Gunderson et al. *(10)* performed a retrospective review of second-look laparotomies performed at the University of Minnesota over a two-decade period up to 1971. Most patients in the study were at high risk for recurrence, because of lymph node positivitity. Patients who had obvious distal recurrence were not reexplored, representing a bias in the reporting of failure patterns in this retrospective review. Also of note, this study was conducted before computed tomography (CT) scanning was available. The intra-abdominal pattern of spread was reported on 105 patients who had a second-look laparotomy. Fifty-five percent recurred in the stomach bed, 42% in the peritoneal cavity, and 40% in lymph nodes. Intra-abdominal failure at multiple sites was recorded in 69%. Extra-abdominal failure was reported in 13%. In two postmortem series, the incidence of local-regional failure was 40–80% *(8–9)*. In particular, peritoneal relapse was a commonly occurring event. Distal spread was found in 20–40% of patients. The second-look laparotomy series and the autopsy series clearly underscore the potential utility of a regional-based therapy, given the high risk of abdominal failure of GC.

Western and Japanese investigators have explored the role of ip treatment with mitomycin (MMC) *(26–29)*, 5-fluorouracil (5-FU) or its analogs *(30,31)*, or cisplatin *(32–34)*, after curative resections in GC.

3. PHASE II MSKCC ADJUVANT IP CHEMOTHERAPY EXPERIENCE

IP chemotherapy has been extensively investigated at MSKCC for a number of gastrointestinal and other cancers. In colon cancer, ip therapy has focused on FUDR and leucovorin; the early studies in GC focused on a combination of ip cisplatin and 5-FU and iv 5-FU. More recent ip studies in GC have utilized the FUDR and leucovorin combination.

The initial experiences with ip therapy in GC at MSKCC has been reported by Atiq et al. *(25)*. Thirty-five patients with high-risk GC were treated with PO adjuvant ip cisplatin (25 mg/m^2) on d 1–4 and ip 5-FU (750 mg/m^2), given as a combined ip dose, and iv 5-FU (750 mg/m^2) on d 1–4, on a monthly basis for five cycles. Therapy was commenced within 14–28 d after gastric resection.

All patients had transmural (T3) tumors, and 29 patients had N1 or N2 nodal disease (stage III). With follow-up of over 3.5 yr, 40% of patients are free of recurrence. Myeleosuppression was the most commonly occurring toxicity, but only two patients had neutropenic fever requiring hospitalization. An interesting side effect of sclerosing encapsulating peritonitis (SEP) was observed in 15% of patients. The latter was attributed to the alkalinity of 5-FU solutions, resulting in hydrolysis of cisplatin to an alkylating agent in the alkaline environment. Subsequent patients were treated by administering cisplatin and 5-FU in separate solutions, with no further occurrences of SEP noted.

Overall, in this study, PMs occurred less frequently than in historical controls, but still with considerable frequency. This study paved the way for the current MSKCC phase II neoadjuvant gastric study, which is discussed in some detail in subheading 10 of this chapter.

4. PHASE III WORLDWIDE ADJUVANT IP CHEMOTHERAPY EXPERIENCE

There have been a number of small phase III studies with ip chemotherapy administered in the adjuvant setting for GC, conducted by several Western and a number of

Table 1
GC: Phase III IP Adjuvant Trials

Study (ref.)	Treatment	No. patients	Median survival	2-yr survival (%)
Hagiwara et al., 1989 (27)	Surgery	25	14 mo	26.9
	Surgery + MMC	24	>3 yr	68.6
Schiessel et al., 1989 (28)	Surgery	33	15 mo	
	Surgery + cisplatin	31	15 mo	38
Hamazoe et al., 1994 (26)	Surgery	40	–	52.5
	Surgery + MMC	42	–	64.3
Sautner et al., 1994 (29)	Surgery	34	16 mo	–
	Surgery + cisplatin	33	17.3 mo	–
Rosen et al., 1998 (30)	Surgery	45		
	Surgery + MMC	46		

Japanese investigators (Table 1). Hamazoe et al. (26) conducted a phase III random-assignment trial in high-risk GC, in which patients received either surgery alone ($n = 40$) or surgery and ip therapy ($n = 42$). The surgery-and-ip group received ip MMC via continuous hyperthermic peritoneal perfusion (CHPP) immediately postoperatively. There was a nonstatistical difference in 5-yr survival favoring ip therapy (64.3 vs 52.5%). Peritoneal failures were seen more commonly in the surgery-alone group (59 vs 39%), although the difference was not statistically significant.

Hagiwara et al. (27) conducted a similar randomized study of surgery alone ($n = 25$) and surgery and adjuvant MMC administered intraperitoneally ($n = 24$), in a high-risk resected population. MMC was administered immediately after surgery, using a carbon-containing adsorbant. Early follow-up at 2 yr showed a striking difference in survival of 68.6 vs 26.91% for the group receiving adjuvant ip therapy. The rationale for the carbon adsorbant related to prolonged retention of MMC within the peritoneal cavity.

In a third study, Schiessel et al. (28), in a multicenter German trial, administered ip 90 mg/m^2 cisplatin and iv thiosulfate within 4 wk of surgery, to 31 patients randomized to receive adjuvant therapy. The major difference in this study, contrasting with the previous two, is that a proportion of the patients had residual disease (R2), undergoing only palliative resections. No difference in outcome was appreciated between the surgery-alone and surgery-and-ip therapy groups in this study.

Sautner et al. (29) randomized 67 patients either to surgery alone or to surgery and 90 mg/m^2 cisplatin as a single dose administered on a monthly basis. Similarly, in this study, no survival difference was detected between the two groups. As in the study by Schiessel et al., some patients with PMs were also included. A fifth study, recently reported by Rosen et al. (30), randomized patients to surgery alone ($n = 45$) or to surgery and ip 50 mg MMC bound to a carbon adsorbant ($n = 46$). In contrast to the other studies, a significantly higher rate of PO complications was noted for the group that received ip therapy, (35 vs 16%), compared to surgery alone. Also, early mortality was higher in the adjuvant arm (11 vs 2%), and no differences were noted in overall or disease-free survival between the control and adjuvant arm. This study was terminated early.

The conclusions from the five small random-assignment trials of surgery alone vs surgery and adjuvant ip chemotherapy, using a variety of different drugs and schedules, suggest that there may be a small survival benefit, and possibly a decrease in PMs, for adjuvantly treated patients, although the most modern study, by the Austrian group *(30)*, impels caution because of the excess morbidity and mortality and lack of survival difference in the adjuvant arm. This underscores the point that adjuvant PO ip chemotherapy remains experimental, and should not be administered outside the context of a clinical trial.

5. CONTINUOUS HYPERTHERMIC PERITONEAL PERFUSION

This technique utilizes the fact that hyperthermia may increase the efficacy of chemotherapy, as well as the favorable pharmacokinetic advantage of ip chemotherapy. This approach has been advocated mostly by Japanese investigators *(26,31,32)*. Patients who are at high risk for regional failure, and patients with small-volume PMs, were the initial targeted populations of this approach. MMC is the chemotherapeutic agent most commonly employed.

A number of adjuvant studies have looked at the efficacy of CHPP as an immediate adjuvant treatment in GC. Koga et al. *(33)* reported on 47 patients with resected transmural tumors: The patients who received adjuvant CHPP had a slight nonstatistical survival advantage over surgery alone. However, another cohort of patients in the same study did have a survival advantage, compared to historical controls. In another study, by Fujimoto et al. *(34)*, the overall survival of patients treated with CHPP was superior, and was evident in patients with and without PMs. In another randomized study of surgery alone vs surgery and CHPP and surgery and nonhyperthermic peritoneal perfusion in patients with T3 tumors, the overall survival was better in the two perfusion groups.

6. PALLIATIVE IP CHEMOTHERAPY

A high proportion of patients present with small-volume peritoneal metastases, often not evident on CT imaging, but found during laparoscopic staging of GC. There is a very limited body of data advocating an aggressive approach of systemic chemotherapy followed by surgical resection of the primary, and regional chemotherapy postsurgery. Preliminarily, it appears that a small number of patients may benefit from this approach, although it should be emphasized that this represents a highly selected patient population, and certainly is not a universally applicable approach. Similarly, a small proportion of patients with recurrent small-volume PMs or ascites may be effectively temporarily palliated with ip chemotherapy that maximizes dose and mitigates some of the systemic toxicity associated with ip chemotherapy *(34,35)*. CHPP may also provide an effective method of disease palliation, not only from GC, but in recurrent intra-abdominal malignancies from any primary site.

7. RATIONALE FOR NEOADJUVANT CHEMOTHERAPY IN GC

Neoadjuvant chemotherapy refers to chemotherapy given prior to definitive surgery. Induction chemotherapy can induce tumor regression, favorably influence local-regional disease control, and may treat early micrometastatic disease *(36,37)*. Additionally, neoadjuvant chemotherapy may identify a group of patients who have a higher likelihood of responding to PO therapy (Table 2).

Given the high risk of systemic relapse in GC, early systemic therapy intuitively makes sense. On the obverse side, induction chemotherapy may delay effective local control, drug resistance may emerge, and some patients may overtly progress during

Table 2
Selected Neoadjuvant Chemotherapy Trials

Study (ref.)	Regimen	No. patients	Operable n (%)	Resected n (%)	Median survival (mo)	2-Yr survival (%)
Ajani et al. (17)	EAP	48	41 (85)	37 (77)	16	42
Rougier et al. (18)	Cis/5-FU	30	23 (77)	18 (60)	16	42
Ajani (17)	Inf. 5-FU	30	28 (97)	23 (79)	16	NS
Crookes (40)	Cis/5-FU	38	35 (92)	29 (76)	17+	NS
	IP FUDR/Cis	59	56 (95)	40 (71)	52	64 (Est)
Kelsen (38)	FAMTX IP Cis/5-FU	56	50 (89)	34 (61)	15	40

EAP = Etoposide, doxorubicin, cisplatin; Cis/5-FU = cisplatin/5-fluorouracil; Inf 5-FU = infusional 5-fluorouracil; FUDR/Cis = floxuridine/cisplatin; FAMTX = 5-fluorouracil, doxorubicin, methotrexate; NS = not stated; Est = estimate.

neoadjuvant chemotherapy. Although the latter appear to be disadvantageous, it may actually spare a number of patients from surgery in which the outcome is destined to be unfavorable, because of occult established metastases at diagnosis.

8. PHASE II MSKCC COMBINED NEOADJUVANT AND ADJUVANT IP CHEMOTHERAPY EXPERIENCE

Two major trials using neoadjuvant chemotherapy, followed by surgery and IP chemotherapy, have been conducted and published. Kelsen et al. (38), from MSKCC, conducted a phase II neoadjuvant study of three cycles of preoperative 5-FU, doxorubicin, and methotrexate (FAMTX), followed by surgery and PO ip cisplatin and 5-FU and concurrent iv 5-FU in patients with high-risk GC.

The end points assessed included the resectability rate and disease-free and overall survival. The treatment program involved three cycles of induction FAMTX, followed by a D2 radical lymph node resection (planned for wk 11–12). Patients who were resected received three cycles of PO ip cisplatin, 5-FU, and systemic 5-FU. Fifty-six patients were enrolled. This phase II study commenced in July 1991, and closed to accrual in December 1993. The following paragraphs summarize the outcomes.

8.1. Response

Typically, in GC, the primary tumor is not easily measurable or evaluable, thus, objective response to preoperative (pre-op) chemotherapy was difficult to assess. However, clinical benefit, as judged by appetite, weight gain, relief of pain, and so on, was seen in about 50% of patients.

8.2. Toxicity

Myelosuppression was the major pre-op toxicity. Fifty-seven admissions occurred, in 40 patients (67% of all enrollees) with neutropenic fever, and one patient died of neutropenic sepsis. In contrast, myelosuppression resulted much less frequently from PO chemotherapy. Postoperatively, six patients were admitted with neutropenic fever, one of whom ultimately died, although that patient had evidence of carcinomatous meningitis at autopsy.

8.3. Surgery

Of the 56 evaluable patients, 50 (89%) underwent surgical exploration and 34 (61%) had a curative resection performed. Four patients (7%) had evidence of metastatic disease prior to surgery. In retrospect, 3 of 4 patients, on review of initial staging scans, had evidence of metastatic disease at presentation: One had pulmonary nodules, a second hepatic lesions, initially felt to be cysts, and the third an ovarian mass. The fourth patient developed malignant ascites. Overall, 9% of patients developed clinical progression during the induction period, and one patient (2%) developed metastases not previously identified during the pre-op chemotherapy.

8.4. Resectability

Eighty-nine percent had a surgical exploration, of whom 61% had curative and 20% palliative resections. Perioperative morbidity was assessed by comparing a noncontrol group of patients proceeding directly to surgery, and by retrospective comparison to other GC patients. No difference in 30-d operative mortality was appreciated. However, there was a slightly higher occurrence of anastomotic leaks in the patients receiving pre-op therapy, but, mostly, these were of little clinical significance. As a comparison during the same period that this study was conducted (July 1991 to September 1993), 223 nonstudy patients underwent exploration. In the T3/4 group, only 53 of 153 (35%) had curative resections. Thus, the 61% resectability rate in this institutional group compares favorably with concurrent controls.

8.5. Survival and Patterns of Failure

The commonest sites of initial failure were the liver and peritoneum. Peritoneal failure occurred in 16%. The overall survival for all patients was 15 mo. For the group who underwent curative surgery, it was 34 mo. Sixteen of 34 patients who had an R0 resection are free of recurrence.

8.6. Summary

This study demonstrated that the toxicity of induction and PO adjuvant chemotherapy was tolerable, although the major toxic side effect of myelosuppression, leading to hospitalization with neutropenic fever, occurred in 60%. The operability rate was high, at 89%, and the resectability rate was also high, at 74%, with curative resections performed in 61% and palliative surgery in the remainder. There was no significant increase in either operative morbidity or mortality. Additionally, ip chemotherapy was safely delivered, with acceptable toxicity, and there appeared to be a reduction in the rate of intra-abdominal recurrences. Early follow-up is encouraging, with a 2-yr survival of 40%.

9. OTHER PHASE II U.S. COMBINED NEOADJUVANT AND ADJUVANT IP CHEMOTHERAPY EXPERIENCES

A second phase II study of neoadjuvant and adjuvant ip chemotherapy, conducted in patients with resectable GC, was originally published by Leichman et al. *(39),* and was recently updated by Crookes et al. *(40).* This trial utilized different induction and adjuvant regimens, compared to the MSKCC study.

Fifty-nine patients with localized GC were enrolled, of whom 58 completed two induction cycles of 100 mg/m^2 cisplatin on d 1, infusional 200 mg/m^2/d 5-FU for 21 d, and weekly 20 mg/m^2 leucovorin, cycled on a monthly basis. Forty patients (68%)

Table 3
Pilot Neoadjuvant/IP U.S. Studies

Study	Preoperative treatment	Postoperative treatment	Enrolled	Target accrual
Kelsen ( )	Cisplatin/5-FU × two cycles	IP FUDR/leucovorin d 1–3 × three cycles	24	30
Ajani (17)	Cisplatin, inf. 5-FU, leucovorin × two combined ChemoRT	None	30	41
ECOG ( )	Cisplatin/paclitaxel	Chemoradiation with 5-FU/leucovorin	–	–

ChemoRT = combined chemoradiation.

subsequently underwent potentially curative gastric surgery, of whom 35 (60%) received 1–2 cycles of PO ip chemotherapy with 3000 mg FUDR on d 1–3, and 200 mg/m^2 cisplatin and iv sodium thiosulfate on d 4.

At the time of the updated report, the median follow-up was 43 mo, and 53% (31 of the 59 patients) were alive. The median survival was estimated at 52 mo, 95% CI 25–76 mo, and the estimated 2-yr survival was high, at 64%. The median survival for this group of patients was in excess of 4 yr, which was considerably longer than historical controls might predict. There was also a low rate of peritoneal relapse, with only 3 of 9 recurrences within the peritoneal cavity. Those authors attributed the latter to the administration of ip chemotherapy, and the overall favorable median survival to the combination of neoadjuvant and ip chemotherapy, rather than to the surgery per se.

In the MSKCC study (36), a higher-risk population was treated because of the requirement for endoscopic ultrasound staging (EUS), which was not incorporated into the study by Leichman et al. (39), suggesting that a number of patients with earlier-staged disease, and an inherently better prognosis, were included. Laparoscopic staging was not required for participation in either of the two studies; however, laparoscopy is mandated for all ongoing neoadjuvant U.S. studies. Other differences between these two studies relate to demographics: Specifically, there was a higher proportion of White patients with proximal gastric tumors in the MSKCC study, in contrast to the higher frequency of distal cancers in a predominantly Asian and Hispanic population in the study by Leichman et al.

10. ONGOING COMBINATION NEOADJUVANT/IP PHASE II U.S. TRIALS

Three pilot phase II trials are underway in the United States, looking at neoadjuvant chemotherapy and/or radiation and/or adjuvant ip chemotherapy in patients with locally advanced, but resectable, GC (Table 3). It is anticipated that the most promising of these three trials will become the experimental arm in a major future intergroup study, testing these concepts against surgery alone for high-risk, surgically resectable patients.

These trials have in common the following themes: They test some of the most innovative concepts in the treatment of GC (neoadjuvant chemotherapy, neoadjuvant PO adjuvant chemoradiation, and adjuvant ip chemotherapy) in varied combinations; they share the use of cisplatin and fluoropyrimidine- or paclitaxel-based chemotherapy, although designs in individual studies differ; and they all mandate laparoscopic staging prior to enrollment.

The first of these trials is a phase II study of neoadjuvant cisplatin/5-FU followed by PO ip FUDR and leucovorin, which is being conducted by Kelsen et al. at MSKCC.

The primary objectives of this study include assessments of toxicity, resectability, and operative morbidity and mortality, as well as determination of failure patterns and disease-free and overall survival. An additional component of this study involves snap-freezing fresh tumor obtained at the time of gastric surgery, for the determination of the following molecular markers: thymidylate synthetase (TS), dihydropyrimidine dehydrogenase (DPD), excision repair cross-complementing gene I (*ERCC-1*), and *p53* status. All of these markers will be correlated with stage of disease and outcome, and may allow individualization of therapy in the future. Additionally, quality of life data, in relation to both chemotherapy and surgery, is being recorded for all patients.

Eligibility requirements include T2 or T3 gastric tumors, with or without local lymph node involvement (N0 or N1–2), but with no evidence of other intra-abdominal, peritoneal, or hepatic tumor spread at laparoscopic staging. Other requirements include no prior chemotherapy, radiation, or other active malignancy within the preceding 5 yr.

The treatment plan involves two cycles of induction cisplatin and 5-FU, dosed at 20 mg/m^2 cisplatin on d 1–5 and 1000 mg/m^2 5-FU on d 1–5, as a continuous iv infusion, cycled on a 28-d basis for two cycles. Following a restaging CT of the abdomen/pelvis, patients proceed to definitive surgery. The third phase of the study, the PO portion, involves three cycles of 1,000 mg/m^2 5-FU ip on d 1–3 and 240 mg/m^2 leucovorin on d 1–3 every 14 d. PO ip chemotherapy is scheduled to start within 5–10 d of gastric resection. The ip regimen chosen for this study represents a divergence from ip chemotherapy used in previous MSKCC-based gastric studies. The rationale for the current choice is based on the tolerability of the regimen, the effectiveness in colon cancer, the known activity of fluoropyrimidines in GC, and the synergism of FUDR and leucovorin. Following completion of all therapy, patients are monitored every three months with physical examinations, laboratory studies, and CT scans.

As of July 1998, 24 patients have been enrolled. Five patients are currently receiving treatment on the study. Nine patients have completed all planned therapy, with the follow-up ranging from 1 to 10 mo. This study continues to accrue, with a target accrual of 26–30 patients. As yet, no meaningful inferences can be made, other than to note that there have been no pathologic complete responses to cisplatin–5-FU chemotherapy (which is as anticipated).

Some patients have noted symptomatic improvement in their presenting symptoms following induction cisplatin–5-FU, although this is difficult to correlate with objective response, given the difficulty in evaluating response in the primary tumor with standard CT imaging. A small pilot study is underway, to assess whether position emission tomography PET scanning pre- and postinduction chemotherapy may help predict response to chemotherapy in the primary tumor, and thus provide a more valuable objective measurement in determining merit from pre-op chemotherapy.

It is unclear whether the surgical morbidity of gastric resection is enhanced by perioperative chemotherapy. The ability to deliver the planned PO ip chemotherapy is a notable end point that will be attentively assessed. Further follow-up is awaited before meaningful data analyses can be performed.

The second ongoing trial is a multi-institutional, neoadjuvant study, which is being performed at the M.D. Anderson Cancer Center *(41)*.

Eligibility includes patients with GCs staged as T2–T3, any N, and M0. All patients were staged with laparoscopy and endoscopic ultrasonography. The treatment program involves two cycles of 200 mg/m^2 5-FU on d 1–21 and 20 mg/m^2 leucovorin iv bolus on d 1, 7, 14, and 21. The second cycle of induction chemotherapy is administered on d 28. On d 56, patients receive combined modality chemoradiation with 45 Gy (25 fractions over 5 wk to the primary site and local lymph nodes), and 300 mg/m² 5-FU as a continuous infusion 5 d/wk for the 5 wk of radiation. Patients are then restaged, and undergo surgery 5–6 wk postcompletion of this therapy. No PO chemotherapy is administered.

To date, 19 patients, of a planned 41, have been enrolled. The median age is 60 yr, median Zubrod performance status is 1, range 0–2. Ten patients have had proximal GCs, and four have had distal tumors. Eighteen patients have been staged with EUS, 16 having a T3 tumor, and 12 with N1 nodal disease. One patient withdrew consent after one cycle of therapy, and two additional patients had progression in the liver on pre-op therapy. Eight have proceeded to surgery: Four have had a pathological complete remission, and one a pathological partial remission (>90% necrosis). Five of 18 patients (28%) have experienced grade 4 toxicities. Further data is awaited, but the results are preliminarily encouraging, although the number of patients with progression prior to surgery is disconcerting, considering the extensive invasive upfront staging that is required for participation in this protocol.

The third study, being coordinated by the Eastern Co-operative Oncology Group, is in the advanced planning stage. The tentative program involves neoadjuvant cisplatin and paclitaxel, followed by surgery and PO chemoradiation with 5-FU and leucovorin. Data is awaited.

11. CONCLUSIONS

Adjuvant iv chemotherapy alone, neoadjuvant iv chemotherapy alone, and PO adjuvant ip chemotherapy alone remain experimental, even in high-risk resected GC patients. Similarly, although there is sound scientific rationale for neoadjuvant therapy in combination with adjuvant ip chemotherapy, this concept remains investigational. The former has the virtues of early impact on micrometastatic disease, as well as downstaging the primary cancer and facilitating resectability, and the latter is targeted on administration of high doses of chemotherapy to the major sites of known relapse. However, its merit remains to be determined in a future random assignment trial vs surgery alone, which continues to be the current standard of care for patients with resectable GC.

Another major development is the soon-to-be ubiquitous use of molecular prognostic determinants, such as TS levels, DPD levels, *ERCC1* levels, *p53* status, and so on, to predict both prognosis and response to a given chemotherapeutic agent *(42–45)*. The latter concept is currently undergoing phase II testing for fluoropyrimidine therapy in colon cancer. A recent abstract *(43)*, reported at the 1998 ASCO meeting, has shown that, for virtually all patients with high TS levels (>4.0) and high DPD levels, almost no responses were noted to 5-FU-based therapy in colon cancer. It is anticipated that such markers will be utilized for individualization of chemotherapy for GC in the near future.

One of the most difficult issues relating to neoadjuvant therapy is determination of response to pre-op therapy. Clearly, a high proportion of patients, probably in excess of 50%, experience symptomatic benefits to induction chemotherapy. Despite this, it is very difficult to provide objective verification of response, even with sophisticated CT imaging or other standard radiologic tools *(7)*. PET may provide a useful method for correlating symptomatic benefits with chemotherapy response *(46)*, but, further research is clearly needed.

The concepts of induction chemotherapy and/or chemoradiation and adjuvant ip chemotherapy are promising, but probably the most limiting factor to successful long-term outcome in GC is the relative inefficacy of current standard chemotherapy drugs. Short of earlier diagnosis, it does not appear that future developments in surgical technique will impact on long-term outcome, because even gastroectomy with extended lymph node dissection (D2) *(47,48),* an aggressive surgical approach, remains unproven. A number of new drugs, such as irinotecan *(49,50),* paclitaxel *(51,52),* docetaxel *(53,54),* and, possibly also gemcitabine *(55,56),* have recently been shown to have activity in metastatic GC. Large European and U.S. multi-institutional studies will examine a number of these drugs in combination with, and vs, a current standard combination of cisplatin–5-FU, in the metastatic setting. Perhaps more active systemic therapy for advanced disease will be identified, which can then be translated to the neoadjuvant and ip setting in patients with potentially resectable, and thus curable, GC. Identification of chemotherapeutic agents with greater activity, above all else, is destined to have the greatest impact on the cure rate of GC.

REFERENCES

1. Cameron AJ, Ott BJ, and Payne WS. Incidence of adenocarcinoma in columnar-lined (Barrett's) esophagus, *N. Engl. J. Med.,* **313** (1985) 857–859.
2. Hesketh PJ, Clapp RW, Doos WG, and Spechler SJ. Increasing frequency of adenocarcinoma of the esophagus, *Cancer,* **64** (1989) 526–530.
3. Blot WJ, Devesa SS, Kneller RW, and Fraumeni JF Jr. Rising incidence of adenocarcinoma of the esophagus and gastric cardia, *JAMA,* **265** (1991) 1287–1289.
4. Landis SH, Murray T, Bolden S, and Wingo PA. Cancer statistics, *CA. Cancer J. Clin.,* **48** (1998) 6–29.
5. Noguchi Y, Imada T, Matsumoto A, Coit DG, and Brennan MF. Radical surgery for gastric cancer. A review of the Japanese experience, *Cancer,* **64** (1989) 2053–2062.
6. Wanebo HJ, Kennedy BJ, Chmiel J, Steele G Jr., Winchester D, and Osteen R. Cancer of the stomach. A patient care study by the American College of Surgeons, *Ann. Surg.,* **218** (1993) 583–592.
7. Botet JF, Lightdale CJ, Zauber AG, et al. Preoperative staging of gastric cancer: comparison of endoscopic US and dynamic CT, *Radiology,* **181** (1991) 426–432.
8. Wisbeck WM, Becher EM, and Russell AH. Adenocarcinoma of the stomach: autopsy observations with therapeutic implications for the radiation oncologist, *Radiother. Oncol.,* **7** (1986) 13–18.
9. McNeer G, Vanderberg H, and Donn F. Critical evaluation of subtotal gastrectomy for the cure of the stomach, *Ann. Surg.,* **134** (1951) 1–7.
10. Gunderson LL and Sosin H. Adenocarcinoma of the stomach: areas of failure in a re-operation series (second or symptomatic look) clinicopathologic correlation and implications for adjuvant therapy, *Int. J. Radiat. Oncol. Biol. Phys.,* **8** (1982) 1–11.
11. Landry J, Tepper JE, Wood WC, Moulton EO, Koerner F, and Sullinger J. Patterns of failure following curative resection of gastric carcinoma, *Int. J. Radiat. Oncol. Biol. Phys.,* **19** (1990) 1357–1362.
12. Fujimoto S, Takahashi M, Mutou T, et al. Improved mortality rate of gastric carcinoma patients with peritoneal carcinomatosis treated with intraperitoneal hyperthermic chemoperfusion combined with surgery, *Cancer,* **79** (1997) 884–891.
13. Yashiro M, Chung YS, Nishimura S, Inoue T, and Sowa M. Peritoneal metastatic model for human scirrhous gastric carcinoma in nude mice, *Clin. Exp. Metastasis,* **14** (1996) 43–54.
14. Nakajima T. Review of adjuvant chemotherapy for gastric cancer, *World J. Surg.,* **19** (1995) 570–574.
15. Hermans J, Bonenkamp JJ, Boon MC, et al. Adjuvant therapy after curative resection for gastric cancer: meta-analysis of randomized trials, *J. Clin. Oncol.,* **11** (1993) 1441–1447.
16. Ajani JA, Ota DM, and Jackson DE. Current strategies in the management of locoregional and metastatic gastric carcinoma, *Cancer,* **67 (Suppl 1)** (1991) 260–265.
17. Ajani JA, Mayer RJ, Ota DM, et al. Preoperative and postoperative combination chemotherapy for potentially resectable gastric carcinoma, *J. Natl. Cancer Inst.,* **85** (1993) 1839–1844.
18. Rougier P, Mahjoubi M, Lasser P, et al. Neoadjuvant chemotherapy in locally advanced gastric carcinoma: a phase II trial with combined continuous intravenous 5-fluorouracil and bolus cisplatinum, *Eur. J. Cancer,* **9** (1994) 1269–1275.

19. Archer S and Gray B. Intraperitoneal 5-fluorouracil infusion for treatment of both peritoneal and liver micrometastases, *Surgery,* **108** (1990) 502–507.

20. Markman M. Intraperitoneal chemotherapy for malignant diseases of the gastrointestinal tract, *Surg. Gynecol. Obstet.,* **164** (1987) 89–93.

21. Kelsen DP, Saltz L, Cohen AM, et al. Phase I trial of immediate postoperative intraperitoneal floxuridine and leucovorin plus systemic 5-fluorouracil and levamisole after resection of high risk colon cancer, *Cancer,* **74** (1994) 2224–2233.

22. Sugarbaker PH. Early postoperative intraperitoneal adriamycin as an adjuvant treatment for advanced gastric cancer with lymph node or serosal invasion, *Cancer Treat. Res.,* **55** (1991) 277–284.

23. Sugarbaker PH. Peritoneal carcinomatosis: natural history and rational therapeutic interventions using intraperitoneal chemotherapy, *Cancer Treat. Res.,* **81** (1996) 149–168.

24. Sugarbaker PH. Mechanisms of relapse for colorectal cancer: implications for intraperitoneal chemotherapy, *J. Surg. Oncol.,* **2 (Suppl),** (1991) 36–41.

25. Atiq OT, Kelsen DP, Shiu MH, et al. Phase II trial of postoperative adjuvant intraperitoneal cisplatin and fluorouracil and systemic fluorouracil chemotherapy in patients with resected gastric cancer, *J. Clin. Oncol.,* **11** (1993) 425–433.

26. Hamazoe R, Maeta M, and Kaibara N. Intraperitoneal thermochemotherapy for prevention of peritoneal recurrence of gastric cancer. Final results of a randomized controlled study, *Cancer,* **73** (1994) 2048–2052.

27. Hagiwara A, Takahashi T, Sawai K, Yamaguchi T, Iwamoto A, and Yoneyama C. Intraoperative chemotherapy against peritoneal dissemination of gastric cancer with intraperitoneal activated carbon particles adsorbing mitomycin C, *Gan. To Kagaku Ryoho.,* **16** (1989) 187–192.

28. Schiessel R, Funovics J, Schick B, et al. Adjuvant intraperitoneal cisplatin therapy in patients with operated gastric carcinoma: results of a randomized trial, *Acta. Med. Austriaca.,* **16** (1989) 68–69.

29. Sautner T, Hofbauer F, Depisch D, Schiessel R, and Jakesz R. Adjuvant intraperitoneal cisplatin chemotherapy does not improve long-term survival after surgery for advanced gastric cancer, *J. Clin. Oncol.,* **12** (1994) 970–974.

30. Rosen H, Jatzko G, Repse R, et al. Adjuvant intraperitoneal chemotherapy with carbon-adsorbed mitomycin in patients with gastric cancer: results of a randomized multicenter trial of the Austrian working group for surgical oncology, *J. Clin. Oncol.,* **16** (1998) 2733–2738.

31. Inoue Y, Yamashiro H, Sawada T, et al. Therapeutic results and pharmacokinetics of combined used anticancer drug in intraperitoneal hyperthermo-chemotherapy (CHPP), *Gan. To Kagaku Ryoho.,* **17** (1990) 1551–1554.

32. Fujimoto S, Takahashi M, Metou T, et al. Improved mortality rate of gastric carcinoma patients with peritoneal carcinomatosis treated with intraperitoneal hyperthermic chemoperfusion combined with surgery, *Cancer,* **79** (1997) 884–891.

33. Koga S, Kaibara N, Iitsuka Y, Kudo H, Kimura A, and Hiraoka H. Prognostic significance of intraperitoneal free cancer cells in gastric cancer patients, *J. Cancer Res. Clin. Oncol.,* **108** (1984) 236–238.

34. Fujimoto S, Takahashi M, Kobayashi K, Kasanuki J, and Ohkubo H. Heated intraperitoneal mitomycin C infusion treatment for patients with gastric cancer and peritoneal metastasis, *Cancer Treat. Res.,* **81** (1996) 239–245.

35. Takahashi T, Hagiwara A, Shimotsuma M, Sawai K, and Yamaguchi T. Prophylaxis and treatment of peritoneal carcinomatosis: intraperitoneal chemotherapy with mitomycin C bound to activated carbon particles, *World J. Surg.,* **19** (1995) 565–569.

36. Kelsen DP. Adjuvant and neoadjuvant therapy for gastric cancer, *Semin. Oncol.,* **23** (1996) 379–389.

37. Ajani JA, Mansfield PF, and Ota DM. Potentially resectable gastric carcinoma: current approaches to staging and preoperative therapy, *World J. Surg.,* **19** (1995) 216–220.

38. Kelsen D, Karpeh M, Schwartz G, et al. Neoadjuvant therapy of high-risk gastric cancer: a phase II trial of preoperative FAMTX and postoperative intraperitoneal fluorouracil-cisplatin plus intravenous fluorouracil, *J. Clin. Oncol.,* **14** (1996) 1818–1828.

39. Leichman L, Silberman H, Leichman CG, et al. Preoperative systemic chemotherapy followed by adjuvant postoperative intraperitoneal therapy for gastric cancer: a University of Southern California pilot program, *J. Clin. Oncol.,* **10** (1992) 1933–1942.

40. Crookes P, Leichman CG, Leichman L, et al. Systemic chemotherapy for gastric carcinoma followed by postoperative intraperitoneal therapy: a final report, *Cancer,* **79** (1997) 1767–1775.

41. Ajani JA, Mansfield PF, Janjan N, et al. Preoperative chemoradiation therapy in patients with potentially resectable gastric carcinoma: a multi-institutional pilot, *Proc. Am. Soc. Clin. Oncol.,* **16** (1998) 1089.

42. Fata F, Baylor L, Karpeh M, et al. Thymidylate synthetase (TS) is not an independent predictor of outcome in patients with operable gastric cancer, *Proc. Am. Soc. Clin. Oncol.,* **16** (1998) 1079.

43. Danenberg K, Salonga D, Park JM, et al. Dihydropyrimidine dehydrogenase (DPD) and thymidylate synthetase (TS) gene expressions identify a high percentage of colorectal tumors responding to 5-fluorouracil (5-FU), *Proc. Am. Soc. Clin. Oncol.,* **16** (1998) 992.

44. Saltz L, Danenberg K, Paty P, et al. High thymidylate synthetase (TS) expression does not preclude activity of CPT-11 in colorectal cancer, *Proc. Am. Soc. Clin. Oncol.,* (1998) 1080.

45. Metzger R, Leichman CG, Danenberg K, et al. ERCC1 mRNA levels complement thymidylate synthase mRNA levels in predicting response and survival for gastric cancer patients receiving combination cisplatin and fluorouracil chemotherapy, *J. Clin. Oncol.,* **16** (1998) 309–316.

46. Watanabe A. Evaluation of therapeutic effect on lung cancer and mediastinal tumor by 18f-fluoro-2-deoxy-d-gluocose (FDG) positron emission tomography, *Proc. Am. Soc. Clin. Oncol.,* **16** (1998) 1943.

47. Bonenkamp JJ, Songun I, Hermans J, et al. Randomised comparison of morbidity after D1 and D2 dissection for gastric cancer in 996 Dutch patients, *Lancet,* **345 (8952)** (1995) 745–748.

48. Smith JW, Shiu MH, Kelsey L, and Brennan MF. Morbidity of radical lymphadenectomy in the curative resection of gastric carcinoma, *Arch. Surg.,* **126** (1991) 1469–1473.

49. Futatsuki K, Wakui A, Nakao I, et al. Late phase II study of irinotecan hydrochloride (CPT-11) in advanced gastric cancer. CPT-11 Gastrointestinal Cancer Study Group, *Gan To Kagaku Ryoho.,* **21** (1994) 1033–1038.

50. Shirao K, Shimada Y, Kondo H, et al. Phase I-II study of irinotecan hydrochloride combined with cisplatin in patients with advanced gastric cancer, *J. Clin. Oncol.,* **15** (1997) 921–927.

51. Ajani JA, Ilson DH, Kelsen DP. Paclitaxel in the treatment of patients with upper gastrointestinal carcinomas, *Semin. Oncol.,* **23 (Suppl. 12)** (1996) 55–58.

52. Ilson DH and Kelsen DP. Adjuvant postoperative therapy of gastrointestinal malignancies, *Oncology,* **8** (1994) 75–83, 88–90,95.

53. Sulkes A, Smyth J, Sessa C, et al. Docetaxel (Taxotere) in advanced gastric cancer: results of a phase II clinical trial. EORTC Early Clinical Trials Group, *Br. J. Cancer* **70** (1994) 380–383.

54. Kaye SB. Docetaxel (Taxotere) in the treatment of solid tumors other than breast and lung cancer, *Semin. Oncol.,* **22 (Suppl 4)** (1995) 30–33.

55. Christman K, Kelsen D, Saltz L, and Tarassoff PG. Phase II trial of gemcitabine in patients with advanced gastric cancer, *Cancer,* **73** (1994) 5–7.

56. Sessa C, Aamdal S, Wolff I, et al. Gemcitabine in patients with advanced malignant melanoma or gastric cancer: phase II studies of the EORTC Early Clinical Trials Group, *Ann. Oncol.,* **5** (1994) 471–472.

16 Regional Therapy for Gastric Cancer with and without Peritoneal Metastasis by Intraperitoneal Hyperthermic Chemoperfusion

Shigeru Fujimoto and Makoto Takahashi

CONTENTS

1. INTRODUCTION

Although the death rate from gastric cancer (GC) has been decreasing over the past few decades, GC is still a common disease throughout the world. In Japan, 32,000 men and 18,000 women died of GC in 1995 *(1)*. However, Japanese emigrants to the United States show a marked decrease in the occurrence of GC, and second-generation Japanese living in the United States show a more than 50% reduction in occurrence, compared with first-generation immigrants *(2)*. These findings suggest that environmental factors play a role in the etiology of GC.

GC may arise at any age in either sex, but, it rarely appears in persons under 30 yr. In 1995, in Japan, only 151 patients under 30 yr died from GC, where about 80% of GC patients are above the age of 60 yr, and the most frequent occurrence is from 65 to 75 yr *(1)*.

From: *Current Clinical Oncology: Regional Chemotherapy: Clinical Research and Practice*
Edited by: M. Markman © Humana Press Inc., Totowa, NJ

Table 1
Comparison of Histology of Primary Lesion Between
Advanced GC Patients with and without Peritoneal Metastasis

	Without peritoneal metastasis (n = 448)	With peritoneal metastasis (n = 66)	P value
Age (yr)[a]	60.1 ± 12.8	52.7 ± 9.1	0.0000215
Gender (m/f)	290/158	37/29	0.172
Histology			0.00255
Well dif AC	93 (20.8%)	6 (9.1%)	
Moderately dif AC	123 (27.5%)	11 (16.7%)	
Poorly dif AC	232 (51.8%)	49 (74.2%)	
Sum	448	66	

[a]Mean ± SD.
dif AC = differentiated adenocarcinoma.

Prognosis of patients with GC depends mostly on the disease stage, and the recent improvement in the prognosis for GC patients in Japan chiefly results from a considerable increase in the number of GC patients treated at an early stage. Although the prognosis for early GC is favorable, and the screening division of Social Insurance Funabashi Central Hospital (SIFCH) has carried out GC mass screenings of thirty-thousand/year, many patients with advanced GC still visit the hospital. Early GCs amount to only about 40% of the patients with GC who were treated surgically in this hospital.

For the remaining 60% of patients, extensive nodal resection, as well as the simultaneous resection of the surrounding invaded organs and primary lesion, were primarily carried out. In the case of a GC patient with serosal invasion, however, it is not clear whether extensive nodal resection contributes effectively toward an improvement in the clinical results of surgical treatment for GC, because the most likely pattern of recurrence is postoperative (PO) peritoneal metastasis (PM).

Iitsuka et al. (3) reported that cancer cells were detected in the abdominal cavity, even in GC patients who have no macroscopic evidence of PM just after laparotomy. The peritoneum when harmed during a surgical operation, provides a likely spot on which cancer cells can implant and grow.

To improve the prognosis of advanced GC patients with existing peritoneal metastasis, and to prevent PM in the near future, therapeutic countermeasures should be found for patients with advanced GC.

2. PATHOLOGIC BACKGROUND CONCERNING PM

Cancer cells generated in the gastric mucosa invade the submucosal layer, and, subsequently, the majority of these cells infiltrate toward the serosal surface and disseminate in the abdominal cavity. Between 1982 and 1993, 861 Japanese patients with GC underwent gastric resection at SIFCH. Among these 861 patients, 773 patients underwent curative gastrectomy: Of these, 325 patients had an early GC, and the remaining 448 had an advanced GC (4). Between 1986 and 1994, 66 gastric cancer patients with PM were treated in this hospital (5).

Table 1 shows a comparison of the histology of the primary lesion between the patients with and without PM. Many of the 448 patients without PM (about 48%) had moderately- or well-differentiated adenocarcinoma; a large majority (about 74%) of

Table 2
Relation Between Positive IP Cytology
and Area of Serosal Invasion in GC Patients

Area of serosal invasion (cm²)	Patients with positive cytology (%)
−10	22 (24/109 pts)
10–20	24 (11/46 pts)
20–	72 (44/61 pts)

Adapted with permission from ref. 6.

the 66 patients with PM had poorly differentiated adenocarcinoma. The two patient groups were significantly different regarding the histologic pattern ($P = 0.00255$), as well as age ($P = 0.0000215$). In other words, in the case of poorly differentiated adenocarcinoma, even if the primary lesion does not involve adjacent organs, it is still common for such cancer cells to extend to the serosal surface, and to present a high risk of peritoneal seeding.

Regarding the relation between the extent of cancerous serosal invasion in the stomach and the detection rate of intraperitoneal (ip) free cancer cells, Kaibara et al. (6) reported (in a study of the intraoperative cytology in peritoneal lavage of 216 patients with histopathologic evidence of malignant cells on the gastric serosal surface) that 72% of the cases with serosal invasion larger than 20 cm² (diameter 5 cm) were positive for ip free cancer cells (Table 2).

3. FUNDAMENTAL DATA ON ANTICANCER EFFICACY OF IP CHEMOTHERAPY AND HYPERTHERMIA

PM refractory to treatment (no matter where its primary focus may be) has a very poor prognosis in cases of conventional intravenous (iv) treatment. However, many cases with GC and PM are characterized by the tendency of the metastasis to stay confined to the peritoneal cavity, and, consequently, local control within the peritoneal cavity is an important and challenging problem.

The traditional standard treatment for advanced GC is comprised of surgery and iv and oral chemotherapy with mitomycin C (MMC), cisplatin, 5-fluorouracil (5-FU), methotrexate, or alkylating agents: This traditional treatment has obtained 5-yr survival rates of 10–30 % (6,7). To improve this dismal prognosis, it is necessary to prevent or eliminate PO peritoneal recurrence, which occurs most frequently in such patients (8). The ideal goal is decisive antitumor treatment at the site of GC cells exfoliated from the primary and metastatic foci.

3.1. IP Chemotherapy

The mechanism underlying the peritoneal transport of water-soluble molecules was established by the pharmacokinetic studies of Dedrick et al. (9). A major portion of an antitumor drug absorbed through the peritoneal membrane is carried to the liver, and is resolved there. The remainder of the absorbed drug is delivered into the systemic circulation. Like 5-FM, MMC is primarily metabolized in the liver (10), and, when administered intraperitoneally, about half of the MMC exits the abdominal cavity within 15 min (11). However, the ip concentration of MMC at 60 min after the ip administration of 10 µg/mL (40 mg/4 L) is equivalent to the peak plasma concentration after an iv injection of MMC at 15 mg/m^2 *(10,11)*.

IP chemotherapy, like every type of treatment, has its potential shortcomings, including limitation of drug penetration, uneven distribution caused by ip adhesion in a patient undergoing abdominal surgery, and the presence of extra-abdominal lesions. Even by the iv or intra-arterial administration routes, a drug has difficulty reaching the center of a bulky tumor, and it is even more difficult for the drug to reach the tumor center, or within the tumor, when the ip administration depends on drug penetration by diffusion. Thus, free-floating cells, cells on the peritoneal surface, and cells just beneath the peritoneum, at the deepest, are attacked by a high concentration of the drug. In the ip treatment of ovarian cancer, Markman *(12)* reported that the drug penetration of cisplatin is limited, ranging from several cell layers to perhaps 1–3 mm from the tumor surface. Thus, advantageous factors for the ip administration of antitumor drugs are ip floating cells; tumors with small diameters, confined to the peritoneal surface; a drug with high plasma clearance and low peritoneal absorption; and the abdominal cavity free of adhesion or hindrance for ip free circulation.

3.2. IP Hyperthermia

Hyperthermia has a direct anticancer effect, and a synergistic anticancer activity with several kinds of anticancer drugs. The destructive activity of hyperthermia depends on the temperature and duration used. The thermal death time is defined as the minimal time of heating that irreversibly damages the malignant tissue at a given temperature. The thermal death times reported to date were obtained from various transplantable tumors of rabbits and rodents. In addition, because these transplanted experimental tumors thrive on regional blood flow from the host, the lethal temperature-exposure factor changes with the posthyperthermic regional blood flow, i.e., with the vascularity within and around transplanted tumor. In the case of ip hyperthermic perfusion, cancer cells floating in the abdominal effusion have no vascularity. The authors have reported the thermal temperature-exposure factor assessed in a suspended-type experiment, with human GC cells serially transplanted into nude mice *(13)*.

BALB/c *nu/nu* mice, aged 5–6 wk, and a human GC (H-23) were used. In the in vitro experiments, fragments (about 1 mm^3) of H-23 tumors were incubated at 37–47°C for various times, and subsequently were assessed by light microscopy. In the in vivo experiments, four incubated tumor fragments were transplanted in the bilateral hind legs of nude mice, and the transplantability and growth delay were then studied, based on the assumption that the hyperthermia-treated GC cells survived posthyperthermically.

3.3. Transplantability

As shown in Table 3, the rates of successful transplantation at 37°C were 92.1% (35 of 38) and 91.9% (34 of 37), without spontaneous tumor regression. There was no difference in transplantability between 37 and 39°C; however, there were notable differences between 37 or 39 and 41°C, for 60 min or longer incubation times. No transplantability was observed at 43°C for 120 min. At 45°C for 15 min, 11% transplantability was seen (Table 3).

3.4. Delay in Tumor Growth

In the group at 37°C, the incubated tumors became palpable 13.4 ± 1.3 d after inoculation. In four subgroups treated at 39°C, there was no growth delay (Fig. 1). At 41°C for 60, 90, and 120 min, the growth delay was 12.0, 10.7, and 23.3 d, respectively,

Table 3
Relation between Incubation Thermal Dose and Tumor Transplantability

Incubation time (min)	37°C	39°C	41°C	43°C	45°C	47°C
15	ND	ND	ND	ND	11.1	0
30	ND	87.5	73.3	62.5	0	0
60	92.1	100	52.9	18.8	0	0
90	ND	87.5	50.0	8.3	ND	ND
120	91.9	88.9	42.1	0	ND	ND

ND = not done.
Numbers in table are the percentage of successfully transplanted tumors of tumors inoculated.

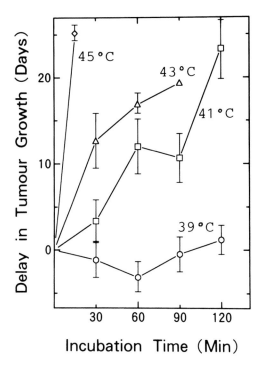

Fig. 1. Relation between incubation thermal dose and time, as well as delay in tumor growth of human GC fragments transplanted into nude mice. Each plot and vertical bar represents the mean and SE, respectively. A symbol without vertical bars indicates that the SE was smaller than the symbol.

with significant differences, compared with the control group. In the case of incubation at 43 and 45°C, the growth delay was significant.

3.5. Histologic Findings

The histopathologic findings of tumor fragments did not change in any of the groups incubated at 39°C, or in a group incubated at 41°C for 30 min, compared with the findings of the control group (37°C). In the remaining three subgroups at 41°C, as well as in three subgroups at 43°C for 30, 60, and 90 min, partial detachment from the basal membrane, scattered pyknosis, cytoplasmic degeneration, and intercellular edema were observed (Fig. 2). In the thermal-dose groups at 43°C for 120 min and 45°C for 30 min, complete destruction of the grandular structure, pyknosis, karyorrhexis, and

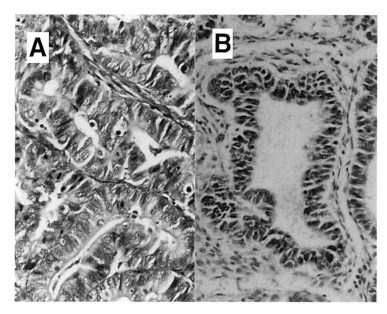

Fig. 2. Histologic changes of GC fragments following exposure to hyperthermia. **(A)** Histologic findings in tumor fragment specimens incubated at 37°C for 120 min. Glandular structures are intact and mitotic figures are evident (H&E ×100). **(B)** Section of fragments at 43°C for 60 min. The glandular structure is maintained, but interstitial edema and partial detachment from the basal membrane are evident. Nuclear condensation and cytoplasmic degeneration are present (H&E, ×100).

cytoplasmic disappearance occurred in almost all of the fragments (Fig. 3A). With thermal doses more than the aforementioned doses, coagulative degeneration and destruction of the glandular and nuclear structures occurred in all of the fragments (Fig. 3B).

4. IP HYPERTHERMIC CHEMOPERFUSION

In the previous subheading, IP chemotherapy and hyperthermia were briefly explained. In the primary stage of peritoneal implants of cancer, these implants are usually microscopic, and located on, or just under, the peritoneal surface. Thus, the most effective anticancer treatment for that stage should be selected, to prevent the spread of the PM all over the peritoneoserosal surface.

It is well known that the cytotoxicity of most commonly used antitumor drugs is considerably intensified at elevated temperatures. This finding has raised the possibility that hyperthermia can be used clinically to heighten the anticancer efficacy of systemically or locally administered chemotherapeutic drugs. Spratt et al. *(14)* reported encouraging results of ip hyperthermic chemoperfusion (IHCP) for a patient with pseudomyxoma peritonei from the pancreas. The therapeutic design reported by Spratt et al. is regarded as the best treatment for preventing or healing peritoneal metastasis from gastrointestinal cancer, because the efficacy of IHCP is excellent for superficial tumors, and because the water used in this design is a good heat conductor. The authors have reported a clinical trial of surgery and subsequent IHCP for advanced GC patients *(15,16),* as described below.

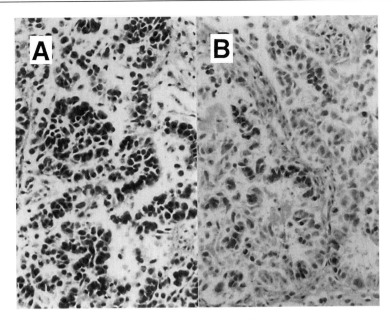

Fig. 3. Histologic findings of gastric tumor fragments following exposure to hyperthermia. **(A)** Histologic changes in specimens incubated at 43°C for 120 min. Glandular structures are markedly damaged, and pyknosis and karyolysis are widely spread (H&E, ×100). **(B)** Histologic changes induced by incubation at 45°C for 60 min. Complete destruction of the glandular structure is seen, and almost all areas are necrotic and dotted with irreversibly damaged cells, in which there is shrinkage of the nuclei and condensation of the chromatin into structureless masses (H&E, ×100).

4.1. Protocol Used at SIFCH

4.1.1. Surgical Treatment

For all patients, extensive tumor resection was carried out, and subsequently the reconstruction of the alimentary tract was done. When tumorous metastatic foci were present on the peritoneoserosal surface, a partial resection of the peritoneum or segmental resection of the small and/or large intestine was performed. When direct invasion to the pancreas, spleen, and/or transverse colon was detected, a pancreatico-duodenectomy, a left upper abdominal exenteration, or a total gastrectomy with splenectomy and distal pancreatectomy was done. When ovarian metastasis was observed, an adnexectomy or oophorectomy was carried out.

From July 1989 onward, to prevent posthyperthermic suture leakage of the esophago-jejunostomy or gastrojejunostomy, as well as duodenal stump, a catheter duodenostomy with a Foley catheter (12 or 14 French) was placed in the descending or horizontal portion of the duodenum of every patient (Fig. 4).

4.1.2. Detailed Explanation of IHCP

Under general anesthesia, just before temporary closure of the abdominal wall after the surgical treatment mentioned above, the equipment needed for IHCP was inserted into Douglas' pouch (outflow use) and the upper abdominal cavity (inflow use) (Fig. 5). This IHCP system (Mera HAD 101 type, Senkosha, Tokyo, Japan) was designed to circulate a closed peritoneal perfusate, aseptically, with a variable dynamic flow of 500–3000 mL/min, with the temperature regulated at 39–48°C. Closed IHCP was performed using 3–4 L Maxwell solution-1, a solution for peritoneal dialysis (Fuso

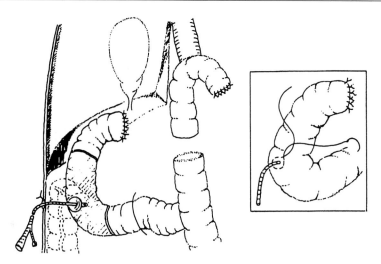

Fig. 4. Catheter duodenostomy with a Foley catheter inserted into the duodenal lumen through connective tissue between the right kidney and transverse colon, for the prevention of post-IHCP suture leakage of the esophagojejunostomy and duodenal stump.

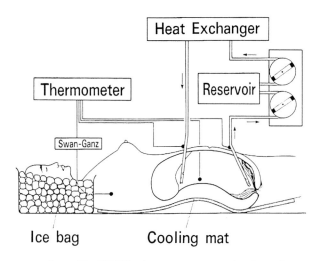

Fig. 5. Schematic presentation of ip (IHCP). Arrows represent the flow direction of the perfusate.

Pharmaceutical Industries, Osaka, Japan), containing 10 µg/mL MMC and/or 15 µg/mL cisplatin.

At the start of the IHCP, the patient's temperature was lowered to 31–32°C, with a cooling mat under the body and icebags around the cervical region, so as not to elevate the pulmonary arterial temperature above 40°C, which was measured with an inserted Swan-Ganz catheter (Baxter Healthcare Corp., Deerfield, IL, USA). Although the inflow temperature was 44–45°C for 2 h, the pulmonary arterial temperature did not exceed 39°C throughout the IHCP. Minor changes in the perfusate volume and concentration of the antitumor drugs were among the adjustments made in a series of IHCP treatments by the authors.

The temperatures of the perfusate at the inflow and outflow sites were maintained at 44–45°C and 43–44°C, respectively. Throughout the IHCP, the perfusate temperature

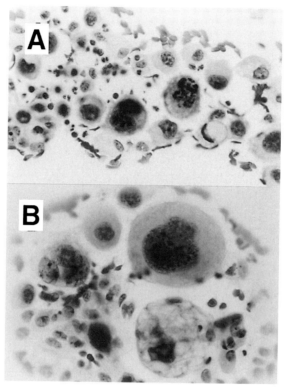

Fig. 6. GC cells in abdominal effusion or lavage just after laparotomy. **(A)** Many GC cells are seen in cluster form, and, among them, GC cells exhibiting prophase and metaphase are seen (Papanicolaou, ×100). **(B)** Typical features of GC cells (Papanicolaou, ×100).

was measured at the following points: the inflow and outflow points, Morison's and Douglas' pouches, and the pulmonary artery.

From October 1989 onward, to prevent scald injury on the peritoneoserosal surface caused by the hot perfusate, a drip-infusion of 50 mg/kg cimetidine was routinely performed just before the IHCP treatment *(17,18)*.

5. ANTITUMOR EFFICACY OF IHCP

The antitumor effect of IHCP on free cancer cells floating in the abdominal effusion was favorable in all gastric and colorectal patients with serosal invasion and/or PM *(5)*. As reported previously by Iitsuka et al. *(4)*, Kaibara et al. *(6)*, and Fujimoto et al. *(15,16)*, even in many GC patients with serosal invasion, many free cancer cells were detected in the abdominal lavage just after laparotomy (Fig. 6) Many GC and colorectal cancer patients with PM, as well as malignant mesothelioma patients, were treated with IHCP treatment plus aggressive surgery, and, although repeated cytologic examinations were performed with the lavage in Douglas' pouch, ip tumor cells were not evident post-IHCP (Fig. 7A), except in two GC patients, as reported previously (Fig. 7B) *(5)*.

Regarding the abdominal effusion in the preoperative stage, regardless of how much ascitic effusion accumulated, the effusion disappeared soon after IHCP (Fig. 8), and thereafter has never reappeared. In recurrent gastrointestinal cancer patients, however, a reaccumulation of the abdominal effusion was seen in some patients at 4–6 mo after IHCP.

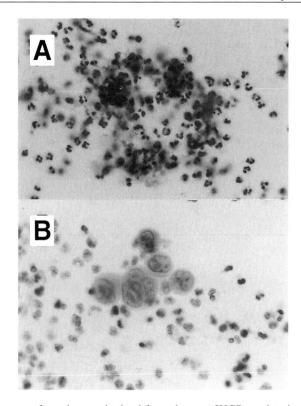

Fig. 7. Light microscopy of specimens obtained from the post-IHCP exudate in the Douglas' pouch. (**A**) Ghost cells surrounded by neutrophils 4 d after IHCP (Papanicolaou, ×100). Generally speaking, dead cells are digested by polymorphonuclear leucocytes or macrophages as a phenomenon of heterolysis. (**B**) Markedly damaged GC cells 5 d after IHCP. These cells are still viable, because they exhibit a fine nuclear membrane and granules, regardless of their low stainability (Papanicolaou, ×100).

6. CLINICAL OUTCOME
FOR GC PATIENTS WITH PM WHO UNDERWENT IHCP

IHCP treatment, combined with aggressive surgery, was carried out at the authors' hospital, on 48 GC patients with PM. During the same period of time, 18 GC patients with PM were treated by surgery alone (control group). These 66 patients were treated with cytoreductive surgery consisting of complete resection of the primary lesion and infiltrated adjacent organs, as well as a thorough resection of metastatic tumors on the peritoneum, small intestine, colon, rectosigmoid, and ovary, i.e., with at least an attempt to extirpate all tumors from the abdominal cavity (Table 4).

In Japan, PM from GC is classified by the Japanese Research Society for Gastric Cancer *(19)* as follows: P_0, no metastasis to the peritoneum; P_1, disseminating metastasis to the adjacent peritoneum (above the transverse colon), including the greater omentum; P_2, several scattered metastases to the distant peritoneum, and ovarian metastasis alone; P_3, numerous metastases to the entire peritoneum.

The antitumor treatment for the control group, (8–10 mg MMC and/or 10–25 mg cisplatin) was administered intraperitoneally; subsequently, about 30 mg MMC and/or 40–50 mg cisplatin were given intravenously by split dosings. Again, picibanil, an immunostimulant derived from *Streptococcus* (Chugai Pharmaceutical, Tokyo, Japan)

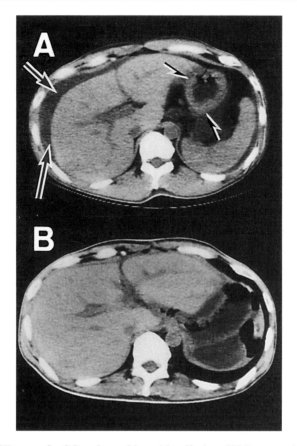

Fig. 8. Abdominal CT scan of a GC patient with ascitic effusion. **(A)** Preoperative CT scan showing the thickened gastric wall (Borrmann IV type: semiarrows) and ascitic effusion (arrows). **(B)** PO CT scan (5 mo after IHCP) shows no retention of effusion.

was given ip weekly at a dose of 10 KE (Klinische Einheit) suspended in 100 mL physiological saline. The total dose of picibanil was 40–60 KE. As PO adjuvant chemotherapy for both groups, a fluoropyrimidine derivative was administered orally for at least 1 yr.

6.1. Survival Rates

The IHCP group consisted of 21 patients with P_1, eight with P_2, and 19 with P_3 metastasis, and the control group consisted of eight patients with P_1 and 10 with P_2 metastasis (Table 4). Before this study, when advanced GC patients with P_3 metastasis underwent the inevitable gastrectomy caused by obstruction, bleeding, and/or perforation of the stomach, all of the patients were hospital fatalities; consequently in this study, GC patients with P_3 metastasis were eliminated from the control group.

The survival curves for the IHCP and control groups are shown in Fig. 9. All 18 patients of the control group died within 494 d. The 1-, 3-, 5-, and 8-yr survival rates for the IHCP group were 54, 42, 31, and 25%, respectively. The survival rate for the IHCP group was significantly superior ($P = 0.00167$) to that for the control group *(5)*.

A comparison of the survival rates of the P_1 patients is shown in Fig. 10. The 1-, 3-, and 6-yr survival rates for the P_1-IHCP group were 84, 73, and 56%, respectively;

Table 4
Clinical Data of GC Patients with Peritoneal Metastasis

Variables	IHCP group (n = 48)			Control group (n = 18)	
	P_1(n = 21)	P_2(n = 8)	P_3(n = 19)	P_1(n = 8)	P_2(n = 10)
Age (yr)[a]	56.9 ± 9.7	48.0 ± 10.6	47.4 ± 8.9	54.0 ± 7.8	56.6 ± 8.5
Gender (m/f)	12/9	3/5	10/9	5/3	7/3
TNM classification[b]					
Primary tumor					
pT3	11	5	9	5	4
pT4	10	3	10	3	6
Nodal metastasis					
pN2	7	4	1	4	4
pN3	12	1	10	4	5
pM LYM	2	3	8	0	1
Type of surgery					
DG	4	2	2	2	3
DG + AOR	4	0	1	1	2
TG + SPL	5	2	8	4	5
TG + SPL + PBT	5	1	0	1	0
TG + SPL + AOR	2	1	6	0	0
TG + OO	0	2	1	0	0
TG + OO + AOR	0	0	1	0	0
PD	1	0	0	0	0
Histology					
Well dif AC	3	1	0	0	2
Moderately dif AC	3	1	4	2	1
Poorly dif AC	15	6	15	6	7

P_1, P_2, P_3 = classification of peritoneal metastasis; *see* text for details.

[a]Mean ± SD.

[b]Union Internationale Centre le Cancer (UICC). TNM Classification of Malignant Tumours. Sobin LH, Wittekind CH (eds), 5th ed., Wiley-Liss, Inc., New York (1997) pp. 59–62.

LYM = lymph; DG = digital gastrectomy; AOR = adjacent organs resection; TG = total gastrectomy; SPL = splenectomy; PBT = body and tail pancreatectomy; OO = oophorectomy; PD = pancreaticoduodenectomy; dif AC = differentiated adenocarcinoma.

all eight patients in the P_1-control group died within 494 d. The 21 patients of the P_1-IHCP group had a better survival rate, compared with that of the eight patients of the P_1-control group ($P = 0.000817$) (5).

Figure 11 illustrates a comparison of survival curves between the P_2-IHCP and control groups. All 10 patients of the P_2-control group died within 358 d; the 1-, 3-, and 6-yr survival rates for the P_2-IHCP group were 62, 62, and 21%, respectively. The median survival duration for the P_2-control group was 110 d; this was 1586 d for the P_2-IHCP group. The P_2-IHCP group's survival rate was significantly better than that of the control group ($P = 0.00937$) (5).

The survival curve for the P_3-IHCP group is shown in Fig. 12. All of the patients died within 673 d, regardless of the IHCP treatment. A survival comparison among the P_1-IHCP, P_2-IHCP, and P_3-IHCP groups is shown in Fig. 13. The survival outcomes between the P_1-IHCP and P_2-IHCP groups did not differ significantly ($P = 0.271$), and

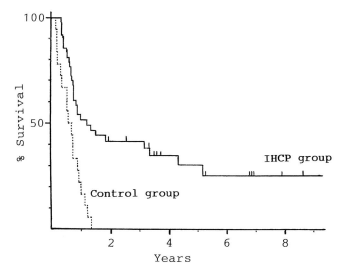

Fig. 9. Overall survival curves of GC patients with peritoneal metastasis. There was a significant difference between the IHCP ($n = 48$) and control ($n = 18$) groups ($P = 0.00167$).

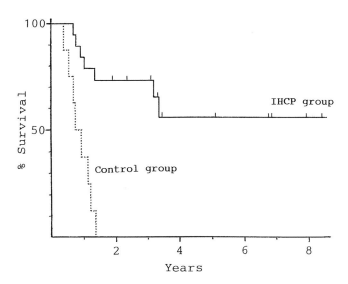

Fig. 10. Survival curves of 29 GC patients with P_1 metastasis. The difference between the IHCP ($n = 21$) and control ($n = 8$) groups was significant ($P = 0.000817$).

the clinical results of the P_3-IHCP group were inferior to those of the other two groups in terms of survival rate *(5)*.

6.2. Cause of Death

Table 5 shows the causes of death in the 66 patients with PM. In the control group, 17 of 18 patients (94%) died of the exacerbation of PM, as did 13 of 48 patients (27%) in the IHCP group. A significant difference between the two groups was noted ($P =$

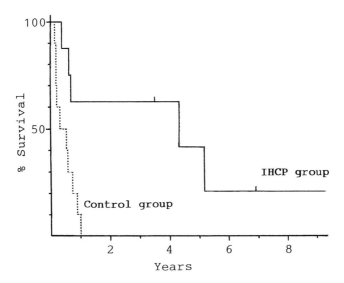

Fig. 11. Survival curves for the IHCP and control groups of gastric cancer patients with P_2 metastasis. The difference between these groups was significant ($P = 0.00937$).

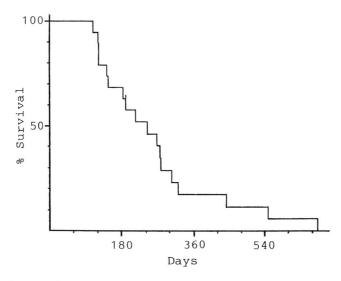

Fig. 12. Survival curve of the 19 GC patients with P_3 metastasis treated with IHCP. The median survival duration was 243 d.

7.08×10^{-7}). There was no significant difference in other causes of death between the IHCP and control groups.

7. PROPHYLACTIC EFFICACY
OF IHCP ON PO SURVIVAL OF GC PATIENTS

As noted in the first and second subheading, the ip free cancer cells act as a spearhead of peritoneal recurrence, and an effective strategy is required to eradicate these floating cancer cells, i.e., to counteract the possibility of peritoneal recurrence. The authors also have applied the IHCP treatment to GC patients with serosal invasion, from which GC cells exfoliate to the abdominal cavity.

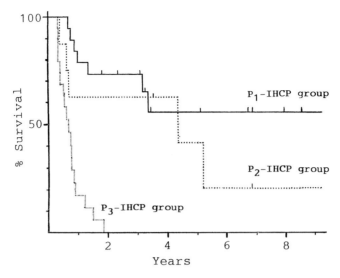

Fig. 13. Comparison of survival curves of the P_1-, P_2-, and P_3-IHCP groups ($n = 21$, 8, and 19, respectively).

Table 5
Causes of Death in IHCP
and Control Groups of GC Patients with Peritoneal Metastasis

	IHCP group			Control group		P value
Variables	P_1 (n = 21)	P_2 (n = 8)	P_3 (n = 19)	P_1 (n = 8)	P_2 (n = 10)	*IHCP vs control*
Cause of death						
Peritoneal rec	2	4	7	7	10	7.08×10^{-7}
Pleural rec	2	1	6	1	0	0.186
Pericardial rec	0	0	1	0	0	
Hepatic rec	1	0	4^a	0	0	
Miscellaneous	2	0	0	0	0	
Postoperative positive cytology	0	0	2	8	10	8.78×10^{-15}

Of four patients, two had hepatic metastases preoperatively.
^{a}rec = recurrence.

The aforementioned IHCP and surgical treatment was carried out randomly on 141 GC patients with macroscopic serosal invasion. However, GC patients with macroscopic peritoneal, ovarian, and/or hepatic metastases and cardiorespiratory lesion were excluded from this project. In this study, 71 patients underwent IHCP combined with surgery (IHCP group), and the remaining 70 underwent surgery alone (control group) (Table 6). As shown in Table 6, there were no significant differences in age, gender, nodal metastasis, type of surgery, histologic type of cancer, and histologic curability between the groups. Gastric wall invasion, however, was significantly more advanced in the IHCP group than the control group ($P = 0.0405$).

7.1. Clinical Outcome

The survival curves for the IHCP and control groups are shown in Fig. 14. The 2-, 4-, and 8-yr survival rates for the IHCP group were 88, 76, and 62%, respectively;

Table 6
Clinical Data of IHCP and Control Groups of GC Patients with Serosal Invasion

Variables	IHCP group (n = 71)	Control group (n = 70)	P value
Age (yr)[a]	58.5 ± 8.1	59.2 ± 9.1	0.629
Gender (m/f)	50/21	51/19	0.753
TNM classification			
Primary tumor			0.0405
pT2	9	15	
pT3	25	33	
pT4	37	22	
Nodal metastasis			0.111
pN1	3	8	
pN2	68	62	
Types of surgery			0.362
DG	33	38	
TG	38	32	
Histology			0.521
Well dif AC	8	10	
Moderately dif AC	12	16	
Poorly dif AC	51	44	
Histologic curability			0.725
Curative surgery	67	65	
Noncurative surgery	4	5	

[a]Mean ± SD; DG = distal gastrectomy; TG = total gastrectomy; dif AC = differentiated adenocarcinoma.

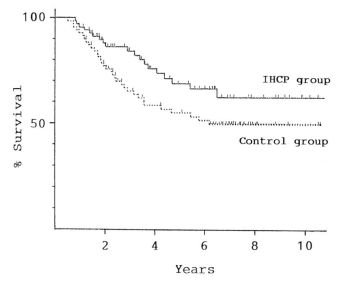

Fig. 14. Survival curves of 141 GC patients with serosal invasion. A significant difference was revealed between the IHCP (*n* = 71) and control (*n* = 70) groups at *P* = 0.0362.

Table 7
Recurrence and Mortality in the IHCP
and Control Groups of GC Patients with Serosal Invasion

Cause of death	Site of recurrence	IHCP group (n = 71)	Control group (n = 70)	P value
Gastric cancer	Peritoneum	1	16	0.0000847
	Liver	6	5	0.769
	Pleura	3	1	0.325
	Lymph node & local	8	9	0.769
Diseases other than gastric cancer		1	2	0.559
Sum		19	33	

those for the control group were 77, 58, and 49%, respectively. The survival rates for the IHCP group were significantly better (*P* = 0.0362) than those for the control group *(20)*.

The recurrence and mortality rates of these two groups are listed in Table 7. Peritoneal recurrence was seen significantly more frequently (*P* = 0.0000847) in the control group, compared with the IHCP group. The incidence of other recurrences did not differ significantly between the two groups *(20)*.

Regarding PO morbidity after the IHCP treatment, the incidence of hematologic and hepatic dysfunction was extremely low, and, even when they occurred, the levels returned to the normal range within about 10 d after the IHCP.

Among the 70 patients in the control group, only two patients suffered minor leakage of the duodenal stump, and that was completely cured without reoperation. As mentioned in the previous subheading, in the IHCP group, the catheter duodenostomy was placed in the descending or horizontal portion of the duodenum in every patient, in order to prevent anastomotic breakdown (Fig. 4).

8. PREVENTIVE MEASURES FOR PO MORBIDITY AFTER IHCP

As mentioned in the previous subheading, the genesis of PM is full-thickness cancer invasion of the gastric wall and exfoliation of cancer cells into the free abdominal cavity. In addition, at the time of resection of the primary lesion, transection of lymphatic vessels, and bleeding from the drainage vein of the primary focus, cancer cells leak into the abdominal cavity.

Because the goal of abdominal surgery is to remove all microscopic and visible evidence of malignancy within the abdominal cavity, IHCP combined with surgery, has been performed. However, hyperthermia has a marked cytotoxicity, not only for malignant cells, but also for normal cells. Above all, in the case of IHCP treatment, because the peritoneal perfusate at 44°C flows throughout the abdominal cavity for 2 h and the inflow site is the upper abdominal cavity, scald injury on the peritoneoserosal surface (particularly on the peritoneoserosal surface of the transverse colon and upper jejunum) presents a major problem.

In order to prevent thermal injury of the peritoneoserosal surface caused by IHCP treatment, 50 mg/kg cimetidine was administered via a drip infusion just prior to IHCP *(17,18)*. The preventive efficacy of cimetidine was confirmed histologically *(21)*.

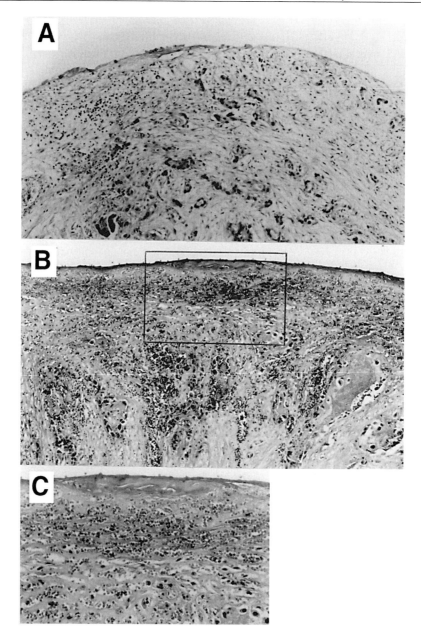

Fig. 15. Light microscopy of peritoneal metastasis from GC. (**A**) Pre-IHCP mesojejunum penetrated by GC cells. GC cells are alive and proliferate in the mesojejunum (H&E, ×40). (**B**) Post-IHCP mesojejunum without cimetidine (H&E, ×40). The mesojejunal surface thickens, and many dilated capillaries in the subserosal layer are seen packed with numerous erythrocytes. This is a distinctive feature of the first-degree scald injury; however, almost all cancer cells are damaged, and are led into pyknosis or karyolysis. (**C**) A higher magnification of the boxed area (×100).

Figures 15A,B show pre- and post-IHCP specimens of the mesojejunum, respectively. Fig. 15A shows that GC cells have invaded the mesojejunum and proliferated within the mesojejunum. Figure 15B shows the distinctive features of the first-degree scald injury of a patient who underwent IHCP treatment without cimetidine, and illustrates an erythema without blistering. As shown in Fig. 15C, many dilated capillaries in the

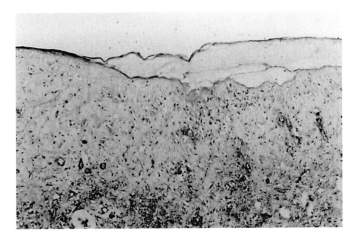

Fig. 16. Post-IHCP mesocolon adjacent to the inflow point of the hot perfusate in a patient who underwent IHCP without cimetidine (H&E, ×40). A small blister swelling is seen on the surface of the mesocolon; it is a second-degree scald injury.

subserosal layer were filled with numerous erythrocytes. Figure 16 shows a post-IHCP specimen of the transverse mesocolon of a patient without cimetidine. Because the transverse mesocolon is situated in the upper abdominal cavity, and in the vicinity of the inflow point of the hot perfusate, a fluid-like-substance-filled vesicle was seen on the surface of the mesocolon. This was considered to be a second-degree thermal injury caused by the hot perfusate.

Figure 17A shows histologic findings obtained in a patient who underwent IHCP with cimetidine. As shown in Figs. 17A,B, the subserosal layer had many dilated capillaries, within which erythrocytes were not found. With respect to antitumor efficacy, whether thermal injury occurred or not, almost all of the nuclei of the cancer cells were pyknotic and karyolytic in the patients, with and without cimetidine, as shown in Figs. 15B,C, and 17A,B.

9. DISCUSSION

Many studies have reported the antitumor effects of moderate hyperthermia in the range of 42.0–44.5°C alone, or in combination with radiation or cancer chemotherapy, based on reliable evidence of selective thermal sensitivity of cancer cells in this temperature range *(5,13,22–24)*. Higher temperatures may be of great therapeutic benefit, but, with temperatures above 45°C, irreversible damage to both normal and cancer tissues occurred in a linear temperature–time relationship *(13,22,23)*. When viewed from another angle, however, many solid tumors suffer more serious damage, compared with the contiguous normal tissue, because their neovascularity is incapable of augmented blood flow in proportion to the increase in temperature *(25,26)*.

Treatment with IHCP + aggressive surgery reduced peritoneal metastasis, and the authors found that second-look surgery resulted in more patients free of cancer. Of course, no patients with P_3 metastasis could be made disease-free by this treatment *(5)*. Unlike colorectal cancer, because GC has an uneven histologic pattern, about 20% of GC patients with P_3 metastasis have no tendency to stay confined to the peritoneal cavity, i.e., they have simultaneous metastases to the peritoneal surface and to the liver, as shown in Table 5.

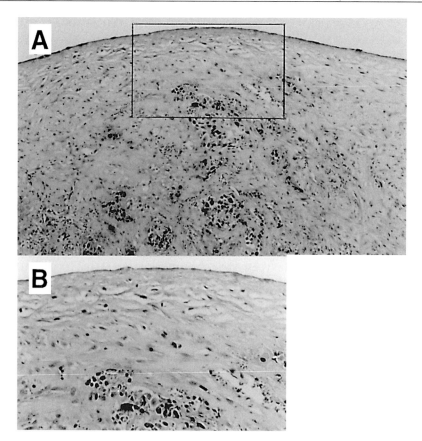

Fig. 17. Light microscopy of post-IHCP mesojejunum of a patient treated with cimetidine. (**A**) The subserosal layer has many dilated capillaries, but they are not packed with erythrocytes, and the mesojejunal surface does not thicken as seen in Fig. 15B,C. Almost all cancer cells in the mesojejunum are damaged, and are led into pyknosis or karyolysis (H&E, ×40). (**B**) A higher magnification of the boxed area (H&E, ×100).

In patients treated with IHCP without cimetidine, marked hyperemia with capillary dilatation, i.e., a first-degree scald injury, was observed on the peritoneomesenterial surface. When a high thermal dose of perfusate was used without cimetidine, a second-degree scald injury occurred on the serosal surface of the transverse colon. These injuries may contribute to post-IHCP morbidity.

Another cause of PO morbidity after the author's IHCP treatment is an inordinate increase in the internal pressure of the duodenum and upper jejunum. In advanced GC patients treated with the IHCP treatment, subtotal or total gastrectomy, with a thoroughgoing lymphadenectomy, may be performed; subsequently, these surgical treatments always considerably delay the recovery of the PO intestinal peristalsis. Thus, the accumulation of intestinal fluids results in the increased internal pressure of the upper alimentary tract and contributes to the high risk of leakage of the duodenal stump and esophagojejunostomy. Catheter duodenostomy can ensure a decompression in the upper alimentary tract, and can eliminate the PO morbidity from the authors' IHCP treatment combined with aggressive surgery.

The data from the author's studies, and others *(28–30),* suggest that peritoneal metastasis from alimentary tract cancer may be treated with IHCP + surgery. A promising start is to thoroughly remove all visible evidence of the tumor within the abdominal cavity.

REFERENCES

1. Health and Welfare Statistics Association. Statistics table in Japan, *J. Health Welfare Stat.,* **44** (1997) 401–434.
2. Haenszel W. Migrant Studies. In Schottenfeld D, Fraumeni JF (eds), *Cancer Epidemiology and Prevention,* Saunders, Philadelphia (1982) pp. 194–207.
3. Iitsuka Y, Kaneshima S, Tanida O, et al. Intraperitoneal free cancer cells and their viability in gastric cancer, *Cancer,* **44** (1979) 1476–1480.
4. Fujimoto S, Takahashi M, Mutou T, et al. Clinicopathologic characteristics of gastric cancer patients with cancer infiltration at surgical margin at gastrectomy, *Anticancer Res.,* **17** (1997) 689–694.
5. Fujimoto S, Takahashi M, Mutou T, et al. Improved mortality rate of gastric carcinoma patients with peritoneal carcinomatosis treated with intraperitoneal hyperthermic chemoperfusion combined with surgery, *Cancer,* **79** (1997) 884–891.
6. Kaibara N, Iitsuka Y, Kimura A, et al. Relationship between area of serosal invasion and prognosis in patients with gastric carcinoma, *Cancer,* **60** (1987) 136–139.
7. Maehara Y, Oiwa H, Oda S, et al. Surgical treatment and prognosis for patients with gastric cancer lesions larger than ten centimeters in size, *Oncology,* **52** (1995) 35–40.
8. Yamada S and Okajima K. Gastric cancer: surgical treatment. In *Cancer Therapy Manual,* Nippon Rinsho, Osaka (1988) pp. 534–538 (in Japanese).
9. Dedrick RL, Myers CE, Bungay PM, et al. Pharmacokinetic rationale for peritoneal drug administration in the treatment of ovarian cancer, *Cancer Treat. Rep.,* **63** (1978) 1–11.
10. Fujita H. Clinical pharmacology of mitomycin C. In Taguchi T (ed), *Mitomicin C,* Kyowa-Kikaku, Tokyo (1984) pp. 213–235 (in Japanese).
11. Fujimoto S, Shrestha RD, Kokubun K, et al. Pharmacokinetic analysis of mitomycin C for intraperitoneal hyperthermic perfusion in patients with far-advanced or recurrent gastric cancer, *Reg. Cancer Treat.,* **2** (1989) 198–202.
12. Markman M. Intraperitoneal chemotherapy, *Semin. Oncol.,* **18** (1991) 248–254.
13. Fujimoto S, Takahashi M, Kiuchi S, et al. Hyperthermia-induced antitumor activity in human gastric cancer cells serially transplanted into nude mice, *Anticancer Res.,* **14** (1994) 67–72.
14. Spratt JS, Adcock RA, Muskovin M, et al. Clinical delivery system for intraperitoneal hyperthermic chemotherapy, *Cancer Res.,* **40** (1980) 256–260.
15. Fujimoto S, Shrestha RD, Kokubun M, et al. Intraperitoneal hyperthermic perfusion combined with surgery effective for gastric cancer patients with peritoneal seeding, *Ann. Surg.,* **208** (1988) 36–41.
16. Fujimoto S, Shrestha RD, Kokubun M, et al. Clinical trial with surgery and intraperitoneal hyperthermic perfusion for peritoneal recurrence of gastrointestinal cancer, *Cancer,* **64** (1989) 154–160.
17. Fujimoto S, Kokubun M, Shrestha RD, et al. Prevention of scald injury on the peritoneo-serosal surface in advanced gastric cancer patients treated with intraperitoneal hyperthermic perfusion, *Int. J. Hyperthermia,* **7** (1991) 543–550.
18. Fujimoto S, Takahashi M, Kokubun M, et al. Clinical usefulness of cimetidine treatment for prevention of scald injury on the peritoneo-serosal membrane in intraperitoneal hyperthermic perfusion for patients with advanced gastric cancer, *Reg. Cancer Treat.,* **6** (1993) 1–6.
19. Japanese Research Society for Gastric Cancer. General rules for the gastric cancer study in surgery and pathology. I. Clinical classification, *Jpn. J. Surg.,* **11** (1981) 127–139.
20. Fujimoto S, Takahashi M, Mutou T, et al. Successful intraperitoneal hyperthermic chemoperfusion for the prevention of postoperative peritoneal recurrence in advanced gastric cancer, *Cancer,* **85** (1999) 529–534.
21. Fujimoto S, Takahashi M, Kobayashi K, et al. Histologic evaluation of preventive measures for scald injury on the peritoneo-serosal surface due to intraoperative hyperthermic chemo perfusion for patients with gastric cancer and peritoneal metastasis, *Int. J. Hyperthermia,* **14** (1998) 75–83.
22. Cavaliere R, Ciocatto EC, Giovanella BC, et al. Selective heat sensitivity of cancer cells: biochemical and clinical studies, *Cancer,* **20** (1967) 1351–1381.
23. Giovanella BC, Morgan AC, Stehlin JS, and Williams LJ. Selective lethal effect of supranormal temperatures on mouse sarcoma cells, *Cancer Res.,* **33** (1973) 2568–2578.
24. Hahn GM. Potential for therapy of drugs and hyperthermia, *Cancer Res.,* **39** (1979) 2264–2268.

25. Storm FK, Harrison WH, Elliot RS, and Morton DL. Normal tissue and solid tumor effects of hyperthermia in animal models and clinical trials, *Cancer Res.,* **39** (1979) 2245–2251.
26. Fujimoto S, Kobayashi K, Takahashi M, et al. Effects of tumour microcirculation in mice of misonidazole and tumour necrosis factor plus hyperthermia, *Br. J. Cancer,* **65** (1992) 33–36.
27. Fujimoto S, Takahashi M, Mutou T, et al. Survival time and prevention of side effects of intraperitoneal hyperthermic perfusion with mitomycin C combined with surgery for patients with advanced gastric cancer, *Reg. Cancer Treat.,* **7** (1994) 71–74.
28. Jacquet P, Stephens AD, Sugarbaker PH, et al. Analysis of morbidity and mortality in 60 patients with peritoneal carcinomatosis treated by cytoreductive surgery and heated intraoperative intraperitoneal chemotherapy, *Cancer,* **77** (1996) 2622–2629.
29. Yonemura Y, Ninomya I, Sugiyama K, et al. Prophylaxis with intraoperative chemohyperthermia against peritoneal recurrence of serosal invasion-positive gastric cancer, *World J. Surg.,* **19** (1995) 450–455.
30. Hamazoe R, Maeta M, Kaibara N. Intraperitonal thermochemotherapy for prevention of peritoneal recurrence of gastric cancer, *Cancer,* **73** (1994) 2048–2052.

17 Intraperitoneal Chemotherapy in Management of Peritoneal Mesothelioma

Maurie Markman

CONTENTS

1. JUSTIFICATION FOR INTRAPERITONEAL THERAPY OF PERITONEAL MESOTHELIOMA

Although there is far less experience employing intraperitoneal (ip) drug delivery in the management of peritoneal mesothelioma, compared to the treatment of ovarian cancer (OC), there is a strong rationale for considering this method of treatment for a carefully selected group of individuals with this devastating malignancy (median life expectancy, 15 mo) *(1–6)*.

Approximately 10–30% of patients with mesothelioma will have peritoneal involvement as the exclusive or major manifestation of their malignancy. Peritoneal mesothelioma remains principally confined to the peritoneal cavity for the majority of its natural history, at least regarding overt clinical symptomatology.

As with OC, it is possible in many patients for surgeons to surgically remove the large volume of cancer present within the peritoneal cavity, so that only microscopic disease, or largest residual tumor nodules <0.5–1 cm in maximal diameter, remain, prior to the initiation of chemotherapy.

However, in standard clinical practice, such a strategy has not generally been employed, or justified, in peritoneal mesothelioma. This is because of the absence of a demonstrated definite survival advantage associated with aggressive surgery, or the availability of a subsequent therapeutic strategy that relies on the surgeon's ability to successfully carry out optimal tumor debulking.

From: *Current Clinical Oncology: Regional Chemotherapy: Clinical Research and Practice*
Edited by: M. Markman © Humana Press Inc., Totowa, NJ

In addition, there is currently no accepted standard chemotherapeutic strategy in the management of peritoneal mesothelioma *(4,7)*. In fact, the role of chemotherapy in mesothelioma has been seriously questioned, because of the limited therapeutic benefits of currently available treatments *(8)*. Therefore, the use of innovative therapies is certainly justified in this clinical setting.

2. LIMITATIONS OF CLINICAL STUDIES EXAMINING IP CHEMOTHERAPY IN MANAGEMENT OF PERITONEAL MESOTHELIOMA

It is often difficult to make a definitive diagnosis of peritoneal mesothelioma in the absence of clear involvement of the pleural cavity. This is particularly an issue in female patients, in whom the diagnosis of OC, or primary carcinoma of the peritoneum, must be considered in the differential diagnosis. In the presence of diffuse involvement of the peritoneal cavity, even finding the ovaries at the time of surgery, to exclude this organ as the primary site of the cancer, may be problematic.

Tumor markers, such as CA-125, are nonspecific, and may be elevated in OC, primary carcinoma of the peritoneum, peritoneal mesothelioma, and a variety of gastrointestinal cancers. Because 20–40% of patients with OC and primary carcinoma of the peritoneum fail to respond to platinum-based systemic chemotherapy *(9)*, absence of tumor regression cannot be used as an indication that the patient has peritoneal mesothelioma.

Expert pathology review is often required to make a definitive diagnosis, including special stains and electron microscopy studies. If there remains a question of the exact diagnosis of the cancer in a female patient, it is most appropriate to treat the individual as though she has OC or primary carcinoma of the peritoneum (including use of a platinum agent and paclitaxel), because of the major prognostic implications associated with a response to this therapy. The objective responses and prolonged survival reported with regional chemotherapy of peritoneal mesothelioma in female patients must be evaluated with this background in mind.

3. CLINICAL TRIALS OF IP CHEMOTHERAPY FOR PERITONEAL MESOTHELIOMA

Over the past decade, several groups have systematically examined a role for ip chemotherapy in the management of peritoneal mesothelioma. Investigators at the University of California, San Diego (UCSD), Cancer Center explored the use of high-dose ip cisplatin, with sodium thiosulfate rescue *(10–12)*. Previous work by this group had demonstrated that it was possible to escalate the dose of ip cisplatin to 200 mg/m^2, if sodium thiosulfate was administered simultaneously intravenously, to neutralize the toxic effects of cisplatin leaving the peritoneal cavity *(13)*.

With this approach, the peritoneal cavity was shown to be exposed to 20-fold higher concentrations of cisplatin than the systemic compartment. At the same time, cytotoxic concentrations of cisplatin were still found within the circulation, despite the use of the neutralizing drug. This presumably resulted from the sodium thiosulfate concentration within the kidney, and was capable to inactivating platinum within this organ (preventing cisplatin-induced nephrotoxicity), but insufficient concentrations of the neutralizing drug were present in the circulation to inactivate significant quantities of the cytotoxic agent.

This strategy had been successfully employed by the UCSD group in the treatment of OC *(13–15)*. Those investigators theorized that the high concentrations of cisplatin present within the peritoneal cavity might convert a marginally active agent in peritoneal mesothelioma into a more useful drug in the treatment of this difficult malignancy. Over a period of several years, a number of patients with peritoneal mesothelioma were treated by the UCSD investigators with high-dose ip cisplatin (along with sodium thiosulfate nephroprotection *(10–12)*. Clinical responses were observed in a number of patients participating in these trials. Most impressive was the control of malignant ascites in patients experiencing this symptom as their major manifestation of disease. Control of ascites was observed in individuals, even when there was no evidence of shrinkage of measurable or evaluable tumor masses.

Several explanations can be proposed for the control of malignant ascites formation in the absence of objective tumor regression. It is possible the ip cisplatin merely acted as a sclerosing agent, reducing the ability of the peritoneal cavity to accommodate the fluid volume. Other cytotoxic agents (including bleomycin) have actually been employed specifically for this purpose. Although this possibility cannot be definitively eliminated, several points can be made against this argument. First, extensive experience administering cisplatin by the ip route has demonstrated that it rarely produces significant abdominal discomfort *(13,16,17)*, and, although adhesion formation is possible, such adhesions are generally limited in extent. Second, surgical assessments performed following treatment with ip cisplatin in OC have confirmed the lack of a severe sclerosing potential for this agent delivered regionally *(17)*. Finally, bowel obstruction is also a very rare occurrence following treatment with ip cisplatin. Thus, it is likely that the control of ascites in patients with peritoneal mesothelioma treated with ip cisplatin, at least in part, resulted from a direct antineoplastic effect of the cytotoxic agent. Because it is now well established that the actual depth of penetration of antineoplastic agents directly into tumor tissue (including cisplatin) is limited (perhaps on the order of several millimeters) *(18,19)*, it is not surprising that larger tumor masses failed to exhibit any shrinkage from the regionally delivered drug.

In contrast, tumor cells circulating in the cavity, which may have been responsible for ascites formation, might have been significantly influenced by the high concentration of cisplatin achievable within the peritoneal cavity following regional delivery. Their clearance may have led to a reduction in ascites formation.

From the important perspective of symptom control, a reduction of malignant ascites accumulation can be viewed as a legitimate aim of ip cisplatin treatment of peritoneal mesothelioma, even in the absence of evidence of regression of large tumor masses. This is a particularly relevant point, considering the limited therapeutic options available for the treatment of this malignancy.

In the UCSD trial, a number of individuals appeared to experience prolonged survival. Unfortunately, in the absence of data from randomized trials, which are extremely difficult to perform in this uncommon malignancy, it remains uncertain if this favorable survival in a subset of individuals reflects the influence of treatment or the heterogenesis natural history of disease in peritoneal mesothelioma.

Investigators at the Memorial Sloan-Kettering Cancer Center (MSKCC), following the lead of UCSD researchers, initiated a trial of ip cisplatin and mitomycin (MMC) in patients with histologically proven peritoneal mesothelioma *(20,21)*. The two-drug combination was based on preclinical data suggesting the potential for synergy between these two agents in peritoneal mesothelioma, and on limited clinical data demonstrating modest activity for the two drugs in pleural mesothelioma *(22–24)*.

The cisplatin dose in this trial was 100 mg/m² with MMC delivered at 5 or 10 mg for each treatment. Because of concern for potential unfavorable interactions between cisplatin and MMC within the peritoneal cavity if the agents were delivered together, cisplatin was administered on d 1 and MMC on d 8 of each 21–28 d treatment cycle. MMC was initially administered at a dose of 5 mg. If unacceptable toxicity was not encountered, the dose was escalated to 10 mg.

As in the UCSD trial, a number of objective responses to the ip treatment program were observed, including control of malignant ascites formation. However, in contrast to the UCSD study, there is greater concern that ascites control might have been influenced by the sclerosing potential of MMC. Long-term disease-free survival (>2–3 yr) was noted in a number of individuals with histologically documented peritoneal mesothelioma treated on this trial. Again, the influence of natural history of disease vs an effect of treatment remains an open question.

In the MSKCC trial, patients with significant tumor bulk were offered an attempt at maximal surgical tumor debulking prior to the initiation of the ip treatment program. The goal was to leave the patient with as small an ip tumor volume as possible, prior to delivery of the regional chemotherapy program.

Although the impact of this strategy on survival of this small patient population remains uncertain, the hypothesis on which it is based appears reasonable. This statement is supported by solid data in OC, in which responses to second-line ip cisplatin are limited to those individuals with microscopic disease only or small-volume macroscopic disease when the ip treatment program is initiated *(16,17).*

A third group of investigators examined a somewhat different strategy in the use of ip cytotoxic drug delivery in the management of peritoneal mesothelioma *(25–27).* Recognizing the poor outcome in this malignancy, and the importance of small-volume disease when regional therapy is employed, researchers at the Dana-Farber Cancer Institute utilized an aggressive multimodality approach in the treatment of peritoneal mesothelioma *(25–27).* Patients underwent an attempt at maximal surgical tumor cytore-duction, followed by a regimen of ip cisplatin and doxorubicin. The ip chemotherapy was followed by whole abdominal radiation therapy.

As might have been anticipated, toxicity of this treatment program was considerable. However, in a small number of individuals with limited disease at the initiation of the regional treatment, impressive survival was noted (6 of 10 patients were reported to be free of disease 19–78+ mo following diagnosis). It will be important for this novel strategy to be examined in a larger series of patients with peritoneal mesothelioma, to determine the relative significance of treatment vs the selection of individuals for this aggressive therapeutic regimen who had a relatively good prognosis independent of therapy.

Also, because of the multimodality approach, it is unclear which components of the treatment program were most important to the observed survival outcome. Of particular concern was the potential local toxicity of doxorubicin, previously documented by others *(14),* and whole-abdominal radiation treatment following ip drug delivery *(28).*

4. CONCLUSION

Experience with ip therapy of peritoneal mesothelioma remains very limited, particularly in comparison with OC. Further exploration of a role for this therapeutic strategy is hampered by the relative rarity of the malignancy, and by the overall ineffectiveness of cytotoxic chemotherapy in the condition.

However, a reasonable rationale for regional drug delivery in peritoneal mesothelioma exists, and further examination of the approach is warranted in appropriately selected individuals who have the malignancy. This includes patients with a good performance status, to justify an attempt at maximal surgical cytoreduction prior to the administration of chemotherapy, and individuals whose major manifestation of disease is the presence of symptomatic malignant ascites, in which a reduction in malignant fluid reaccumulation would have a significant, favorable impact on overall quality of life.

REFERENCES

1. Elmes PC and Simpson MJC. Clinical aspects of mesothelioma, *Q. J. Med.,* **179** (1976) 427–449.
2. Antman K, Shemin R, Ryan L, et al. Malignant mesothelioma: prognostic variables in a registry of 180 patients, the Dana-Farber Cancer Institute and Brigham and Women's Hospital experience over two decades, 1965–1985, *J. Clin. Oncol.,* **6** (1988) 147–153.
3. Antman KH, Blum RH, Greenberger JS, et al. Multimodality therapy for malignant mesothelioma based on a study of natural history, *Am. J. Med.,* **68** (1980) 356–362.
4. Antman KH, Pomfret EA, Aisner J, et al. Peritoneal mesothelioma: natural history and response to chemotherapy, *J. Clin. Oncol.,* **1** (1983) 386–391.
5. Lerner HJ, Schoenfeld DA, Martin A, et al. Malignant mesothelioma. The Eastern Cooperative Oncology Group (ECOG) experience, *Cancer,* **52** (1983) 1981–1985.
6. Plaus WJ. Peritoneal mesothelioma, *Arch. Surg.,* **123** (1988) 763–766.
7. Aisner J. and Wiernik PH. Chemotherapy in the treatment of malignant mesothelioma, *Semin. Oncol.,* **8** (1981) 335–343.
8. Alberts AS, Falkson G, Goedhals L, et al. Malignant pleural mesothelioma: a disease unaffected by current therapeutic maneuvers, *J. Clin. Oncol.,* **6** (1988) 527–535.
9. Cannistra SA. Cancer of the ovary, *N. Engl. J. Med.,* **329** (1993) 1550–1559.
10. Pfeifle CE, Howell SB, and Markman M. Intracavitary cisplatin chemotherapy for mesothelioma, *Cancer Treat. Rep.,* **69** (1985) 205–207.
11. Markman M, Cleary S, Pfeifle CE, et al. Cisplatin administered by the intracavitary route as treatment for malignant mesothelioma, *Cancer,* **58** (1986) 18–21.
12. Kirmani S, Cleary SM, and Mowjy J. Intracavitary cisplatin for malignant mesothelioma: an update, *Proc. Am. Soc. Clin. Oncol.,* **7** (1988) 273 (abstract).
13. Howell SB, Pfeifle CE, Wung WE, et al. Intraperitoneal cisplatin with systemic thiosulfate protection, *Ann. Intern. Med.,* **97** (1982) 845–851.
14. Markman M, Howell SB, Lucas WE, et al. Combination intraperitoneal chemotherapy with cisplatin, cytarabine, and doxorubicin for refractory ovarian carcinoma and other malignancies principally confined to the peritoneal cavity, *J. Clin. Oncol.,* **2** (1984) 1321–1326.
15. Markman M, Howell SB, Cleary S, et al. Intraperitoneal chemotherapy with high dose cisplatin and cytarabine for refractory ovarian carcinoma and other malignancies principally involving the peritoneal cavity, *J. Clin. Oncol.,* **3** (1985) 925–931.
16. Markman M. Intraperitoneal therapy of ovarian cancer, *Semin. Oncol.,* **25** (1998) 356–360.
17. Alberts DS, Liu PY, Hannigan EV, et al. Intraperitoneal cisplatin plus intravenous cyclophosphamide versus intravenous cisplatin plus intravenous cyclophosphamide for stage III ovarian cancer, *N. Engl. J. Med.,* **335** (1996) 1950–1955.
18. Los G, Mutsaers PHA, van der Vijgh WJF, et al. Direct diffusion of cis-diamminedichloroplatinum (II) in intraperitoneal rat tumors after intraperitoneal chemotherapy: a comparison with systemic chemotherapy, *Cancer Res.,* **49** (1989) 3380–3384.
19. Ozols RF, Locker GY, Doroshow JH, et al. Pharmacokinetics of adriamycin and tissue penetration in murine ovarian cancer, *Cancer Res.,* **39** (1979) 3209–3214.
20. Markman M. and Kelsen D. Intraperitoneal cisplatin and mitomycin as treatment for malignant peritoneal mesothelioma, *Reg. Cancer Treat.,* **2** (1989) 49–53.
21. Markman M. and Kelsen D. Efficacy of cisplatin-based intraperitoneal chemotherapy as treatment of malignant peritoneal mesothelioma, *J. Cancer Res. Clin. Oncol.,* **118** (1992) 547–550.
22. Chahinian AP, Norton L, and Holland JF. Experimental and clinical activity of mitomycin C and cis-diamminedichloroplatinum in malignant mesothelioma, *Cancer Res.,* **44** (1984) 1688–1692.
23. Mintzer DM, Kelsen D, and Frimmer D. Phase II trial of high-dose cisplatin in patients with malignant mesothelioma, *Cancer Treat. Rep.,* **69** (1985) 711–712.

24. Bajorin D, Kelsen D, and Mintzer DM. Phase II trial of mitomycin in malignant mesothelioma, *Cancer Treat. Rep.,* **71** (1987) 857–858.

25. Antman KH, Klegar KL, Pomfret EA, et al. Early peritoneal mesothelioma. A treatable malignancy, *Lancet,* **2** (1985) 977–980.

26. Lederman GS, Recht A, Herman T, et al. Combined modality treatment of peritoneal mesothelioma, *NCI Monogr.,* **6** (1988) 321–322.

27. Lederman GS, Recht A, and Herman T. Long-term survival in peritoneal mesothelioma: the role of radiotherapy and combined modality treatment, *Cancer,* **59** (1987) 1882–1886.

28. Shelly WE, Starreveld AA, Carmichael JA, et al. Toxicity of abdominopelvic radiation in advanced ovarian carcinoma patients after cisplatin/cyclophosphamide therapy and second-look laparotomy, *Obstet. Gynecol.,* **71** (1988) 327–332.

18 Intravesical Therapy for Superficial Bladder Cancer

Kerry L. Kilbridge and Eric A. Klein

1. INTRODUCTION

The bladder is an ideal organ for the application of regional chemotherapy. The urethra provides easy and relatively noninvasive access for the introduction of therapeutic agents, the urothelium provides a protective barrier that prevents the systemic absorption of the most commonly used intravesical agents, the intact ureterovesical junction prevents reflux of these agents into the upper urinary tracts, voluntary control of the external urinary sphincter allows a prolonged dwell time for maximal tumor contact, and the agents are discarded from the bladder during micturition, without the need for further instrumentation. The chief limitations of the regional approach for bladder cancer (BC) are that the depth of penetration of available agents is limited to a few millimeters, restricting use to those patients with superficial tumors; the production of urine during a prolonged dwell time may dilute the concentration of the agent, and therefore its therapeutic effect; variations in urine pH may effect the antitumor efficacy of some agents; and some agents produce a substantial local toxicity.

The use of regionally applied agents in the management of superficial BC is well established, based on multiple empiric clinical trials (1). In general, the treatment of BC is dictated by several important clinical observations that describe its natural history: Most invasive BC presents that way; most superficial tumors are noninvasive and stay noninvasive; only 10–15% of superficial tumors progress to muscle invasion; some carcinoma *in situ* (CIS) is destined to remain CIS.

From: *Current Clinical Oncology: Regional Chemotherapy: Clinical Research and Practice*
Edited by: M. Markman © Humana Press Inc., Totowa, NJ

Currently available evidence suggests that different genetic pathways are responsible for the genesis and progression of papillary tumors from normal mucosa to muscle invasion, compared to the pathway for CIS *(2)*. In addition, current genetic and clinical evidence raises questions about whether all transitional cell carcinomas (TCCs) are the result of a multifocal field defect, or may arise as monoclonal tumors that spread to adjacent areas within the bladder *(3)*. These observations have potential significance for therapeutic intervention, as well as for understanding the basic biological mechanisms underlying tumor progression.

2. STAGING

Superficial bladder tumors are defined as tumors confined to the mucosa and submucosal layers of the bladder, and which do not invade into the underlying muscularis propria. More than 95% of these tumors are of transitional cell origin, and grow either as flat, moss-like lesions with the histologic appearance of CIS, or, most commonly, as frondular papillary structures based on a fibrovascular stalk. Tumors that are confined to the mucosa are termed "noninvasive," and those that exhibit growth into the submucosal lamina propria, "superficially invasive." The American Joint Committee on Cancer TNM staging system assigns the T category for superficial tumors, based on both tumor morphology and depth of invasion *(4)*: Ta refers to noninvasive papillary tumors, Tis to CIS, and T1 to tumors that invade subepithelial connective tissue (i.e., lamina propria). T1 tumors may be of either flat or papillary morphology. In common clinical practice, tumors of grade 1 or 2 are generally considered low-grade, and tumors of grade 3 are high-grade. Most T1 tumors are histological grade 3, and recent evidence suggests that the depth of invasion into the lamina propria may have prognostic significance, leading several investigators to propose substaging T1 tumors into T1a (superficial invasion of lamina propria) and T1b (deep invasion to the level of muscularis mucosa) *(5,6)*. Intravesical therapy has no established role in the treatment of tumors that invade the muscularis propria (clinical stage T2 or greater).

3. NATURAL HISTORY

The majority of superficial bladder tumors are low-grade papillary tumors of clinical stage Ta confined to the mucosa. The natural history of these tumors is characterized by multiple recurrences in time and space, with approx 60–70% of patients experiencing recurrence within 3 yr of initial diagnosis. These recurrences are not life-threatening, but their management is a nuisance, requiring repeated cystoscopic evaluations, transurethral resections, and upper-tract imaging studies. Progression to muscle-invasive disease is rare, occurring in only 5–15% of patients. However, in contrast to noninvasive recurrences, invasive tumors can be life-threatening, and their treatment requires cystectomy, systemic chemotherapy, radiation treatments, or a combination of these therapies. These observations highlight several central questions in the management of superficial tumors:

1. Do available intravesical agents prevent tumor recurrence?
2. Is the likelihood of progression to muscle-invasive disease predictable at the time of initial diagnosis?
3. Do available intravesical agents prevent progression to muscle invasive disease?

This chapter focuses on the efficacy and toxicity of available intravesical agents in preventing recurrence and progression. A detailed discussion of predicting the risk of progression is beyond the scope of this discussion, and, although most low-grade Ta

Table 1
Goals of Intravesical Therapy for BC

Tumor Status	Goals of Therapy
Low-grade, papillary (Ta)	Prevent recurrence
High-grade, papillary (Ta or T1)	Prevent or delay progression
CIS	Eradicate existing disease and prevent progression

tumors do not progress, and high-grade T1 tumors are considered potentially life-threatening, at present it is not possible to predict with certainty the likelihood of progression for an individual patient.

4. PRINCIPLES OF INTRAVESICAL THERAPY

The initial management of a patient with superficial disease is designed to establish the number, location, size, extent, grade, and depth of invasion (T stage) of the tumors; to determine whether CIS is present concomitantly with papillary tumors; and to assess the upper urinary tract for renal function, obstruction, anatomic abnormalities, and the presence of upper tract tumors. Initial evaluation should include voided cytology, intravenous urogram (IVU) or retrograde pyelograms, and visual endoscopic mapping of tumor extent by cystoscopy. The presence of hydronephrosis on IVU usually indicates the presence of muscle-invasive disease (T2 or greater) or an invasive ureteral tumor. Complete excision of all visible tumor by transurethral resection of bladder tumor (TURBT) should be attempted, to ensure complete tumor sampling for establishing T stage. For papillary tumors, complete TURBT is also an important therapeutic maneuver, with older trials demonstrating the inability of intravesical chemotherapy to eradicate unresected tumors, and many randomized trials demonstrating a substantial therapeutic benefit to TURBT alone *(7)*. Random biopsy of normal-appearing mucosa is advocated by some, to detect the presence of "invisible" CIS. A postresection voided cytology may also be helpful in determining whether all tumor has been removed endoscopically. For patients with diffuse CIS, complete resection is usually not possible, and biopsies from multiple sites should be obtained, to assess tumor extent and depth of invasion.

The decision to proceed with intravesical therapy is dictated by the clinical characteristics of the tumor. Patients with small, solitary, first-time Ta tumors of low-grade are at lowest risk of recurrence and progression, and toxicity of therapy may outweigh any clinical benefit. Patients with multiple recurrences of low-grade Ta tumors, those with concomitant CIS, those with T1 tumors, and those with diffuse CIS are more likely to achieve a therapeutic benefit with intravesical treatment. The value of a single intravesical instillation of a chemotherapeutic agent immediately following TURBT, to prevent implantation of tumor cells liberated by resection, remains controversial *(8)*. Before deciding on whether to proceed with a more prolonged course of intravesical therapy, and which agent to use, it is useful to keep in mind the goals of therapy for each clinical situation (Table 1).

Additional general principles for intravesical therapy apply for all agents, once the decision to proceed with therapy has been made. Therapy should not begin until the bladder has healed from the effects of TURBT (usually 7–10 d later), to prevent systemic absorption. Most treatment regimens dictate intravesical instillation on a weekly basis for 6–8 wk, sometimes with additional maintenance therapy given at more prolonged intervals. In each instance, a urinalysis should be performed prior to instillation. The urine should be uninfected, and therapy should be delayed until an adequate course of antibiotics has been administered if infection is present. The patient should limit fluid intake for 8–12 h prior to instillation, to minimize dilution of the instilled agent. The efficacy of some agents, such as mitomycin C (MMC) and doxorubicin (DOX) may be affected by urine pH, and some regimens include pharmacologic manipulation of urinary pH prior to instillation *(9)*. The bladder should be emptied of urine, both by micturition and catheterization, prior to instillation, again, to minimize dilution. No agent should be instilled under high pressure, especially if a traumatic catheterization has occurred. Severe systemic illness and death have been reported with systemic absorption of bacille Calmette-Guérin vaccine (BCG) given following urethral trauma from catheter passage *(10)*. Most regimens dictate a dwell time of 2 h, after which patients may resume oral intact and normal voiding habits. A follow-up cystoscopy 12 wk after initiation of therapy is indicated in all patients, to assess tumor response.

5. ASSESSING OUTCOMES

5.1. Recurrence

The most common end point used in the evaluation of intravesical therapies is tumor recurrence. At least three different measures of tumor recurrence exist, and are useful for comparing agents: recurrence-free interval (median time to tumor recurrence), recurrence rate, and mean time between recurrences. Recurrence-free interval is the time between intravesical therapy and evidence of tumor recurrence. This measure can be analyzed and represented graphically by the Kaplan-Meier method. It is equivalent to the disease-free survival (DFS) used to compare many other oncologic interventions. Directly related to time to tumor recurrence is the median time to tumor recurrence, which reflects the median time for which patients remain disease-free after treatment. It is an important aggregate measure of the benefit of an intravesical agent, which can help both physicians and patients gage an average benefit of treatment. For instance, if an intravesical therapy is being used as a prophylactic treatment to prevent symptomatic tumor recurrence, and requires 12 weekly instillations, but results in only a 4-wk gain in median time to tumor recurrence compared to TURBT, it may not be a clinically worthwhile intervention, even if the result is statistically significant. Another measure of tumor recurrence is the recurrence rate, defined as the number of follow-up cystoscopic studies at which recurrence is noted, divided by the total months of follow-up. This result is then multiplied by 10 to simplify presentation. Although useful for detecting differences between therapies, recurrence rates may be more difficult to translate into clinical benefit for individual patients. Last, the mean interval between recurrences represents the time intervals between treatment and tumor recurrence, combined with the intervals between subsequent recurrences. The difference between this measure and disease-free interval comes from including time from first to second recurrence and time from second to third recurrence, and so on. For studies with lengthy follow-up, mean interval between tumor recurrences captures long-term efficacy of an intravesical therapy that may not be reflected in the disease-free interval.

5.2. Progression

Another end point reported for many studies of intravesical therapy is tumor progression. The definition of tumor progression varies, but usually refers to progression from superficial TCC stage Ta or T1, any grade, with or without CIS, to the development of muscle-invasive or metastatic tumor, stage T2 or greater. However, many studies will define progression as any increase in stage or grade. By this criterion, a patient who starts with a stage Ta TCC, and subsequently develops a T1 tumor, or a patient with a Ta grade 1 tumor who develops a Ta grade 2 tumor, are both considered to have disease progression.

The prognosis for muscle-invasive or metastatic tumor bears a direct impact on life expectancy, that may not result from progression to a Ta grade 2 superficial tumor. It is important, therefore, to avoid comparison of tumor progression between studies of intravesical therapies that have employed different definitions of progression. Similarly, tumor recurrence is not necessarily correlated with development of muscle-invasive or metastatic disease. Superficial TCC recurs frequently with another superficial tumor, but rarely progresses to stage T2 or greater. There are numerous trials in the literature that demonstrate a statistically significant decrease in tumor recurrence for an intravesical agent, and fail to show a decrease in tumor progression to muscle-invasive or metastatic disease *(11–13)*. As a result, it is not clear whether reduction in tumor recurrence by an intravesical agent translates directly into a decrease in invasive or metastatic tumor, with an improvement in long-term survival. Nevertheless, a decrease in tumor recurrence may be a clinically important end point, even in the absence of a demonstrable survival benefit, for those patients who tolerate TURBT poorly, or who have symptomatic superficial tumor recurrences.

5.3. Cost-effectiveness

The cost-effectiveness of a medical intervention has gained emphasis with the advent of managed care and capitated health insurance. Although the term is frequently used as a loose description of good, but not costly, medical care, it has a precise meaning that deserves definition. The cost-effectiveness ratio of a medical intervention refers to its dollar cost/year of life saved, compared to the next best alternative treatment. By virtue of its definition, cost-effectiveness requires comparison between two or more medical interventions, regarding both costs and life expectancy. Most well-accepted medical interventions have cost-effectiveness ratios less than or equal to $50,000/yr of life saved. Although there is no strict cutoff for the cost-effectiveness ratio of a treatment to be considered worthwhile, controversial medical interventions usually have cost-effectiveness ratios greater than $100,000/yr of life saved.

In the case of intravesical therapy for superficial BC, most agents would be evaluated in comparison to TURBT alone. Both strategies entail TURBT for tumor recurrence, cystectomy for muscle-invasive progression, and chemotherapy for metastatic disease. Thus, the cost-effectiveness of intravesical therapy depends on the added expense of the treatment, including physician visits; the degree to which costs are decreased by avoiding TURBT, cystectomy, and chemotherapy; and the degree to which therapy increases life expectancy.

The more successful intravesical therapy prevents cancer death, the more expensive it can be and still be cost-effective, compared to alternative treatments. Unfortunately, it can be difficult to estimate cost-effectiveness based on the recurrence rates most frequently reported for studies of these agents. Specifically, because a statistically significant decrease in tumor recurrence may not change the rate of tumor progression and, in turn, alter life expectancy, intravesical therapy must result in a dramatic difference in the costs of care in order to be cost-effective. When tumor progression to muscle-invasive or metastatic disease is reported for an agent, however, some estimate of cost-effectiveness can be made, because progression directly influences life expectancy and the costs of medical care: Preventing progression avoids the costs of cystectomy or radiation therapy and chemotherapy. Only a single cost-effectiveness study of intravesical agents has been performed for BCG therapy *(14)*. Preliminary results of the analysis are reviewed subsequently. Doubtless these considerations will assume increasing importance with further penetration of managed care into the field of urological oncology.

6. AGENTS AND DOSING

Intravesical therapies include chemotherapeutic agents and a growing list of immunotherapies. The distinction between the two types of therapies is that chemotherapy has a direct cytotoxic effect on neoplasia, while immunotherapy has an indirect effect on tumor tissue that is mediated by numerous biologic response modulators, only a few of which have been defined. The most frequently used intravesical chemotherapies include thio-TEPA, MMC, DOX, and epirubicin (EPI). BCG is the most commonly used intravesical immunotherapy, but trials of interferon (IFN), interleukin (IL)-2, and several other new agents have been reported.

In 1961, Jones and Swinney *(15)* were the first to suggest that thio-TEPA could decrease superficial tumor recurrence, when used as an intravesical chemotherapy directly instilled into the bladder. The drug's mechanism of action is thought to be through DNA crosslinking, but at least one investigator *(16)* has suggested that it may act by reducing cell adherence and increasing mucosal permeability. Several large randomized studies support the idea that intravesical thio-TEPA results in a statistically significant decrease in tumor recurrence. Shulman et al. *(11)* of the European Organization for Research and Treatment of Cancer (EORTC), randomized over 300 patients with primary or recurrent Ta and T1 tumors to receive thio-TEPA, VM26, or TURBT alone. The group found no change in the time to first recurrence, but documented a significantly lower recurrence rate in patients treated with thio-TEPA than TURBT alone. Similarly, Prout et al. *(12)* and Zincke et al. *(17)* randomized patients to thio-TEPA or TURBT alone. Both studies documented a statistically significant decrease in tumor recurrence. Although thio-TEPA may delay time to tumor recurrence, the single analysis with long-term follow-up shows that thio-TEPA's effect is not durable *(12)*. Ultimately, just as many treated patients experience tumor recurrence as patients undergoing TURBT alone. The delivery of thio-TEPA is complicated by its small mol wt, which allows significant systemic and dose-dependent absorption across bladder epithelium. Consequently, the drug's major side effects are leukopenia and thrombocytopenia. Recent work by Masters et al. *(18),* however, has shown that, by decreasing the volume of instillate, but maintaining the dose of thio-TEPA to increase its concentration, it is possible to increase the dose to the bladder epithelium without increasing systemic toxicity. Thio-TEPA is well known to be leukemogenic when given systemically, and there have been numerous reports of secondary leukemias and myelodysplasias associated with intravesical therapy that probably reflect systemic absorption *(19)*. The most commonly used dosing regimen is 30–60 mg thio-TEPA in an equal volume of instillate weekly for four treatments, then monthly for no more than 1 yr, to avoid the myelosuppression that has been observed with higher doses over repeated instillations.

MMC is an alkylating agent derived from *Streptomyces caespitous*. Its proposed mechanism of action is through DNA binding, resulting in strand breakage and inhibition of protein synthesis *(20),* but some investigators have suggested that DNA breaks occur through free-radical production *(21)*. Because MMC has a relatively high mol wt, there is little systemic absorption after intravesical instillation, and its side effects are predominantly local. Chemical cystitis and contact dermatitis are the most frequent side effects reported. Less often, reduced bladder capacity and allergic hypersensitivity reactions have been observed *(19)*. At least two large randomized prospective trials have demonstrated a decrease in superficial tumor recurrence after treatment with MMC. Niijima et al. *(22)* of the Japanese Urological Cancer Research Group, randomized 278 patients who had primary or recurrent superficial TCC, to 20 mg MMC in 40 cc, instillate twice weekly for 4 wk or to TURBT alone. These investigators found a significant increase in DFS at 1 yr for patients treated with MMC. Tolley et al. *(13)* of the Medical Research Council (MRC) randomized 502 patients who had primary Ta or T1 tumors, to 40 mg MMC in 40 cc instillate immediately after TURBT, the same dose after TURBT, and at each 3-mo check cystoscopy for 1 yr (five instillations altogether), or to TURBT only. Initial results from the trial, at a median follow-up of 12 mo, revealed an increase in the time to first recurrence for patients who received five instillations of MMC, compared to patients treated with TURBT alone. Tumor recurrence rates for patients who received either schedule of MMC were significantly lower than controls. These results were confirmed at 7-yr follow-up *(23)*. MMC resulted in decreased recurrence rates and increased recurrence-free survival. Data suggested, but did not show, a conclusive advantage for five instillations of MMC compared to a single treatment at the time of TURBT. Niijima et al. *(22)*, however, failed to demonstrate a durable increase in recurrence-free survival with longer follow-up.

6.1. DOX

DOX is an anthracycline antibiotic processed from *Streptomyces peucetius caesius*. Its activity has been attributed to both DNA intercalation *(24)* and cell surface cytotoxicity *(25)*. Like MMC, DOX exhibits negligible systemic absorption, so that its most common complication is chemical cystitis. Occasional reports of mild nausea and vomiting have been noted, and the drug has rarely been associated with systemic hypersensitivity *(19)*. Two randomized studies performed in the 1980s, support a significant decrease in tumor recurrence with the use of intravesical DOX *(17,22)*. In the same trial that explored the efficacy of MMC, Niijima et al. *(22)* compared two doses of DOX twice weekly for 4 wk, 30 mg in 30 cc, instillate, or 20 mg, in 40 cc instillate, to TURBT only, in patients with Ta or T1 primary and recurrent superficial TCC. At 15 mo follow-up, both regimens showed a statistically significant increase in recurrence-free survival, compared to controls. However, by 1.5 y follow-up, there was no indication that either DOX regimen provided lasting improvement in DFS. Dysuria and hematuria appeared to be worse with the higher dose of DOX. Zincke et al. *(17)* examined tumor recurrence at 3-mo cystoscopic exam, following a single dose of DOX, 50 mg in 60 cc distillate, at the time of TURBT, compared to TURBT only. The group noted a significant decrease in tumor recurrence for patients who received intravesical therapy, although only 31 patients received treatment, and results of long-term follow-up were not reported.

A growing interest in EPI, an anthracycline derivative of DOX, with less toxicity when given intravenously, has led to randomized prospective trials of intravesical therapy over the past several years. Okamura et al. *(26)* randomized 119 patients with superficial tumors to TURBT alone, or to EPI, 40 mg in 40 cc instillate, immediately after resection, then once the first week, weekly for 4 wk, and monthly for a full year of treatment. Both the time to first recurrence and recurrence rate per year were significantly improved in treated patients. Most recently, Ali-el-dein et al. *(27)* random-ized 253 patients with Ta or T1 tumors to a four-armed trial comparing 50 or 80 mg EPI vs 50 mg DOX vs TURBT alone. Intravesical therapy was administered weekly for 8 wk then monthly for the next 10 mo. The investigators confirmed results of previous DOX studies, with a significant decrease in tumor recurrence rates and increased time to first recurrence for patients treated with either chemotherapy. The rate of tumor recurrence was significantly lower in patients treated with EPI, compared to patients treated with DOX.

The impact of intravesical chemotherapies overall was examined in a meta-analysis conducted by the EORTC and the MRC *(28)*. Investigators combined results of four EORTC trials using several different agents (thio-TEPA, VM26, DOX, epodyl, EPI, and pyridoxine) with two MRC trials using thio-TEPA and MMC. Results from over 2500 patients were considered. A statistically significant effect on prolonged recurrence-free survival was documented for the use of adjuvant intravesical chemotherapy vs no adjuvant therapy (TURBT alone). Even in aggregate, however, no improvement in overall survival or progression to muscle-invasive or metastatic disease was observed in the patients treated with intravesical therapy.

6.2. BCG

Despite the encouraging results achieved with intravesical chemotherapy in decreas-ing tumor recurrence, no trial has shown a statistically significant decrease in tumor progression, or prolonged survival caused by these agents. Only BCG immunotherapy has shown a decrease in tumor progression, with a resulting increase in disease-specific and overall survival. However, because BCG is an attenuated strain of tuberculin bacillus, significant side effects and complications are seen with therapy. At its worst, BCG has been associated with systemic infection, sepsis, and death from overwhelming infection. Lesser infections have also been observed, with granulomatous prostatis, epididymitis, pneumonitis, hepatitis, or upper urinary tract infections occurring in 0.5–1% of patients, and requiring 3–6 mo of antituberculous therapy *(10)*. The exact pathway by which BCG prevents tumor recurrence and progression remains obscure, but IL-2 and IL-6 appear to be involved, among many other urinary cytokines, and their levels have been correlated with BCG response in a recent study *(29)*. These tests have yet to be proven of clinical benefit, however, and are not available on a routine basis. Regardless of its mechanism, BCG causes an exuberant local immune reaction that usually results in irritative symptoms and a flu-like syndrome. Fevers may accompany administration, and granuloma formation is usually apparent on subsequent bladder biopsies. On reviewing BCG regimens and trials, it should be known that BCG doses may not be directly comparable, because the number of organisms per weight and volume vary among BCG strains.

Herr et al. *(30,31)* were the first investigators to show a statistically significant reduction in tumor progression from BCG intravesical immunotherapy. The group randomized 86 patients with multiple recurrent high-grade Ta or T1 tumors, with and without CIS, to receive 120 mg BCG intravesically and an intradermal BCG dose (5 × 107 U) weekly for 6 wk vs TURBT alone. Both progression to muscle-invasive or metastatic disease and overall survival were significantly improved in the patients who received BCG therapy. These results have been confirmed at 10- *(31)* and 15-y *(32)* follow-up. At 10-yr follow-up, 62% of BCG-treated patients and 37% of controls were alive without progression. Ten BCG-treated patients (23%) and 17 control patients

(40%) had died of BC. Luftnegger et al. *(33)* have subsequently shown, in a randomized prospective trial with 154 patients, that intradermal BCG does not add to the efficacy of intravesical BCG. The observations by Herr et al. were corroborated in a later trial by Pagano et al. *(34),* reported in 1991. In this study, 133 patients with recurrent superficial TCC were randomized to a lower dose of 75 mg BCC, weekly for 6 wk, followed by monthly for 1 yr, and quarterly for the next year, vs TURBT. After a mean follow-up of 21 mo, patients treated with BCG experienced a significantly lower recurrence rate than controls (3.7 and 12.3, respectively). Progression to muscle-invasive or metastatic disease was also significantly lower: 4 vs 17% in BCG-treated patients vs controls, respectively.

These two trials firmly established the benefit of BCG treatment in comparison with TURBT. In an analogous investigation, Lamm et al. *(35)* addressed the relative merit of intravesical BCG immunotherapy vs intravesical chemotherapy. This study randomized 262 patients, with CIS or rapidly recurrent Ta or T1 tumors, to 120 mg BCG weekly for 6 wk and 3, 6, 12, 18, and 24 mo after enrollment, or 50 mg DOX mg, weekly for 4 wk then monthly for a full year. After median follow-up of 65 mo, 45% of BCG-treated patients without CIS, and 37% of BCG-treated patients with CIS, were disease-free, compared to 18% of DOX-treated patients without CIS, and 17% of DOX-treated patients with CIS ($P < 0.015$ for patients with or without CIS). The estimated median times to recurrence or progression for both subgroups were substantially improved with BCG treatment; 10 vs 23 mo for patients without CIS treated with DOX or BCG, respectively, and 5 vs 39 mo for patients with CIS treated with DOX or BCG, respectively. No difference in overall survival was observed. It is clear from these three analyses that BCG offers a highly effective and durable benefit to patients with superficial BC who are at high risk of progression. A similar advantage for patients with less aggressive tumors (stage Ta grade 1–2 without evidence of CIS) has never been established. Given the substantial risk of infectious side effects, BCG therapy should be used judiciously in low-risk populations, in the absence of proven benefit.

At least one study has addressed the cost-effectiveness of BCG immunotherapy vs TURBT in high-grade recurrent superficial TCC with or without CIS. Preliminary results by Kilbridge et al. *(14)* indicate that a six weekly course of intravesical BCG vs TURBT alone is a cost-effective therapy, compared to many other standard oncologic interventions. Combining data from the randomized prospective trial by Herr et al. *(31)* with the large series by Lamm et al. *(10)* on the incidence and treatment of the infectious complications resulting from intravesical BCG, the investigators quantified the risks and benefits of BCG treatment. They used a Markov decision-analytic model to examine the cause of death for a cohort of 1000 men, aged 65 yr with recurrent high-grade TCC treated with six weekly instillations of BCG vs TURBT. Summarizing these studies, it was observed that of 1000 men treated with TURBT alone, 639 died of other causes, 360 died of metastatic disease, and less than 1 in 1000 men died of complications from TURBT and cystoscopy. Of 1000 men treated with BCG, 782 died of other causes, 217 died of BC, and less than 1 in 1000 died of either TURBT or cystoscopy or BCG sepsis. Thus, 143 of 1000 men treated with BCG will be spared death from metastatic BC, which is equivalent to a 40% decrease in the cancer-specific mortality observed in patients treated with TURBT alone. These differences in the cause of death for a cohort of men result in a significant increase in the overall life expectancy of the average patient treated with BCG. Treating a 65-yr-old man with BCG, including infectious complications, costs $9100 over the course of his lifetime vs $7700 lifetime costs for treatment with TURBT alone. BCG results in a 6-mo gain in life expectancy, for an incremental cost-effectiveness ratio of $2800/yr of life saved. In contrast, autologous bone marrow transplant for limited-stage metastatic breast cancer costs $115,000/yr of life saved, chemotherapy for node-negative breast cancer costs $50,000/yr of life saved, propranolol for moderate hypertension costs $33,000/yr of life saved, and adjuvant chemotherapy for Duke's C colon cancer costs $3000/yr of life saved. For patients with high-grade recurrent TCC with or without CIS, BCG treatment compares well to many other commonly used medical interventions.

6.3. Interferon and Other Agents

Over the past several years, a number of randomized prospective trials have addressed the efficacy of newer immunotherapeutic agents, specifically, IFNs, in relation to BCG. At least three randomized trials have failed to show an advantage for IFN over BCG in the prophylaxis of tumor recurrence (36–38). The largest and most recent study randomized 122 patients to 150 mg, BCG vs 54 million units IFN-α2a, given weekly for the first month, biweekly for 2 mo, then monthly for 9 mo. A significant decrease in the recurrence rate, and increase in the recurrence-free interval, was observed in patients who received BCG compared to IFN, 2.2 vs 5.5 and 19.3 vs 15.3 mo, respectively. However, there was no difference in progression between the two groups. Because IFN has been better tolerated than BCG, with fewer side effects, the minimal difference in time to recurrence may prove to be an important consideration in IFN use, if larger studies with more follow-up confirm that IFN results in an improvement in progression, and in overall survival similar to BCG. Some trials have suggested that IFN may be efficacious when used as salvage therapy for patients who have failed BCG, but this is still under investigation (37). In addition to IFN, keyhole-limpet hemocyanin, IL-2, and tumor necrosis factor have all been used as intravesical immunotherapeutic agents. None of these agents has appeared to be more promising than BCG or IFN in early phase I and phase II trials.

6.4. Maintenance Therapy

The optimal duration of intravesical therapy has never been established. Preliminary results from a randomized prospective trial by the Southwestern Oncology Group, comparing six weekly treatments of 120 mg, BCG to maintenance therapy with three weekly instillations at 3 and 6 mo plus every 6 mo thereafter for 3 yr, suggest an advantage to maintenance therapy (39). Investigators found a statistically significant improvement in recurrence-free survival and median time to recurrence (75 and 36 mo, respectively), for patients who received maintenance BCG. The group also found a significant improvement in worsening disease (defined as progression, cystectomy, or use of systemic or radiation therapy) with the use of maintenance therapy (73 vs 90 events). This apparent benefit must be balanced with the observation that overall survival was not statistically different for the two treatment groups: 26% of patients on maintenance therapy experienced grade 3 or 4 toxicities, and 10% of patients failed to complete the maintenance regimen secondary to toxicity. Final results of the trial are pending. Other investigators in the EORTC have examined the benefit of prolonged intravesical chemotherapy (40). Thirty-one patients were randomized to two parallel studies, comparing 30 mg MMC or 50 mg DOX administered on the day of resection vs 7–15 d after TURBT, and given for 6 vs 12 mo. Their study indicated that recurrence rates were higher in patients who received therapy over the shorter 6-mo vs 12-mo interval. After 4 yr follow-up, there was no difference in progression, overall survival, or the development of second recurrences. Multivariate analysis supported these findings.

7. FOLLOW-UP AFTER THERAPY

Repeat endoscopic evaluation of the bladder following completion of therapy is essential to monitor therapeutic response. Follow-up cystoscopy usually commences 3 mo after the initiation of the first cycle of therapy, although the full effect of therapy with BCG may not be apparent until 6 mo *(41)*. For patients with recurrent Ta tumors who demonstrate no signs of progression in grade or stage, repeat administration of the same drug, instillation of a different drug, or simple repeat TURBT alone are reasonable options. In patients with diffuse CIS who have an incomplete response, an additional 6-wk cycle of BCG is indicated, although some investigators would recommend proceeding directly to radical cystectomy. Patients with recurrent tumors that demonstrate progression from low- to high-grade, or stage from Ta to T1, are at high risk of further progression to muscle-invasive (T2) disease, and should be considered candidates for aggressive definitive therapy, such as cystectomy *(11,42,43)*.

The ideal follow-up interval for patients with nonprogressive, but recurrent, disease is not defined. Usually, these patients are monitored 3–4 ×/yr in the first year after therapy, and at increasingly longer intervals, if recurrences are infrequent. Several adjuncts to voided cytology are under study, which rely on detection of basement-membrane or tumor-associated antigens, and which have demonstrated superior sensitivity for the detection of low-grade tumors, and may eventually supplant the need for some interval cystoscopic examinations *(44,45)*. Virtual cystoscopy, using three-dimensional reconstructions of magnetic resonance images, is also under study, and may also reduce the need for transurethral instrumentation *(46,47)*.

Patients treated with intravesical BCG appear to be at increased risk for developing tumors of the upper urinary tract. Although the overall risk of upper tract tumors is generally believed to be 2–3%, Herr et al. *(48)* reported a 23% rate in 307 patients with high-risk disease followed for a minimum of 10 yr, with cumulative risks of 10, 26, and 34% after 5, 10, and 15 yr, respectively. Cystectomy appeared to have a protective effect in these patients, although the occurrence of upper tract tumors did not affect disease-specific survival. These observations emphasize the need for continued radiographic evaluation of the upper tracts in patients after intravesical therapy.

8. CONCLUSIONS

Patients with superficial BC, at high risk of recurrence or progression, are appropriate candidates for intravesical chemotherapy or immunotherapy. Currently available chemotherapeutic agents are modestly effective in reducing the rate of tumor recurrence, but probably do not prevent tumor progression. BCG immunotherapy appears to delay progression to muscle-invasive disease in a cost-effective manner, but may be associated with significant toxicity. Treated patients require long-term monitoring of the bladder and upper urinary tract, for early detection and therapy of recurrences.

REFERENCES

1. Witjes JA, Oosterhof GON, Debruyne FMJ. Management of superficial bladder cancer Ta/T1/TIS: intravesical chemotherapy, In Volgelzang NJ, et al. (eds), *Comprehensive Textbook of Genitourinary Oncology,* Williams and Wilkins, Baltimore (1996) pp. 416–427.

2. Cordon-Cardo C, Dalbagni G, Sarkis AS, and Reuter VE. Genetic alterations associated with bladder cancer, In Devita VT, Hellman S, Rosenberg SA (eds), Important Advances in Oncology, Lippincott, Philadelphia (1994).

3. Harris AL and Neal DE. Bladder cancer: field vs. clonal origin, *N. Engl. J. Med.,* **326** (1992) 759.

4. *AJCC Cancer Staging Handbook,* 5th ed., Lippincott-Raven, Philadelphia (1998).

5. Hasui Y, Osada Y, Kitada S, and Nishi S. Significance of invasion to the muscularis mucosae on the progression of superficial bladder cancer, *Urology,* **43** (1994) 782–786.

6. Younes M, Sussman J, and True LD. Usefulness of the level of the muscularis mucosae on the progression of superficial bladder cancer, *Cancer,* **66** (1990) 543.

7. Lamm DL, Riggs DR, Traynelis CL, and Nseyo UO. Apparent failure of current intravesical chemotherapy prophylaxis to influence the long-term course of superficial transitional cell carcinoma of the bladder, *J. Urol.,* **153** (1995) 1444.

8. Lamm DL. Long-term results of intravesical therapy for superficial bladder cancer, *Urol. Clin. North Am.,* **19** (1992) 573.

9. Wientjes MG and Badalament RA. Use of pharmacologic data and computer simulations to design an efficacy trial on intravesical mitomycin C therapy for superficial bladder cancer, *Cancer Chemother. Pharmacol.,* **32** (1993) 255.

10. Lamm DL, van der Meijden APM, Morales A, et al. Incidence and treatment of complications of BCG in intravesical therapy in superficial bladder cancer, *J. Urol.,* **147** (1992) 596.

11. Schulman CC, Robinson M, Denis L, et al. Prophylactic chemotherapy of superficial transitional cell bladder carcinoma: an EORTC randomized trial comparing thiotepa, an epidodophyllotoxin (VM26) and TUR alone, *Eur. Urol.,* **8** (1982) 207.

12. Prout GR, Koontz WW, Coombs LJ, et al. Long-term fate of 90 patients with superficial bladder cancer randomly assigned to receive or not to receive thiotepa, *J. Urol.,* **130** (1983) 677.

13. Tolley DA, Hargreave TB, Smith PH, et al. Effect of mitomycin C on recurrence of newly diagnosed superficial bladder cancer: interim report from the Medical Research Council Subgroup on Superficial Bladder Cancer (Urological Cancer Working Party), *Br. Med. J.,* **296** (1988) 1759.

14. Kilbridge KL, Kuntz KM, Kantoff PW, et al. Is bacillus Calmette-Guerin (BCG) immunotherapy cost-effective in recurrent high-grade transitional cell cancer (TCC)?, *J. Urol.,* **157 (Suppl)** (1997) 214.

15. Jones HC and Swinney J. Thiotepa in the treatment of tumours of the bladder, *Lancet,* **2** (1961) 615.

16. Weaver D, Khare N, Haigh J, et al. Effect of chemotherapeutic agents on the ultrastructure of transitional cell carcinoma in tissue culture, *Invest. Urol.,* **17** (1980) 288.

17. Zincke H, Utz DC, Taylor WF, et al. Influence of thiotepa and doxorubicin instillation at the time of transurethral surgical treatment of bladder cancer on tumor recurrence: a prospective, randomized, double-blind, controlled trial, *J. Urol.,* **129** (1983) 505.

18. Masters JR, McDermott BJ, Harland S, et al. ThioTEPA pharmacokinetics during intravesical chemotherapy: the influence of dose and volume of instillate on systemic uptake and dose rate to tumour, *Cancer Chemother. Pharmacol.,* **38** (1996) 59.

19. Thrasher JB and Crawford ED. Complications of intravesical chemotherapy, *Urol. Clin. N. Am.,* **19** (1992) 529.

20. Iyer VN and Szybalski W. Molecular mechanism of mitomycin linking complementary DNA strands, *Proc. Natl. Acad. Sci. USA,* **50** (1963) 355.

21. Lown JW. Molecular mechanism of antitumor action of the mitomycins, In Carter SK, ST Crooke (eds), *Mitomycin C: Current Status and New Developments,* Academic, Orlando (1979).

22. Niijima T, Koiso K, Akaza H, et al. Randomized clinical trial on chemoprophylaxis of recurrence in cases of superficial bladder cancer, *Cancer Chemother. Pharmacol.,* **11 (Suppl)** (1993) S79.

23. Tolley DA, Parmar MK, Grigor KM, et al. Effect of intravesical mitomycin C on recurrence of newly diagnosed superficial bladder cancer: a further report with 7 years follow up, *J. Urol.,* **155** (1996) 1233.

24. Carter SK. Adriamycin: a review, *J. Natl. Cancer Inst.,* **55** (1975) 1265.

25. Tritton TR and Yee G. Anticancer agent Adriamycin can be actively cytotoxic without entering cells, *Science,* **217** (1982) 248.

26. Okamura K, Murase T, Obata K, et al. Randomized trial of early intravesical instillation of epirubicin in superficial bladder cancer. The Nagoya University Urological Oncology Group, *Cancer Chemother. Pharmacol.,* **35** (1994) S31.

27. Ali-el-dein B, el-Baz M, Aly AN, et al. Intravesical epirubicin versus doxorubicin for superficial bladder tumors (stages pTa and pT1): a randomized prospective study, *J. Urol.,* **158** (1997) 68.

28. Pawinski A, Sylvester R, Kurth KH, et al. Combined analysis of European Organization for Research

and Treatment of Cancer, and Medical Research Council randomized clinical trials for the prophylactic treatment of stage TaT1 bladder cancer, *J. Urol.*, **156** (1996) 1934.

29. de Reijki TM, de Boer EC, Kurth KH, et al. Urinary cytokines during intravesical bacillus Calmette-Guerin therapy for superficial bladder cancer: processing, stability and prognostic value, *J. Urol.*, **155** (1996) 477.

30. Herr HW, Laudone VP, Badalament RA, et al. Bacillus Calmette-Guerin therapy alters the progression of superficial bladder cancer, *J. Clin. Oncol.*, **9** (1988) 1450.

31. Herr HW, Schwalb DM, Zhang ZF, et al. Intravesical bacillus Calmette-Guerin therapy prevents tumor progression and death from superficial bladder cancer: ten-year follow-up of a prospective randomized trial, *J. Clin. Oncol.*, **13** (1995) 1404.

32. Cookson MS, Herr HW, Zhang ZF, et al. Treated natural history of high risk superficial bladder cancer: 15-year outcome, *J. Urol.*, **158** (1997) 62.

33. Luftnegger W, Ackermann DK, Futterleib A, et al. Intravesical versus intravesical plus intradermal bacillus Calmette-Guerin: a randomized prospective study in patients with recurrent superficial bladder tumors, *J. Urol.*, **155** (1996) 483.

34. Pagano F, Pierfrancesco B, Milani C, et al. Low-dose bacillus Calmette-Guerin regimen in superficial bladder cancer therapy: is it effective?, *J. Urol.*, **146** (1991) 32.

35. Lamm DL, Blumenstein BA, Crawford ED, et al. Randomized trial of intravesical doxorubicin and immunotherapy with bacille Calmette-Guerin for transitional-cell carcinoma of the bladder, *N. Engl. J. Med.*, **325** (1991) 1205.

36. Kalbe T, Beer M, Mendoze E, et al. BCG vs interferon A for prevention of recurrence of superficial bladder cancer. A prospective randomized study, *Urologe A.*, **33** (1994) 133.

37. Zerbib M, Botto H, Mandel E, et al. Intravesical IFN compared to BCG therapy in "high risk" superficial bladder cancer, results of a prospective multicentric randomized study, *J. Urol.*, **157** (1997) 213.

38. Jimenez-Cruz JF, Vera-Donoso CD, Leiva O, et al. Intravesical immunoprophylaxis in recurrent superficial bladder cancer (stage T1): multicenter trial comparing bacille Calmette-Guerin and interferon-alpha, *Urol.*, **50** (1997) 529.

39. Lamm DL, Blumenstein B, Sarosdy M, et al. Significant long-term patient benefit with BCG maintenance therapy: a Southwest Oncology Group study, *J. Urol.*, **157 (Suppl.)** (1997) 213.

40. Bouffioux C, Kurth KH, Bono A, et al. Intravesical adjuvant chemotherapy for superficial transitional cell bladder carcinoma: results of 2 European Organization for Research and Treatment of Cancer randomized trials with mitomycin C and doxorubicin comparing early versus delayed instillations and short-term versus long-term treatment. European Organization for Research and Treatment of Cancer Genitourinary Group, *J. Urol.*, **153** (1995) 934.

41. Herr HW, Wartinger DD, Fair WR, and Oettgen HF. BCG therapy for superficial bladder cancer: a ten-year follow up, *J. Urol.*, **147** (1992) 1020.

42. Klein EA, Rogatko A, and Herr HW. Management of local BCG failures in superficial bladder cancer, *J. Urol.*, **147** (1992) 601.

43. Herr HW, Klein EA, and Rogatko A. Local BCG failures in superficial bladder cancer. A multivariate analysis of risk factors influencing survival, *Eur. Urol.*, **19** (1991) 97.

44. Soloway MS, Briggman V, Carpinito GA, et al. Use of a new tumor marker, urinary NMP22, in the detection of occult or rapidly recurring transitional cell carcinoma of the urinary tract following surgical treatment, *J. Urol.*, **156** (1996) 363.

45. Grossman HB. New methods for detection of bladder cancer, *Semin. Urol. Oncol.*, **16** (1998) 17.

46. Hussain S, Loeffler JA, Babayan RK, and Fenlon HM. Thin-section helical computed tomography of the bladder: initial clinical experience with virtual reality imaging, *Urology*, **50** (1997) 685.

47. Fenlon HM, Bell TV, Ahari HK, and Hussain S. Virtual cystoscopy: early clinical experience, *Radiol.*, **205** (1997) 272.

48. Herr HW. Long-term results of BCG therapy: concern about upper tract tumors, *Semin. Urol. Oncol.*, **16** (1998) 13.

19 Principles of Intrathecal Chemotherapy

Glen Stevens and David M. Peereboom

1. INTRODUCTION

Delivery of chemotherapy to the leptomeninges is useful for treatment of established leptomeningeal cancer (LC), or for central nervous system (CNS) prophylaxis against certain malignancies with a high propensity for leptomeningeal metastasis *(1)*. The rationale for intrathecal (IT) chemotherapy parallels that for other regional chemotherapies: to achieve high local concentrations of chemotherapy with minimal or no systemic toxicity.

The meninges consist of the dura mater, arachnoid membrane, and the pia mater (*see* Fig. 1). Leptomeninges refers to the arachnoid membrane, the pia mater, and the subarachnoid space between, through which cerebrospinal fluid (CSF) flows. The terms "leptomeninges" and "meninges" are frequently used interchangeably. The terms "leptomeningeal metastasis" and "neoplastic meningitis" refer to any malignancy involving the leptomeninges; "leptomeningeal carcinomatosis" and "carcinomatous meningitis" refer only to epithelial malignancies, such as breast or lung cancer. "Intrathecal delivery" refers to drug administration into the subarachnoid space via lumbar puncture, or by Ommaya reservoir (intraventricular).

Metastases reach the subarachnoid space by hematogenous spread via the choroid plexus or the arachnoid vessels, or by direct extension from tumors within the CNS,

From: *Current Clinical Oncology: Regional Chemotherapy: Clinical Research and Practice*
Edited by: M. Markman © Humana Press Inc., Totowa, NJ

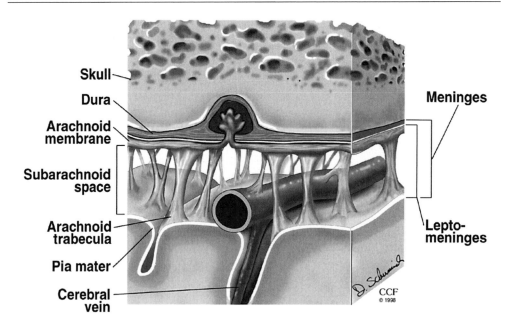

Fig. 1. The meninges.

or from systemic cancers that travel along nerve roots. Cancer cells then spread within the subarachnoid space, with multiple deposits throughout the leptomeninges that can consist of any combination of bulk deposits of tumor, a thin layer of cells rather evenly distributed, or exfoliated cells suspended in the CSF. The heaviest deposits of tumor usually occur along the basilar cisterns, the posterior fossa, and the cauda equina *(2)*.

LC occurs in roughly 5–8% of all patients with metastatic cancer who come to autopsy *(3)*. Among hematologic malignancies, the incidence ranges from less than 5%, in patients with acute myelogenous leukemia, to as high as 30%, in high-risk patients with acute lymphoblastic leukemia who do not receive prophylactic CNS therapy *(4)*. Although LC can arise from almost any solid tumor, approx 5% of patients with breast cancer, and as many as one-quarter of those with small-cell lung cancer, and with melanoma, develop this complication *(4–8)*. Carcinomatous meningitis is becoming more frequent, especially in patients with breast and small-cell lung cancer *(5,9,10)*.

2. HISTORY

Delivery of drugs to the meninges was first used for treatment of infectious meningitis, using percutaneous injection of antibiotics through frontal burr holes *(11)*. The first reported use of IT chemotherapy was reported in 1954 by Sansone *(12)*, who treated patients who had CNS leukemia with antifolates. With the exception of nitrogen mustard, antifolates were the only chemotherapy drugs available at that time. With success against CNS leukemia, investigators extended the use of antifolates to other meningeal malignancies. IT methotrexate (MTX) was first reported as a treatment for meningeal breast carcinomatosis in 1968 *(13)*. Reports of IT cytosine arabinoside (ara-C) and thio-TEPA were first published in the early 1970s *(14,15)*. Combination IT regimens were reported in the 1980s, but have not shown an advantage over single-agent therapy *(16,17)*. Ommaya *(18,19)* developed an implantable reservoir to minimize the morbidity

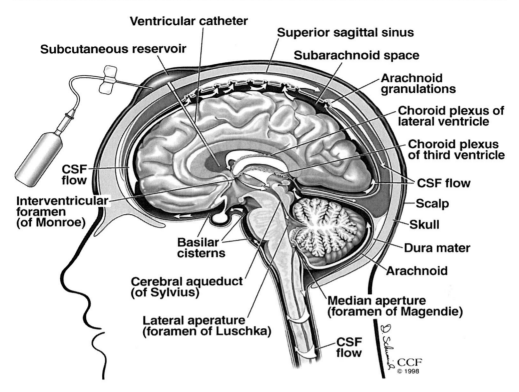

Fig. 2. Cerebrospinal fluid flow dynamics; placement of an Ommaya reservoir for intraventricular administration of chemotherapy.

of intraventricular drug administration. Intraventricular delivery through the Ommaya reservoir remains the method of choice for IT chemotherapy.

3. CSF ANATOMY AND FLOW DYNAMICS

CSF production in the lateral ventricles creates a hydrostatic pressure that forces CSF through the interventricular foramina into the third ventricle, through the cerebral aqueduct into the fourth ventricle (*see* Fig. 2). CSF exits the fourth ventricle via the foramina of Luschka and Magendie to the base of the brain, where a portion flows inferiorly in the spinal subarachnoid space *(20)*. CSF returns to the basilar cisterns, and flows over the cortical convexities to exit the CNS through the arachnoid granulations.

This flow pattern has important implications for the distribution of IT drugs. First, the unidirectional flow of CSF limits the distribution of drug to the ventricles, when given by lumbar puncture. Ventricular MTX levels generally reach less than 10% of simultaneous lumbar concentrations after intralumbar administration *(21)*. This route of administration may result in inadequate drug delivery to the ventricles, and has been associated with inferior treatment outcomes for patients with CNS leukemia *(22)*. Second, leptomeningeal metastases can disrupt the normal CSF flow. Approximately 30–70% of patients have abnormal CSF flow dynamics caused by ventricular outlet obstruction, spinal blocks, or flow disturbances over the cortical convexities *(23–25)*. Such disturbances in CSF flow can lead to marked variations in drug delivery *(23)*, with inadequate delivery to some areas or increased toxicity in regions with stasis of drug-laden CSF. Therefore, patients should have CSF flow assessed by radionuclide

Table 1
Recommended IT MTX Dose by Age

Patient age (yr)	Dose (mg)
<1	6
1	8
2	10
≥3	12

Adapted with permission from ref. *27*.

ventriculography (Indium-111-DTPA CSF flow study) before IT chemotherapy is begun. Those with obstruction of CSF flow should receive radiation therapy (RT) to these sites to restore CSF flow to a more physiologic state before IT chemotherapy is given *(26)*.

In the normal development of the CNS, CSF volume reaches its adult volume of 140 cc by age 3 yr *(27)*. Therefore, unlike intravenous (iv) chemotherapy, IT chemotherapy doses are adjusted by age, not body surface area. Table 1 illustrates an example of age-adjusted doses for MTX.

4. INDICATIONS

Brain and/or other systemic metastases are often present at diagnosis of leptomeningeal carcinomatosis, implying far-advanced disease. The patient may have been heavily pretreated. Therefore, the tumor cells may have inherent or acquired resistance to chemotherapy, and the performance status of the patient is often compromised. These factors limit efficacy and the patient's tolerance of therapy to this region. Despite these limitations, improvements in systemic therapy have led to a growing minority of patients with controlled systemic disease at the time of meningeal relapse *(6,10,28)*.

The goals of treatment for patients with LC are to stabilize or improve neurologic symptoms, and to prolong survival *(29)*. IT chemotherapy alone does not prolong survival for patients with established leptomeningeal metastases. Without therapy, patients die from progressive neurologic dysfunction at an average of 4–6 wk *(30,31)*. Recent studies of patients who had solid tumors treated with IT chemotherapy and RT produced a median survival of 4–7 mo, with occasional patients surviving as long as 2–3 yr *(32,33)*. These survival differences probably reflect selection bias, rather than a true effect of IT chemotherapy. Grossman et al. *(32)* observed that patients who had a particularly short survival (median 8 wk), despite therapy, had one of the following: performance status of 3 (i.e., at bed rest more than 50% of the day), lung cancer, or progressive systemic disease (i.e., outside the CNS) at the start of therapy. Patients with any of these characteristics would probably not benefit from IT chemotherapy. Although most patients with carcinomatous meningitis do not improve symptomatically, some may be spared progressive neurologic deterioration *(32)*. Indeed, several authors have argued that IT chemotherapy for leptomeningeal carcinomatosis adds nothing to systemic chemotherapy and RT *(33,34)*. These conclusions, however, apply only to metastases from solid tumors, and are derived from either small, single-institution series or nonrandomized comparisons of patients treated with systemic chemotherapy and RT, with and without IT chemotherapy. Patients with leptomeningeal metastases from hematologic malignancies are much more likely to have major responses to therapy.

Nonetheless, the appropriate use of IT chemotherapy requires careful patient selection, and a frank discussion with the patient regarding the goals and expectations of therapy.

Treatment of LC is indicated for patients who have controlled systemic disease; a histology that might respond, such as breast cancer, lymphoma, or leukemia, rather than nonsmall-cell lung cancer or melanoma (the latter group especially should be treated on a clinical trial, if IT chemotherapy is felt to be warranted); and minimal neurologic symptoms *(29,32)*. Indications for CNS prophylaxis for hematologic malignancies are described in Chapters 21 and 22.

5. PHARMACOKINETIC CONSIDERATIONS

Despite the relatively high drug concentrations that can be achieved by IT administration *(35)*, preclinical data suggest that the drug penetrates to a maximum depth of only 2–3 mm from the tumor surface *(11,36,37)*. Additional calculations have predicted that nodules over 5 mm in diameter are not adequately treated by local chemotherapy *(38,39)*. These data suggest that bulk deposits of tumor in the leptomeninges, such as nodules apparent on magnetic resonance imaging, would be unlikely to respond to IT chemotherapy alone. Such metastases, especially if symptomatic, are treated more effectively with RT.

Several investigators *(40–42)* have reported protocols for prolonged exposure of IT chemotherapy to CNS. MTX has been studied in this fashion, in an attempt to minimize neurotoxicity, and to exploit the cell cycle specificity of the drug. One study randomized patients with leptomeningeal leukemia to standard 12 mg/m^2 MTX twice weekly, or to 1 mg every 12 h for six doses, with dose adjustments to maintain trough lumbar CSF concentrations greater than 0.5 μmol/I *(40)*. Those authors demonstrated the ability to maintain prolonged CSF MTX concentrations greater than the therapeutic threshold of 1 μmol/L, while avoiding excessive peak concentrations, with attendant neurotoxicity and myelosuppression. This "concentration × time" schedule did reduce the neurotoxicity, but did not increase efficacy. Petit et al. *(41)* reported two patients treated with continuous IT MTX, 10 mg/d × 5 d, via a pump attached to a lumbar catheter. The authors achieved steady-state CSF MTX concentrations greater than 10 μmol/L, with serum concentrations below 0.1 μmol/L. Nakagawa et al. treated 13 patients who had leptomeningeal carcinomatosis, using ventriculolumbar perfusion of MTX (10–30 mg) and ara-C (40 mg) every 8–12 h for 6–9 doses *(42)*. Nine of 13 patients in this pilot study responded, with dramatic neurological improvement in at least five patients. The authors were encouraged by the outcome, but also stated that toxicity of this particular regimen was formidable. This approach to improving the therapeutic index of IT therapy deserves further investigation.

A different method for improving the therapeutic index of IT chemotherapy has involved a depot formulation of cytarabine, DTC 101, which consists of cytarabine contained within spherical particles, each of which contains numerous aqueous chambers bounded by a single lipid membrane *(43)*. As the drug diffuses from the chambers in the periphery of each particle, it is replaced by diffusion of drug from deeper chambers, resulting in a slow release of drug over time. This extended release formulation of cytarabine has 40-fold longer CSF elimination half-life (141 vs 3.4 h), with cytotoxic concentrations maintained in the CSF for 2 wk *(44)*. These pharmacokinetic properties allow dosing every 2 wk. Furthermore, this drug can achieve cytotoxic ventricular concentrations when given by lumbar puncture, thus avoiding the need for placement of an Ommaya reservoir. In a small randomized trial of DTC 101 vs IT MTX, toxicity and cytologic response rate appeared equal, and DTC 101 produced a longer mean time to clinical progression (119 vs 38 d) *(45)*. Extended-release drug formulations may improve the pharmacologic advantage of regional chemotherapy, and could produce a clinically meaningful benefit.

The assumption that cytotoxic CSF concentrations of chemotherapy can be achieved uniquely by IT administration has recently been challenged. A nonrandomized comparison of high-dose iv MTX and IT MTX described pharmacokinetics, response rate, toxicity, and survival data *(46)*. Sixteen patients with neoplastic meningitis received high-dose (8 gm/m^2) iv MTX, and were compared to a contemporaneous group of 15 patients who received standard IT MTX. Patients treated with high-dose iv MTX achieved peak CSF MTX concentrations of 4–55 µmol/L, and maintained cytotoxic concentrations far longer than those treated with IT MTX. Cytologic clearance of the CSF occurred in 81 and 60% of the IV and IT cohorts, respectively. The median survival in the high-dose iv-treated patients was 14 vs 2.3 mo in the IT MTX group. Additional theoretical advantages of high-dose iv chemotherapy over IT administration include more uniform distribution within the neuraxis, especially in patients with abnormal CSF flow dynamics; avoidance of Ommaya reservoir placement; and systemic therapy for certain malignancies *(47)*. These possible advantages, however, entail significant systemic toxicities, and the data cited above need to be validated prospectively.

Although thiotepa has activity when given IT, its extreme lipid solubility causes rapid clearance from the CSF (approx 9 × the rate of bulk CSF flow), limiting exposure of lumbar area after IT administration *(48)*. Furthermore, thio-TEPA is probably a prodrug that is converted to its active metabolite, (TEPA), in the liver *(49)*. Finally, pharmacokinetic studies have demonstrated equal concentrations of TEPA in the serum and CSF after iv administration *(50)*. Therefore, IT thio-TEPA has no advantage over iv administration.

6. METHODS/TECHNIQUES

IT chemotherapy can be delivered by intralumbar or intraventricular techniques. As mentioned in subheading 2, intraventricular administration is the preferred route for several reasons: improved drug distribution *(35)*, fewer device complications than implantable lumbar devices *(51)*, elimination of risk of epidural administration (~10% risk with administration by lumbar puncture *[52]*), and patient convenience. Intraventricular chemotherapy, however, has the disadvantage of requiring a neurosurgical procedure for implantation of an Ommaya reservoir. Although generally safe to implant and maintain, the Ommaya reservoir can become dislodged or infected (*see* subheading 7). Recently, depot formulations of IT drugs with extended CSF half-lives have been demonstrated to maintain cytotoxic concentrations in the ventricles following intralumbar administration *(43)*. Such drugs could allow the use of IT chemotherapy for patients who are not candidates for Ommaya reservoir placement.

7. TOXICITIES/COMPLICATIONS

Toxicities and complications of IT therapy can result from the drugs administered, the device or method of administration, and the addition of RT (Table 2). In addition, toxicities can occur in an acute, subacute, or delayed period after therapy. Chamberlain et al. *(53)* reported on 120 patients who had LC treated with intraventricular chemotherapy. A significant minority of patients experienced complications with intraventricular therapy, although most complications, including catheter-related infections, could be

Table 2
Complications of Intraventricular
Chemotherapy for Leptomeningeal Metastases (120 patients)

Complication	Number of Patients (%)
Aseptic/chemical meningitis	52 (43)
Myelosuppression	21 (18)
Catheter-related infection	9 (8)
Unidirectional catheter obstruction	6 (5)
Intraventricular catheter malpositioning	2 (2)
Ommaya reservoir exposure	2 (2)
Leukoencephalopathy	2 (2)
Chemotherapy-related myelopathy	1 (1)

Adapted with permission from ref. *53.*

managed medically. Seven (6%) patients had major complications requiring surgery. Seven of nine patients with catheter-related infections were treated successfully with intraventricular and systemic antibiotics.

Additional series *(54)* corroborate the fact that aseptic meningitis is the most common form of toxicity with IT MTX, occurring in up to 40% of patients. Patients usually present with fever, lethargy, headache, nausea, vomiting, and stiff neck 2–4 h after administration, and symptoms last 12–72 h. Some investigators have used IT hydrocortisone or oral dexamethasone, 4 mg bid for 5, to prevent the reaction *(45,55)*. Boogerd et al. *(9)* postulated that these patients are at increased risk of developing leukoencephalopathy. IT MTX can also cause a subacute and dose-dependent myelopathy or encephalopathy, which usually resolves in weeks, but can be irreversible in some cases *(20,26)*. Patients present with cranial nerve palsies, limb weakness, bowel and bladder dysfunction, seizures, and coma. Delayed leukoencephalopathy occurs months to years after therapy, and is most common in patients who receive concurrent cranial irradiation. This toxicity presents as a progressive dementing illness. Although the incidence has been estimated at approx 10% *(56–58)*, a recent report in patients with non-AIDS primary CNS lymphoma has found this toxicity to occur as often as 30% in patients treated with IT and iv MTX, iv cytarabine, and whole-brain RT *(59)*. Elderly patients appear to have the highest incidence of this complication *(59)*. Children, however, have a significant risk of leukoencephalopathy, as well, and can present with learning disabilities and personality changes *(60)*. Children cured of leukemia and treated with IT MTX and cranial irradiation have an approx 15-point decline in IQ after treatment *(61)*.

As noted above, IT MTX administration can lead to systemic toxicity, with myelosuppression and mucositis, despite the use of relatively small amounts of drug. Although similar amounts of iv MTX almost never require leucovorin rescue, MTX has a prolonged clearance from third-space fluid collections, and may leach slowly into the systemic circulation from the CSF *(62)*. Furthermore, CSF clearance of MTX may be prolonged in patients with active meningeal disease or obstructive hydrocephalus *(23,63)*. Overall, leucovorin rescue is advisable for patients who have renal insufficiency, or who experience myelosuppression or mucositis with previous courses of IT MTX. Although several regimens have been used, 10 mg leucovorin every 6 h for six doses, starting 24 h after each IT MTX administration, should suffice. Only in rare instances, with severe systemic toxicity, would monitoring of serum MTX concentrations be indicated.

IT MTX overdose has been managed by immediate CSF drainage by lumbar puncture, ventriculostomy with ventriculolumbar perfusion, corticosteroids, and iv leukovorin *(26)*. IT leucovorin is not recommended *(64)*. A newer antidote for IT MTX overdose is carboxypeptidase-G_2, an enzyme that rapidly hydrolyzes MTX to inactive metabolites *(65)*. Carboxypeptidase-G_2 can reduce CSF MTX concentrations 400-fold within 5 min *(66)*. Thus carboxypeptidase-G_2 represents an important advance in the management of IT MTX overdose.

Toxicities of IT cytarabine occur less frequently than those of MTX. Arachnoiditis is the most common complication. Other possible toxicities include seizures, paraparesis, and paraplegia *(67,68)*. Because thio-TEPA diffuses rapidly into the systemic circulation after IT administration, the chief toxicity is myelosuppression.

8. DATA ON TUMORS OTHER THAN BREAST, LYMPHOMA, AND LEUKEMIA

With few exceptions, most reports on IT chemotherapy do not focus on a single tumor type, but rather combine patients with various histologies. In addition, many series are small, single-institution reviews of a given IT regimen, often combined with RT. Several retrospective studies do exist for small-cell lung cancer. Data regarding IT therapy for breast carcinoma, lymphoma, and leukemia are reviewed in Chapters x, y, and z, respectively.

Because most patients receive RT to sites of bulk or symptomatic disease, the efficacy of IT chemotherapy as a single modality is difficult to ascertain. Furthermore, response criteria in the medical literature vary significantly, and have included cytologic responses and symptomatic responses. Some authors have scored stable disease as a response, with the rationale that patients with neoplastic meningitis do not remain neurologically stable without treatment *(16)*. A recent review of liposomal cytarabine by the U.S. Food and Drug Administration's Oncologic Drug Advisory Committee *(69)* questioned whether cytologic responses could serve as a valid surrogate for clinical benefit. Because sites of symptomatic disease are usually treated with RT, neurologic improvement most often cannot be attributed to IT chemotherapy. It is important to evaluate reports of IT chemotherapy in this context. Exceptions may include patients with responsive tumors, such as lymphoma or leukemia, for whom IT therapy can be effective as a single modality. Although imperfect, cytologic response rate is probably the most objective and useful measure of efficacy of IT chemotherapy.

9. SPECIFIC TUMOR TYPES

9.1. Small-Cell Lung Cancer

Small-cell lung cancer is the second most common cause of leptomeningeal carcinomatosis. Table 3 summarizes reports of small-cell lung cancer patients treated with various IT regimens. Approximately one-half of patients with small-cell leptomeningeal metastases respond to therapy, which most often combines MTX and radiation. Despite this response rate, the response duration and median survival is disappointingly short.

9.2. Other Solid Tumors

Other tumor types, such as nonsmall-cell lung cancer, primary brain tumors, melanoma, and cancer of unknown primary site, are described in various reports in small numbers. Response rates for the individual tumor types are only sporadically reported,

Table 3
Leptomeningeal Carcinomatosis in Small-Cell Lung Cancer

No. Patients	No. cytologic responses	No. symptomatic responses	Median survival (wk)	IT Chemo[a]	Ref.
24	12	6	NR	MTX	(6)
13	9	NR	8	MTX ± ARA-C[b]	(17)
10	5	5	11	MTX	(7)
8	4	4	2.5	MTX	(10)
4	NR	NR	NR	DTC 101	(45)
2	1	1	NR	MTX-ara-C–thio-TEPA	(16)

[a]Therapy included radiation to symptomatic sites.
[b]Randomized trial.
   IT = intrathecal; NR = not reported; MTX = methotrexate; ara–C = cytosine arabinoside; DTC 101 = liposomal cytosine arabinoside.

Table 4
Novel IT Chemotherapies

Histology	IT Regimen	Responses	Comment	Ref.
Melanoma	5–20 mg DTIC twice/week	Transient symptomatic	two patients	(70)
Melanoma	[131]I radiolabeled MAb	5/11	Phase I	(71)
Melanoma	rIL-2	NR	15-mo progression-free interval	(72)
Glioma	[131]I radiolabeled MAb	2/23	Phase I	(71)
Glioma	rIL-2 ± IFN	2/3 symptomatic	Phase I	(73)
Any	Gene therapy	NR	Proposed	(74)
Any	Diaziquone	62%	Well tolerated	(75)

   IT = intrathecal; DTIC = dacarbazine; MAb = monoclonal antibodies; rIL-2 = recombinant interleukin-2; IFN = interferon; NR = not reported.

and conclusions based on these numbers are not possible. Patients with these malignancies, however, generally have poorly responsive tumors, and should be offered experimental IT chemotherapy or supportive care. Several examples of novel IT therapies are listed in Table 4.

10. COMBINATION IT CHEMOTHERAPY

Several studies of regional delivery of combination chemotherapy to the cerebrospinal fluid have been reported. Giannone et al. *(16)* reported on 22 patients treated with biweekly intraventricular MTX, cytarabine, and thio-TEPA. Most of the patients received radiation to symptomatic areas, or systemic chemotherapy. Overall, nine patients achieved a partial response lasting 4–24+ mo. The median overall survival for the entire group was 10 wk, and myelosuppression was significant. This combination regimen did not appear to offer an advantage over single-agent therapy in this study.

Few prospective randomized studies of IT chemotherapy have been performed. One study compared MTX to MTX and cytarabine in patients with meningeal carcinomatosis

(17). Forty-four patients entered the study, most of whom had small-cell lung cancer (29% of patients) or breast cancer (25%). Other tumor types included adenocarcinoma of unknown primary site (ACUP), CNS primary, cervix, nasopharynx, and melanoma. As a group, 55% patients responded to therapy, with no significant difference between the treatment arms in response rate, survival, or toxicity, although the study was underpowered. Seven of 44 patients achieved a complete response, defined as improved clinical status, negative CSF cytology, and normalization of CSF biochemistry for at least 4 wk. Response rates according to tumor type were as follows: small-cell lung cancer, 9 of 13 (69%); breast, 4 of 11 (36%); ACUP, 3 of 6 (50%). Responders had an longer median survival than nonresponders (18 vs 7 wk, $P < 0.05$). Although the study was randomized, the numbers of patients with each tumor type were insufficient to detect an advantage of combination therapy over single-agent MTX. This trial was unable to demonstrate an advantage of the combination over MTX alone in this heterogeneous group of patients.

A randomized study by the Eastern Cooperative Oncology Group compared intraventricular MTX to thio-TEPA in previously untreated neoplastic meningitis *(32)*. Fifty-two adults, 90% of whom had primary breast cancer, lung cancer, or lymphoma, were assessable for response. No difference in efficacy, toxicity, or median survival (approx 15 wk) was observed in either treatment arm of this trial. Although 31% of patients converted from positive to negative CSF cytology, no patients had clinically important neurologic improvement, and 75% deteriorated within 8 wk of beginning therapy. Three factors predicted for shorter survival: progressive systemic disease, poor performance status, and significant cranial nerve palsies. These data confirm that standard regional chemotherapy for LC remains limited in its efficacy, and is unable to reverse established neurologic deficits.

11. CONCLUSIONS

IT chemotherapy has a clearly defined role in the CNS prophylaxis of lymphoid leukemia *(1)*, but its role in established leptomeningeal disease remains less well defined, for several reasons. First, the most widely used agents have only modest activity against the major tumor types that cause neoplastic meningitis. More prospective studies need to be performed in single tumor types. Second, the advanced stage of cancer, and compromised performance status of many patients in this situation, creates barriers to the diagnosis and treatment of these patients. Third, response to therapy can be difficult to assess because of fixed neurologic deficits, the lack of radiographically measurable disease, and the necessary use of RT. Future trials of IT therapy should incorporate established tools for the measurement of quality of life. In addition, recent data regarding IV treatment of leptomeningeal metastases suggest the need for prospective, randomized trials of IV vs IT regimens, which measure quality of life, toxicity, and costs, and which incorporate standard measures of response. The application of rational drug development and improved pharmacokinetic properties hold promise for improvements in IT chemotherapy.

REFERENCES

1. Cortes J, O'Brien SM, Pierce S, et al. Value of high-dose systemic chemotherapy and intrathecal therapy for central nervous system prophylaxis in different risk groups of adult acute lymphoblastic leukemia, *Blood,* **86** (1995) 2091–2097.

2. Boyle R, Thomas M, and Adams J. Diffuse involvement of the leptomeninges by tumor: a clinical and pathological study of 63 cases, *Postural Med. J.,* **56** (1980) 149–158.

3. Bleyer WA. Leptomeningeal cancer in leukaemia and solid tumors, *Curr. Prob. Cancer,* **12** (1988) 185–237.

4. DeAngelis LM and Posner JB. Neurologic complications, In Holland JF, et al. (eds), *Cancer Medicine, 4th ed.,* Williams and Wilkins, Baltimore, 1997, pp. 3117–3139.

5. Yap HY, Yap BS, Tashima CK, et al. Meningeal carcinomatosis in breast cancer, *Cancer,* **42** (1978) 283–286.

6. Rosen ST, Aisner J, Makuch RW, et al. Carcinomatous leptomeningitis in small-cell lung cancer: a clinicopathologic review of the National Cancer Institute experience, *Medicine,* **61** (1982) 45–53.

7. Aroney RS, Dalley DN, Chun WK, et al. Meningeal cancer in small cell carcinoma of the lung, *Am. J. Med.,* **71** (1981) 26–32.

8. Amer MH, Al-Sarraf M, Baker LH, and Viatkavicius VK. Malignant melanoma and central nervous system metastases: incidence, diagnosis, treatment and survival, *Cancer,* **42** (1978) 660–668.

9. Boogerd W, Hart AA, van der Sande JJ, and Engelsman D. Meningeal carcinomatosis in breast cancer: prognostic factors and influence of treatment, *Cancer,* **67** (1991) 1685–1695.

10. Nugent LJ, Bunn PA, Matthews MJ, et al. CNS metastases in small cell bronchogenic carcinoma: increasing frequency and changing pattern with lengthening survival, *Cancer,* **44** (1979) 1885–1893.

11. Forman AD and Levin VA. Intraventricular therapy, In Perry MC (ed), *Chemotherapy Source Book,* Williams and Wilkins, Baltimore, 1992, pp. 213–225.

12. Sansone G. Pathomorphosis of acute infantile leukemia treated with modern therapeutic agents, meningoleukemia and Frolich's obesity, *Ann. Pediat.,* **183** (1954) 33–42.

13. McKelvey EM. Meningeal involvement with metastatic carcinoma of the breast treated with intrathecal methotrexate, *Cancer,* **22** (1968) 576–580.

14. Wang JJ and Pratt CB. Intrathecal arabinosyl cytosine in meningeal leukemia, *Cancer,* **25** (1970) 531–534.

15. Gutin PH, Weiss HD, Wiernik PH, et al. Intrathecal N, N', N''-triethylenephosphoramide [Thio-TEPA (NSC 6396)] in the treatment of malignant meningeal disease: phase I–II study, *Cancer,* **38** (1976) 1471–1475.

16. Giannone L, Greco FA, and Hainsworth JD. Combination intraventricular chemotherapy for meningeal neoplasia, *J. Clin. Oncol.,* **4** (1986) 68–73.

17. Hitchins RN, Bell DR, Woods RL, and Levi JA. Prospective randomized trial of single-agent versus combination chemotherapy in meningeal carcinomatosis, *J. Clin. Oncol.,* **5** (1987) 1655–1662.

18. Ratcheson RA and Ommaya AK. Experience with the subcutaneous cerebrospinal fluid reservoir, *N. Engl. J. Med.,* **239** (1968) 161–165.

19. Ommaya AK. Implantable devices for chronic access and drug delivery to the central nervous system, *Cancer Drug Deliv.,* **1** (1984) 169–179.

20. Jayson GC and Howell A. Carcinomatous meningitis in solid tumors, *Ann. Oncol.,* **7** (1996) 773–786.

21. Bleyer WA and Poplack DG. Clinical studies on the central-nervous system pharmacology of methotrexate, In Pinedo HM (ed), *Clinical Pharmacology of Anti-Neoplastic Drugs,* Elsevier/North Holland, Amsterdam, 1978, pp. 115–131.

22. Bleyer W and Poplack D. Intraventricular versus intralumbar methotrexate for central nervous system leukemia: prolonged remission with the Ommaya reservoir, *Med. Ped. Oncol.,* **6** (1978) 207–213.

23. Grossman SA, Trump DL, Chen DCP, et al. Cerebrospinal fluid flow abnormalities in patients with neoplastic meningitis, *Am. J. Med.,* **73** (1982) 641–647.

24. Chamberlain MC. Pediatric leptomeningeal metastasis: ^{111}In-DTPA cerebrospinal fluid flow studies, *J. Child Neurol.,* **9** (1994) 150–154.

25. Chamberlain MC. Comparative spine imaging in leptomeningeal metastases, *J. Neurooncol.,* **23** (1995) 233–238.

26. Blaney SM and Poplack DG. Pharmacologic strategies for the treatment of meningeal malignancy, *Invest. New Drugs,* **14** (1996) 69–85.

27. Bleyer WA. Clinical pharmacology of intrathecal methotrexate: an improved dosage regimen derived from age-related pharmacokinetics, *Cancer Treat. Rep.,* **61** (1977) 1419–1425.

28. Mayer R, Berkowitz R, and Griffiths C. Central nervous system involvement by ovarian carcinoma: a complication of prolonged survival with metastatic disease, *Proc. Am. Assoc. Cancer Res.,* **19** (1978) 318.

29. Wasserstrom WR, Glass JP, and Posner JB. Diagnosis and treatment of leptomeningeal metastases from solid tumors: experience with 90 patients, *Cancer,* **49** (1982) 759–772.

30. Little JR, Dale AJD, and Okazaki H. Meningeal carcinomatosis: clinical manifestations, *Arch. Neurol.*, **30** (1974) 138–143.

31. Olson ME, Chernick NL, and Posner JB. Infiltration of the leptomeninges by systemic cancer: a clinical and pathologic study, *Arch. Neurol.*, **30** (1974) 122–137.

32. Grossman SA, Finkelstein DM, Ruckdeschel JC, et al. Randomized prospective comparison of intraventricular methotrexate and thiotepa in patients with previously untreated neoplastic meningitis, *J. Clin. Oncol.*, **11** (1993) 561–569.

33. Bokstein F, Lossos A, and Siegal T. Leptomeningeal metastases from solid tumors: a comparison of two prospective series treated with and without intra-cerebrospinal fluid chemotherapy, *Cancer*, **82** (1998) 1756–1763.

34. Grant R, Naylor B, Greenberg HS, and Junck L. Clinical outcome in aggressively treated meningeal carcinomatosis, *Arch. Neurol.*, **51** (1994) 457–461.

35. Shapiro WR, Young DF, and Mehta BM. Methotrexate distribution in cerebrospinal fluid after intravenous, ventricular and lumbar injections, *N. Engl. J. Med.*, **293** (1975) 161–166.

36. Axils RF, Locker GO, Doroshow J, et al. Pharmacokinetics of adriamycin and tissue penetration in murine ovarian cancer, *Cancer Res.*, **39** (1979b) 3209–3214.

37. Blasberg R, Patlak C, and Fenstermacher J. Intrathecal chemotherapy. Brain tissue profiles after ventriculo-cisternal perfusion, *J. Pharm. Exp. Therap.*, **195** (1976) 73–83.

38. Flessner MF, Fenstermacher JD, Dedrick RL, and Blasberg RG. Peritoneal adsorption of macromolecules studied by quantitative autoradiography, *Am. J. Physiol.*, **248** (1985) H26–32.

39. Flessner MF, Fenstermacher JD, Dedrick RL, and Blasberg RG. Distributed model of peritoneal-plasma transport: tissue concentration gradients, *Am. J. Physiol.*, **248** (1985) F425–435.

40. Bleyer WA, Poplack DG, and Simon RM. "Concentration × time" methotrexate via a subcutaneous reservoir: a less toxic regimen for intraventricular chemotherapy of central nervous system neoplasms, *Blood*, **51** (1987) 835–842.

41. Petit T, Defour P, Korganov AS, et al. Continuous intrathecal perfusion of methotrexate for carcinomatous meningitis with pharmakokinetic studies: two case studies, *Clin. Oncol.*, **9** (1997) 189–190.

42. Nakagawa H, Fujita T, Kubo S, et al. Ventriculolumbar perfusion chemotherapy with methotrexate and cytosine arabinoside for meningeal carcinomatosis: a pilot study of 13 patients, *Surg. Neurol.*, **45** (1996) 256–264.

43. Kim S, Chatelut E, Kim JC, et al. Extended CSF cytarabine exposure following intrathecal administration of DTC 101, *J. Clin. Oncol.*, **11** (1993) 2186–2193.

44. Chamberlain MC, Kormanik P, Howell SB, and Kim S. Pharmacokinetics of intralumbar DTC-101 for the treatment of leptomeningeal metastases, *Arch. Neurol.*, **52** (1995) 912–917.

45. Jaekle K, Glantz M, Chamberlain M, et al. Treatment of carcinomatous meningitis and lymphomatous meningitis with intra-CSF cytarabine sustained-release liposome injection versus methotrexate, *Blood*, **10(suppl 1)** (1997) 79a.

46. Glantz MJ, Cole BF, Recht L, et al. High dose intravenous methotrexate for patients with nonleukemic leptomeningeal cancer: is intrathecal chemotherapy necessary?, *J. Clin. Oncol.*, **16** (1998) 1561–1567.

47. Seibel NL and Reaman GH. Special considerations of chemotherapy for children with cancer, In Holland JF, et al., *Cancer Medicine*, 4th ed., Williams and Wilkins, Baltimore, 1997, pp. 2922–2923.

48. Strong JM, Collins JM, Lester C, and Poplack DG. Pharmacokinetics of intraventricular and intravenous N,N',N"-triethylenephosphoramide (thiotepa) in rhesus monkeys and humans, *Cancer Res.*, **46** (1986) 6101–6104.

49. Lee JB, Antman K, and Frei E. Evidence for metabolic activation of thioTEPA, *Proc. Am. Assoc. Cancer Res.*, **29** (1988) 487a.

50. Heideman RL, Cole DE, Balis F, et al. Phase I and pharmacokinetic evaluation of thiotepa in the cerebrospinal fluid and plasma of pediatric patients: evidence for dose-dependent plasma clearance of thiotepa, *Cancer Res.*, **45** (1989) 736–741.

51. Obbens D, Leavens M, Beal J, and Lee Y. Ommaya reservoirs in 387 cancer patients: a 15-year experience, *Neurology*, **35** (1985) 1274–1278.

52. Larson SM, Schall GL, and DiChiro G. Influence of previous lumbar puncture and pneumoencephalography on the incidence of unsuccessful radioisotope cisternography, *J. Nucl. Med.*, **12** (1971) 555–557.

53. Chamberlain MC, Kormanik PA, and Barba D. Complications associated with intraventricular chemotherapy in patients with leptomeningeal metastases, *J. Neurosurg.*, **87** (1997) 694–699.

54. Kaplan R and Wiernik P. Neurotoxicity of antineoplastic drugs, *Semin. Oncol.*, **9** (1982) 103–130.

55. Pullen J, Boyett J, Shuster J, et al. Extended triple intrathecal chemotherapy trial for prevention of

CNS relapse in good-risk and poor-risk patients with B-progenitor acute lymphoblastic leukemia: a Pediatric Oncology Group study, *J. Clin. Oncol.,* **11** (1993) 839–849.

56. Shapiro WR, Posner JB, Ushio Y, et al. Treatment of meningeal neoplasms, *Cancer Treat. Rep.,* **61** (1977) 733–743.

57. Sculier JP. Treatment of meningeal carcinomatosis, *Cancer Treat. Rev.,* **12** (1985) 95–104.

58. Bleyer WA. Neurologic sequelae of methotrexate and ionizing radiation: a new classification, *Cancer Treat. Rep.,* **65** (1981) 89–98.

59. Abrey LE, DeAngelis LM, and Yahalom J. Long-term survival in primary CNS lymphoma, *J. Clin. Oncol.,* **16** (1998) 859–863.

60. Ochs J, Mulhern R, Fairclough D, et al. Comparison of neuropsychologic functioning and clinical indicators of neurotoxicity in long-term survivors of childhood leukemia given cranial radiation, *J. Clin. Oncol.,* **9** (1991) 145–151.

61. Butler RW, Hill JM, Steinherz PG, et al. Neuropsychologic effects of cranial irradiation, intrathecal methotrexate, and systemic methotrexate in childhood cancer, *J. Clin. Oncol.,* **12** (1994) 2621–2629.

62. Chabner BA, Stoller DG, Handke K, et al. Methotrexate disposition in humans: case studies in ovarian cancer and following high dose infusion, *Drug Metab. Rev.,* **8** (1978) 107–117.

63. Bleyer WA, Drake JC, and Chabner BA. Neurotoxicity and elevated cerebrospinal fluid methotrexate concentration in meningeal leukemia, *N. Engl. J. Med.,* **289** (1973) 770–773.

64. Jardine LF, Ingram LC, and Bleyer WA. Intrathecal leucovorin after intrathecal methotrexate overdose, *J. Ped. Hematol. Oncol.,* **18** (1996) 302–304.

65. O'Marcaigh AS, Johnson CM, Smithson WA, et al. Successful treatment of intrathecal methotrexate overdose by using ventriculolumbar perfusion and intrathecal instillation of carboxypeptidase G2, *Mayo Clin. Proc.,* **71** (1996) 161–165.

66. Adamson P, Balis F, McCully C, et al. Rescue of experimental intrathecal methotrexate overdose with carboxypeptidase-G$_2$, *J. Clin. Oncol.,* **9** (1991) 670–674.

67. Eden O, Goldie W, Wood T, et al. Seizures following intrathecal cytosine arabinoside in young children with acute lymphocytic leukemia, *Cancer,* **42** (1978) 53–58.

68. Wolff L, Zighelboim J, and Gale R. Paraplegia following intrathecal cytosine arabinoside, *Cancer,* **43** (1979) 83–88.

69. Chiron/Depotech Depocyt. leukemia/lymphoma data requested by FDA Advisory Committee prior to approval; solid tumor indication could be revisited, *Pink Sheet,* **59** (1997) 9.

70. Champagne MA and Silver HKB. Intrathecal dacarbazine treatment of leptomeningeal malignant melanoma, *J. Nat. Cancer Inst.,* **84** (1992) 1203–1204.

71. Bigner DD, Brown M, Coleman RE, et al. Phase I studies of treatment of malignant gliomas and neoplastic meningitis with ^{131}I-radiolabeled monoclonal antibodies anti-tenascin 81C6 and anti-chondroitin proteoglycan sulfate Me1-14 F (ab')$_2$: a preliminary report, *J. Neuro-Oncol.,* **24** (1995) 109–122.

72. Fathalah-Shaykh HM, Zimmerman C, Morgan H, et al. Response of primary leptomeningeal melanoma to intrathecal recombinant interleukin-2. A case report, *Cancer,* **77** (1996) 1544–1550.

73. Salmaggi A, Dufour A, and Silvani A. Immunological fluctuations during intrathecal immunotherapy in three patients affected by CNS tumours disseminating via CSF, *Int. J. Neurosci.,* **77** (1994) 117–125.

74. Oldfield EH, Ram Z, Chiang Y, and Blaese RM. Intrathecal gene therapy for the treatment of leptomeningeal carcinomatosis. GTI 0108. A phase I/II study, *Human Gene Ther.,* **8** (1995) 55–85.

75. Berg SL, Balis FM, Zimm S, et al., Phase I/II trial and pharmacokinetics of intrathecal diaziquone in refractory meningeal malignancies, *J. Clin. Oncol.,* **10** (1992) 143–148.

20 Regional Chemotherapy for Meningeal Involvement with Breast Cancer

Beth A. Overmoyer

1. INTRODUCTION

Leptomeningeal metastasis (LM) most often occurs in the setting of a prior diagnosis of adenocarcinoma *(1–3)*. Among this group of diseases, breast cancer is the most frequently associated malignancy *(2–6)*. Central nervous system (CNS) metastasis from breast cancer follows bone, lungs, and liver as the fourth most common site of disseminated disease *(7,8)*. Unlike patients with other solid tumors, approx 50% of patients with metastatic breast cancer are more likely to die from CNS involvement than from the systemic disease, because of the moderate chemosensitivity of breast cancer *(15–18)*. Approximately 2–5% of breast cancer patients will develop leptomeningeal involvement, which is often associated with other sites of metastatic disease *(4–7,9–14)*. The relative responsiveness of systemic metastasis poses a challenge to the treating physician, because patient survival is primarily dependent on the treatment of the CNS disease *(14,19,20)*. The incidence of LM is also expected to increase, because of the broader application of adjuvant therapy for breast cancer, and the relative impermeability of the CNS to systemic treatment because of the blood–brain barrier *(2,21)*. This chapter will present the accepted therapies for LM, with the understanding that further investigation is needed to determine the optimal treatment strategy.

2. ANATOMY AND PATHOPHYSIOLOGY

The brain is covered by a membrane known as the meninges, which is of mesodermal origin, and is composed of the dura mater (outer layer) and the arachnoid membrane, and pia mater (inner layer). The leptomeninges is defined as the subarachnoid space between the arachnoid and the pia mater. Approximately 600 cc cerebral spinal fluid

From: *Current Clinical Oncology: Regional Chemotherapy: Clinical Research and Practice*
Edited by: M. Markman © Humana Press Inc., Totowa, NJ

(CSF) is produced daily by the choroid plexus in the lateral, third, and fourth ventricles. The CSF flows through the foramen of Magendie and Lusca, traveling through the base of the brain into the spinal subarachnoid space, returning to the basilar cisterns, then flowing over the cortical convexities. The CSF leaves the neuraxis through the arachnoid granulations into the superior sagittal sinus. Contamination of the CSF with adenocarcinoma results in disseminated seeding of the leptomeninges, known as carcinomatous meningitis (1,22,23). Carcinoma and its associated fibrosis, which encompasses meningeal arteries and veins, can diffusely infiltrate the leptomeninges. Multifocal nodular masses of carcinoma are a more common manifestation of LM (2,22,24).

Tumor invasion of the leptomeninges can occur by several mechanisms:

1. Direct extension into the meninges from preexisting parenchymal brain tumors occurs infrequently in patients with breast cancer; direct extension from vertebral metastasis is more common. Breast cancer cells can directly penetrate the leptomeninges via the perivascular spaces, or via the system of intraosseous venous anastomoses. Direct extension can also occur along cranial nerve sheaths (4,24,25).
2. Carcinomatous infiltration of the perineural and perivascular lymphatics can occur by direct invasion, or via cervical lymph node metastasis. These infiltrated lymphatics communicate centrally with the subarachnoid space through the cranial or intervertebral foramina. There may also be carcinomatous involvement of the Virchow-Robin spaces and the choroid plexus (1,2,22,25).
3. Hematogenous spread may occur through Baston's plexus, or through the arterial circulation (1,23,26,27). Carcinoma cells within the meninges spread via the CSF through the brain surface and spinal cords, frequently depositing in the basilar cisterns, posterior fossa, and cauda equina (1,4,24).

Several studies have examined the pathologic correlation with the development of LM from breast cancer. There appears to be a prevalence of lobular carcinoma metastasizing to the meninges, compared with ductal carcinoma, which appears to primarily result in parenchymal CNS metastasis (16,28). Cellular adhesion molecules may play a role in this predisposition for sites of metastasis (6,23). An autopsy series from Yugoslavia (6), involving 226 patients with metastatic breast cancer, demonstrated a 2.6% incidence of leptomeningeal carcinomatosis. Among these patients, lobular carcinoma accounted for 66%. This feature was also demonstrated at the Christie Hospital, Manchester, where 90% of the patients with LM caused by breast cancer (2.7% incidence) had lobular carcinoma as their pathologic diagnosis (15). No other feature appears to be specifically associated with the development of LM from breast cancer, such as age at diagnosis, menopausal status, or disease-free interval (7,15,20,28,29). However, some studies continue to suggest that this pattern of metastatic disease is more common among younger, premenopausal patients, which is suggestive of aggressive disease (20,26,29).

3. SIGNS AND SYMPTOMS

Although LM is rarely the initial presenting feature of breast cancer, this metastasis is not uncommonly the first sign of disease recurrence (3,4,30). Table 1 demonstrates the demographics of patients with LM described in larger published trials. There is great variation in the disease-free interval and overall survival among patients with leptomeningeal carcinomatosis from breast cancer. Some case studies describe a lengthy disease-free interval of 25 yr, and an overall survival of 7 yr following diagnosis (19,27). In general, the overall survival is measured in months, with a median duration of approx 3 mo.

Table 1
Demographics of Patients with LM from Larger Published Studies

Ref.	No. Patients	Age at diagnosis (yr) (Median)	LM only (%)	DFI	OS (Median)
(16)	35	45	14	10.9 mo	77 d
(31)	10	54	10	3.2 yr	6.4 mo
(10)	42	48	38	31.5 mo	12 wk
(14)	44	57	NA	38 mo	12 wk
(13)	22	62.5	5	43 mo	46 d
(3)	29[a]	49	14	2 mo	6 wk
(9)	25	50	4	25 mo	22 wk
(15)	10	51	3	54 wk	27 wk

[a]Study includes nonbreast cancer patients.
DFI = disease-free interval, i.e., time until diagnosis of LM; NA = not available; OS = overall survival.

Table 2
Common Symptoms Associated with LM

Ref.	No. patients	Cerebral headache	Cranial nerve general	visual changes	Spinal motor defect	Pain
(16)	35	10	11	4	3	NA
(31)	10	5	5	3	6	2
(10)	42	19	9	2	17	NA
(11)	23	10	7	NA	2	NA
(14)	44	29	13	NA	26	NA
(5)	21	11	17	7	18	8
(13)	22	4	6	4	4	1
(4)	50[a]	25	47	22	36	32
(3)	29[a]	17	19	12	4	13
(9)	25	13	13	9	7	4
(2)	90[a]	30	35	18	34	23

[a]Study includes nonbreast cancer patients.

The presenting symptoms and signs of LM suggest diffuse involvement throughout the CNS (cerebral, cranial nerve, and spinal) (1,2). Clinical signs of disease are often more severe than the symptoms elicited (2,4,13,24). Table 2 lists the most common symptoms associated with this disease.

In general, headache is the most common symptom encountered, which is thought to be caused by CSF flow obstruction by carcinoma deposits along the meninges, resulting in increased intracranial pressure (2,4,13). Headache is often more severe upon awakening (3). Other symptoms associated with cerebral involvement include dizziness, confusion, nausea, and vomiting (32). Invasion of the cranial nerve roots with carcinoma can result in multiple cranial nerve abnormalities, most commonly involving cranial nerve three, five, six, seven, and eight (3,9,11,30). Spinal manifestations often involve the lower limbs, presumably because of gravitation of the carcinoma into the CSF cul-de-sac (2,3). Characteristics include back pain, weakness, paresthesias, and cauda equina syndrome. In addition to the larger studies presented in Table 2, several case reports mirror the information presented in Table 2 (12,19,22,27,30).

4. DIAGNOSIS

4.1. Cerebral Spinal Fluid

The most important diagnostic test for leptomeningeal carcinomatosis is an examination of the CSF. A positive CSF cytology is diagnostic of disseminated LM, although its absence in the appropriate clinical setting does not rule out the diagnosis (4,33). Initial cytology is positive in 10–50%; however, after three taps, the yield of positive cytology increases to greater than 90% (2–4,15,24). CSF can be obtained by lumbar puncture, cisternal tap, or ventricular tap. The cite of CSF sampling is important, because the content of CSF varies throughout the CNS, and false-negative cytology can occur with sampling from different sites within the same patient. Occasionally, the cytology remains negative after repeated attempts, although it is rare to have a perfectly normal CSF in the presence of leptomeningeal carcinomatosis (2,4,14,22,34,35). False-positive cytology only occurs with CSF involvement with lymphoma, not carcinoma (33). The most common chemical profile in the CSF is a low glucose and high protein level, which is consistent with a large tumor load (3,14,15). A pleocytosis can also occur in this setting (3,5,14,16,31).

Biochemical markers within the CSF may aid in the diagnosis of LM from breast cancer, specifically, in the absence of positive CSF cytology. Carcinoembryonic antigen levels may be elevated in approx 60%, and LDH levels may be elevated in approx 80% of patients (1,2,22,36). Tumor markers, such as tissue polypeptide antigen, and creatine kinase-BB isoenzyme have also been detected within the CSF. Elevated values of these markers have a sensitivity and specificity between 83 and 90% (37,38). Other CSF biochemicals, such as β-glucuronidase, β_2-microglobulin, and CA15-3, are less specific and less sensitive (1,2,22–25,36).

4.2. Neuroimaging

Neuroimaging with computed tomography (CT) and magnetic resonance imaging (MRI) are complementary to the evaluation of the CSF, and, in specific clinical context, may be the only means of establishing the diagnosis of LM (34,39). A gadolinium-enhanced MRI of the brain or spine may demonstrate leptomeningeal enhancement, focal or diffuse dural enhancement, or cranial nerve enhancement in the presence of disease. This technique is associated with 55–60% sensitivity, although it is more likely to be abnormal in cases in which the CSF cytology is positive, thus limiting its value as an independent diagnostic tool (1,22,39,40). Although contrast-enhanced head CT may demonstrate hydrocephalus, it is neither as sensitive nor as specific as gadolinium-enhanced MRI for the diagnosis of leptomeningeal disease (2,22,40).

Myelography is beneficial in demonstrating meningeal disease of the spine, evidenced by irregular filling of the subarchnoid space and nerve roots (2,3). MRI of the spine with gadolinium enhancement has essentially replaced the more invasive myelography.

5. TREATMENT

The purpose of treating leptomeningeal carcinomatosis is to provide stabilization or improvement in neurologic symptoms, and to increase survival. Stabilization of neurologic dysfunction is a goal, because of the inability of the CNS to regenerate once damage occurs, and because the natural history of leptomeningeal carcinomatosis is an unrelenting decline, and any degree of stabilization is beneficial (2,41). Breast cancer patients appear to have a more favorable prognosis following the diagnosis of leptomeningeal disease, compared with other solid tumors, occasionally surviving more than 1 yr following the diagnosis of leptomeningeal carcinomatosis *(4,13,14,19,23,42–44)*.

The clinical course of untreated LM is associated with a median survival of less than 3 mo *(4,9,16,18)*. Several studies have identified specific prognostic features for patients who would benefit from treatment of leptomeningeal disease, and who are expected to continue clinical improvement following an initial trial of therapy. In general, patients with a poor performance status (Karnofsky Performance Status <50%), depressed CSF glucose, and lack of significant disease response, following 2–6 wk of therapy, may not demonstrate a substantial benefit from therapy, and may be better served with a more palliative treatment approach *(14,16,24,31,44–46)*. The ability to clear the CSF of malignant cells is not an independent prognostic indicator for response *(31,41)*.

5.1. Blood–Brain Barrier: Systemic vs Intrathecal Chemotherapy

The blood–brain barrier restricts the entry of water-soluble and charged particles from the systemic circulation to the brain via the circumventricular areas between the epithelial cells lining the brain *(47)*. Although the blood–brain barrier can be disrupted by the growth of metastatic deposits along the leptomeninges, sites of sanctuary remain, where the tumor is protected from the effects of systemic chemotherapy *(48–51)*. Animal models support the relative lack of efficacy with systemic therapy, compared with direct infusion of drug into the CNS *(42,52)*.

Characteristics of systemically administered chemotherapy that determine its ability to penetrate the blood–brain barrier include its free, nonprotein-bound plasma concentration and the rate of cerebral blood flow. Most chemotherapy administered systemically does not result in adequate CNS concentrations *(50,53)*. Studies using chemotherapy known to cross the blood–brain barrier have demonstrated minimal efficacy in the treatment of parenchymal metastasis, and no efficacy in the treatment of leptomeningeal disease *(54–57)*. Intrathecal (IT) chemotherapy can circumvent the blood–brain barrier and deliver higher therapeutic concentrations of drug into the CSF, often with a longer half-life *(41,42,47,58)*. Three chemotherapeutic agents are administered into the CSF: methotrexate (MTX), cytarabine, and thio-TEPA *(46)*.

IT chemotherapy can only penetrate the meninges to a depth of 3–4 mm; therefore, radiation therapy (RT) is used to control tumor nodules often associated with leptomeningeal carcinomatosis *(1,24,42)*. CSF flow studies using indium-111-DTPA demonstrate abnormalities caused by tumor nests. RT, usually whole-brain or spinal radiation, can improve CSF flow by treating areas containing tumor nodules, and facilitate improvement in the distribution of IT chemotherapy *(24,59,60)*. RT of the entire craniospinal neuroaxis is no longer performed, because of myelotoxicity, which compromises the ability to give chemotherapy *(4)*. Whole-brain radiation is commonly given in doses of 24–30 Gy *(23,60)*.

Chemotherapy administered via lumbar puncture is not as effective as direct administration into the lateral ventricles via an Ommaya reservoir. Difficulties may arise in the ability of chemotherapy administered via lumbar puncture to reach nests of carcinoma cells within the choroid plexuses by ascending the spinal subarachnoid space against the flow of the CSF. Additionally, chemotherapy may be erroneously administered into the subdural or epidural space during lumbar puncture *(41,43,47,61,62)*. Leptomeningeal carcinomatosis in the region of the spine may also result in obstruction of CSF flow, interfering with adequate distribution of chemotherapy by lumbar puncture, and resulting in areas of high concentrations of drug associated with increased neurotoxicity *(1,47,59,63–66)*. Although an Ommaya reservoir is the preferred means of delivery of IT chemotherapy, infection and technical complications may occur in up to 15% of cases *(2,14,17,23,42,67,68)*.

5.2. Methotrexate

MTX is the most frequently used IT chemotherapeutic agent *(1,41)*. When MTX is administered intravenously, its concentration ratio of plasma: CSF is 60:1. A therapeutic concentration is $>10^{-7}$ M, and can be maintained for 48 h following IT administration *(1)*. When MTX is administered via lumbar puncture, the CSF concentration is approx 10^{-6} M, and, when administered via an Ommaya reservoir, the concentration is higher, at 10^{-4} M *(23,41)*. Calcium leucovorin is often administered systemically following MTX treatment, in order to reduce the systemic toxicity. Leucovorin does not increase the CSF folate levels appreciably, therefore, its administration does not interfere with the efficacy of IT MTX *(41,69)*.

The optimal dose of IT MTX is not known *(70)*. There appears to be less variability in CSF drug levels when the dose of MTX is standardized, rather than based upon the patient's body surface area. This reflects the drug's volume of distribution within the CSF, and takes into account the reduced metabolism that occurs with advancing age *(71)*. In general, the recommended dose of MTX is 12 mg/m^2 (or 15 mg standard dose). Treatment schedules also vary greatly. Studies that administer a lower dose of MTX more frequently, in order to maintain a therapeutic CSF concentration, i.e., over a "concentration × time" schedule, have not been found to offer a significant treatment benefit, although the toxicity may be reduced *(14,18,47,72,73)*. This treatment schedule is also cumbersome, and not conducive to the palliative goal of therapy. The majority of studies use a dosing schedule of 2–3× each week, until CSF response, followed by maintenance therapy weekly, then monthly. No standard schedule recommendations exist, and the decision to pursue maintenance therapy should be individualized. Treatment with IT MTX increases the overall survival to approx 6 mo or longer, although much variation exists *(2,5,17,18,31,42,74)*. Results from representative studies are listed in Table 3.

5.3. MTX in Combination

Failure to successfully treat leptomeningeal carcinomatosis from breast cancer may result from ineffective drug distribution throughout the CNS, most commonly caused by CSF blocks from tumor infiltration, or by drug resistance of the primary carcinoma. MTX has been combined with cytarabine and thio-TEPA in an attempt to overcome drug resistance. Therapies that have included all three drugs (MTX, thio-TEPA, cytarabine), two-drug combinations (MTX and cytarabine, MTX and thio-TEPA) have demonstrated feasibility, but not necessarily increased efficacy, from the combination of drugs (Table 4; *43,75,77*). Currently, most clinicians use each drug sequentially, changing agents once disease relapse occurs.

5.4. Thio-TEPA

Thio-TEPA is an alkylating agent whose lack of cell-cycle specificity was thought to be efficacious in the treatment of the slowly dividing malignancy within the CNS. Early studies examined the efficacy of thio-TEPA in hematologic malignancies. The dose range is 2–10 mg/m^2, but common dosing excludes the body surface area, and

Table 3
Studies of IT MTX for Treatment
of Leptomeningeal Carcinomatosis in Breast Cancer Patients

Ref.	No. Patients	MTX dose	Route	Response (%)	Median OS (mo)
(2)	46[a]	7 mg/m^2 × 2 wk × 5 wk Then every 1–4 wk	Ommaya	61	7.2
(5)	21[a]	0.25 mg/kg 3 × wk × 6 wk, then maintenance	LP	60	5.9
(42)	15[a]	6.25 mg/m^2 2 × wk or every 2 d × 5, then maintenance	Ommaya	68	5.0
(18)	19	5 mg given to maintain CSF levels > 10^3 nmol/L	Ommaya	79	6.0
(17)	33[a]	12.5 mg 2 × wk × 3 wk, then maintenance	Ommaya	55	6.0
(74)	17[a]	7.5 mg/m^2 to 15 mg (max) 2 × wk, then maintenance	Ommaya/LP	55	5.7

[a]Includes whole-brain radiation
MTX = methotrexate; OS = overall survival.

Table 4
Studies Using Combination IT Chemotherapy

Ref.	No. patients	Chemotherapy	Response (%)	Median OS
(43)[a]	11	MTX 15 mg	67	NA
		MTX 15 mg/cytarabine 50 mg	25	NA
(75)[a]	16	TT 10 mg d 1 MTX 10 mg d 4	68	23 wk
(76)	10	MTX 12 mg/cytarabine 40 mg/ TT 15 mg	60	10 wk
(77)[a]	3	MTX 15–20 mg/cytarabine 75–100 mg/ TT 7.5–10 mg	91	38 wk

[a]Includes whole-brain radiation
ara-C = cytarabine; MTX = methotrexate; NA = not available; OS = overall survival; TT = thio-TEPA.

uses 10–12 mg *(78,79)*. Thio-TEPA does not appear to have a therapeutic advantage, compared to MTX *(46)*.

5.5. Cytarabine

Cytarabine is cell-cycle specific, resulting in cell kill during DNA synthesis *(80,81)*. IT cytarabine is most commonly used in hematologic malignancies, although it is effective against leptomeningeal disease caused by solid tumors. The optimal drug delivery schedule is a daily infusion into the subarachnoid space, which is impractical. Therefore, the commonly used dosing schedule is 20–50 mg/m^2 given 1–3×/wk *(23,41)*. An extended release form of cytarabine (DTC-101) has been investigated in patients with leptomeningeal carcinomatosis, including that from metastatic breast cancer, and it has demonstrated a longer half-life of 141 h, compared with 3.4 h with standard cytarabine. DTC-101 is a cytarabine encapsulated into lipid spheres, and it may optimize the efficacy of cytarabine in the treatment of leptomeningeal carcinomatosis *(80–82)*. DTC-101 is currently investigational.

5.6. Other Therapies

Other investigational IT chemotherapeutic agents include diaziquone, an alkylating agent originally designated to be given systemically, having properties of penetrating the blood–brain barrier, and ACNU, a nitrosourea given intrathecally. These agents have not been proven beneficial for the treatment of leptomeningeal involvement with breast cancer *(83,84)*. Future studies may expand on the role of monoclonal antibodies and their utility in targeting chemotherapy or radiation to sites of leptomeningeal involvement with metastatic disease *(30,85–87)*.

Although studies have demonstrated higher CNS concentrations of tamoxifen and its metabolites, most information comes from studies of parenchymal metastasis, excluding LM *(27,88)*. There does not appear to be any efficacy of using tamoxifen or another hormone therapy in the treatment of this disease *(89–95)*.

5.7. Toxicity

Treatment of leptomeningeal carcinomatosis often results in acute arachnoiditis, manifested by headache, fever, back pain, nausea, and vomiting. Although this entity is associated with MTX use in 50% of cases, it may occur with other IT chemotherapy, and lasts 1–2 d *(2)*. Symptoms spontaneously resolve, and are reduced by corticosteroids. Although steroids have commonly been used in parenchymal metastasis, they reduce the inflammation associated with metastatic carcinoma to the meninges. Dosing is usually 16 mg/d, rapidly tapered to 4 mg/d, until symptoms resolve, then the steroids are discontinued *(96–98)*. Delayed neurologic toxicity may present as a myelopathy or encephalopathy *(14,18,41,43,99)*.

Myelosuppression is a common toxicity related to concurrent systemic chemotherapy administration, RT, and IT chemotherapy *(18,43,76)*. Citrate leucovorin is often used to reduce the incidence of myelosuppression and mucosis associated with MTX *(17,41)*.

Narcotizing leukoencephalopathy presents from 3–15 mo after treatment, and is a serious complication associated with the combination of whole-brain radiation and IT chemotherapy *(2)*. All IT agents can contribute to this toxicity. Leukoencephalopathy may occur in as many as 60% of treated patients, and does not appear to be related to CNS tumor load, or CSF drug level *(70,79,99)*. CT scans demonstrate periventricular hypodensities *(14,18)*. Pathologically, there is multifocal necrosis, demyelination, and axonal swelling of the cerebral periventricular white matter *(41,99)*. The clinical presentation can mimic progressive disease, which makes the diagnosis of treatment-related toxicity difficult. Rarely, blindness, coma, and death may occur from treatment *(100)*.

6. CONCLUSIONS

Leptomeningeal carcinomatosis from metastatic breast cancer is associated with a rapidly progressive decline of the patient. In the past, systemic metastasis was the major cause of tumor-related deaths; however, the advent of more aggressive forms of systemic treatment has resulted in more patients dying of CNS involvement. The current treatment recommendations for LM include whole-brain radiation and insertion of an Ommaya reservoir for the administration of IT chemotherapy. Single-agent MTX is the commonly used agent. Future research should focus on producing less toxic and more effective regional chemotherapy for the treatment of metastatic breast cancer to the leptomeninges.

REFERENCES

1. Grossman S and Moynihan T. Neoplastic meningitis, *Neurol. Clin.,* **9** (1991) 843–856.
2. Wasserstrom W, Glass J, and Posner J. Diagnosis and treatment of leptomeningeal metastases from solid tumors: experience with 90 patients, *Cancer,* **49** (1982) 759–772.
3. Little J, Dale A, and Okazaki H. Meningeal carcinomatosis, *Arch. Neurol.,* **30** (1974) 138–143.
4. Olson M, Chernik N, and Posner J. Infiltration of the leptomeninges by systemic cancer, *Arch. Neurol.,* **30** (1974) 122–137.
5. Theodore W and Gendelman S. Meningeal carcinomatosis, *Arch. Neurol.,* **38** (1981) 696–699.
6. Lamovec J and Zidar A. Association of leptomeningeal carcinomatosis in carcinoma of the breast with infiltrating lobular carcinoma, *Arch. Pathol. Lab. Med.,* **115** (1991) 507–510.
7. Dixon A, Ellis I, Elston C, and Blamey R. Comparison of the clinical metastatic patterns of invasive lobular and ductal carcinomas of the breast, *Br. J. Cancer,* **63** (1991) 634–635.
8. Patahaphan V, Salazar O, and Riscon R. Breast cancer: metastatic patterns and their prognosis, *South. Med. J.,* **81** (1988) 1109–1112.
9. Yap H, Yap B, Tashima C, DiStefano A, and Blumenschein G. Meningeal carcinomatosis in breast cancer, *Cancer,* **42** (1978) 283–286.
10. Sparrow G and Rubens R. Brain metastases from breast cancer: clinical course, prognosis and influence of treatment, *Clin. Oncol.,* **7** (1981) 291–301.
11. Carty N, Foggitt A, Hamilton C, Royle G, and Taylor I. Patterns of clinical metastasis in breast cancer: an analysis of 100 patients, *Eur. J. Surg. Oncol.,* **21** (1995) 607–608.
12. Forman A. Leptomeningeal carcinomatosis, *Am. J. Clin. Oncol.,* **13** (1990) 536–540.
13. Clamon G and Doebbeling B. Meningeal carcinomatosis from breast cancer: spinal cord vs. brain involvement, *Breast Cancer Res. Treat.,* **9** (1987) 213–217.
14. Boogerd W, Hart A, van der Sande J, and Engelsman E. Meningeal carcinomatosis in breast cancer, *Cancer,* **67** (1991) 1685–1695.
15. Smith D, Howell A, Harris M, Bramwell V, and Sellwood R. Carcinomatous meningitis associated with infiltrating lobular carcinoma of the breast, *Eur. J. Surg. Oncol.,* **11** (1985) 33–36.
16. Jayson G, Howell A, Harris M, Morgenstern G, Chang J, and Ryder W. Carcinomatous meningitis in patients with breast cancer, *Cancer,* **74** (1994) 3135–3141.
17. Pfeffer M, Wygoda M, and Siegal T. Leptomeningeal metastases: treatment results in 98 consecutive patients, *Isr. J. Med. Sci.,* **24** (1988) 611–618.
18. Ongerboer de Visser B, Somers R, Nooyen W, van Heerde P, Hart A, and McVie G. Intraventricular methotrexate therapy of leptomeningeal metastasis from breast carcinoma, *Neurology,* **33** (1983) 1565–1572.
19. Moots P, Harrison M, and Vandenberg S. Prolonged survival in carcinamatous meningitis associated with breast cancer, *South. Med. J.,* **88** (1995) 357–362.
20. DiStefano A, Yap Y, Hortobagyi G, and Blumenschein G. Natural history of breast cancer patients with brain metastases, *Cancer,* **44** (1979) 1913–1918.
21. Kamby C, Vestley P, and Mouridsen H. Site-specific effect of chemotherapy in patients with breast cancer, *Acta. Oncol.,* **31** (1992) 225–229.
22. Gasecki A, Bashir R, and Foley J. Leptomeningeal carcinomatosis: a report of 3 cases and review of the literature, *Eur. Neurol.,* **32** (1992) 74–78.
23. Jayson G and Howell A. Carcinomatous meningitis in solid tumors, *Ann. Oncol.,* **7** (1996) 773–786.
24. Boogerd W. Central nervous system metastasis in breast cancer, *Radiother. Oncol.,* **40** (1996) 5–22.
25. Kokkoris C. Leptomeningeal carcinomatosis: how does cancer reach the pia-arachnoid?, *Cancer,* **51** (1983) 154–160.
26. Patchell R. Treatment of brain metastases, Cancer Invest., **14** (1996) 169–177.
27. Leggett C. Metastases from carcinoma of the breast involving the ventral nervous system, *Aust. NZ. J. Surg.,* **59** (1989) 235–242.
28. Kiricuta I, Kölbl ?, Willner J, and Bohndorf W. Central nervous system metastases in breast cancer, *J. Cancer Res. Clin. Oncol.,* **118** (1992) 542–546.
29. Flowers A and Levin V. Management of brain metastases from breast carcinoma, *Oncology,* **7** (1993) 21–33.

30. Sagar S and Price K. Experimental model of leptomeningeal metastases employing rat mammary carcinoma cells, *J. Neuro-Oncol.,* **23** (1995) 15–21.

31. Schabet M, Kloeter I, Adam T, Heidemann E, and Wiethölter H. Diagnosis and treatment of meningeal carcinomatosis in ten patients with breast cancer, *Eur. Neurol.,* **25** (1986) 403–411.

32. Siegal T, Mildworf B, Stein D, and Melamed E. Leptomeningeal metastases: reduction in regional cerebral blood flow and cognitive impairment, *Ann. Neurol.,* **17** (1985) 100–102.

33. Glass J, Melamed M, Chernik N, and Posner J. Malignant cells in cerebrospinal fluid (CSF): the meaning of a positive CSF cytology, *Neurology,* **29** (1979) 1369–1375.

34. Galassi G, Zonari P, Artusi T, et al. Leptomeningeal carcinomatosis presenting as progressive multineuritis: clinical, pathologic and MRI study, *Clin. Neuropathol.,* **15** (1996) 159–162.

35. Rogers L, Duchesneau P, Nunez C, et al. Comparison of cisternal and lumbar CSF examination in leptomeningeal metastasis, *Neurology,* **42** (1992) 1239–1241.

36. Oschmann P, Kaps V, Völker K, and Dorndorf W. Meningeal carcinomatosis: CSF cytology, immuno-cytochemistry and biochemical tumor markers, *Acta. Neurol. Scand.,* **89** (1994) 395–399.

37. Bach F, Bach F, Pedersen A, Larsen P, and Dombernowsky P. Creatine Kinase-BB in the cerebrospinal fluid as a marker of CNS metastases and leptomeningeal carcinomatosis in patients with breast cancer, *Eur. J. Cancer Clin. Oncol.,* **25** (1989) 1703–1709.

38. Bach F, Bjerregaard B, Sölétormos G, Bach F, and Horn T. Diagnostic value of cerebrospinal fluid cytology in comparison with tumor marker activity in central nervous system metastases secondary to breast cancer, *Cancer,* **72** (1993) 2376–2382.

39. Freilich R, Krol G, and DeAngelis L. Neuroimaging and cerebrospinal fluid cytology in the diagnosis of leptomeningeal metastasis, *Ann. Neurol.,* **38** (1995) 51–57.

40. Chamberlain M, Sandy A, and Press G. Leptomeningeal metastasis: a comparison of gadolinium-enhanced MR and contrast-enhanced CT of the brain, *Neurology,* **40** (1990) 435–438.

41. Sculier J. Treatment of meningeal carcinomatosis, *Cancer Treat. Rev.,* **12** (1985) 95–104.

42. Shapiro W, Posner J, Ushio Y, Chernik N, and Young D. Treatment of meningeal neoplasms, *Cancer Treat. Rep.,* **61** (1997) 733–743.

43. Hitchins R, Bell D, Woods R, and Levi J. Prospective randomized trial of single-agent versus combination chemotherapy in meningeal carcinomatosis, *J. Clin. Oncol.,* **5** (1987) 1655–1662.

44. Grant R, Naylor B, Greenberg H, and Junck L. Clinical outcome in aggressively treated meningeal carcinomatosis, *Arch. Neurol.,* **51** (1994) 457–461.

45. Boogerd W, van den Bent MJ, Koehler P, Haaxma-Relche H, de Visser M, and Tijssen C. Relevance of intraventricular treatment of meningeal carcinomatosis from breast cancer, *J. Neuro-Oncol.,* **21** (1994) 56.

46. Grossman S, Finkelstein D, Ruckdeschel J, et al. Randomized prospective comparison of intraventricular methotrexate and thiotepa in patients with previously untreated neoplastic meningitis, *J. Clin. Oncol.,* **11** (1993) 561–569.

47. Greig N. Optimizing drug delivery to brain tumors, Cancer Treat. Rev., **14** (1987) 1–28.

48. Ushio Y, Shimizu K, Aragaki Y, Aria N, Hayakawa T, and Mogami H. Alteration of blood–CSF barrier by tumor invasion into the meninges, *J. Neurosurg,* **55** (1981) 445–449.

49. Freilich R, Seidman A, and DeAngelis L. Central nervous system progression of metastatic breast cancer in patients treated with paclitaxel, *Cancer,* **76** (1995) 232–236.

50. Boogerd W, Dalesio O, Bais E, and van der Sande J. Response of brain metastases from breast cancer to systemic chemotherapy, *Cancer,* **69** (1992) 972–980.

51. Dethy S, Piccart M, Paesmans M, van Houtte P, and Klastersky J. History of brain and epidural metastases from breast cancer in relation with the disease evolution outside the central nervous system, *Eur. Neurol.,* **35** (1995) 38–42.

52. Ushio Y, Posner J, and Shapiro W. Chemotherapy of experimental meningeal carcinomatosis, *Cancer Res.,* **37** (1997) 1232–1237.

53. Rosner D, Nemoto T, and Lane W. Chemotherapy induces regression of brain metastases in breast carcinoma, *Cancer,* **58** (1986) 832–839.

54. Hug V and Horg. G. Mitomycin for treatment of brain parenchymal disease, *J. Clin. Oncol.,* **6** (1988) 1787.

55. Kaba S, Kyritsis A, Hess K, et al. TPDC-FuHu chemotherapy for the treatment of recurrent metastatic brain tumors, *J. Clin. Oncol.,* **15** (1997) 1063–1070.

56. Lange O, Scheef W, and Haase K. Palliative radio-chemotherapy with ifosfamide and BCNU for breast cancer patients with cerebral metastases, *Cancer Chemother. Pharmacol.,* **26** (1990) S78–S80.

57. Colleoni M, Graiff C, Nelli P, et al. Activity of combination chemotherapy in brain metastases from breast and lung adenocarcinoma, *Am. J. Clin. Oncol.,* **20** (1997) 303–307.

58. Galicich J and Guido L. Ommaya device in carcinomatous and leukemic meningitis, *Surg. Clin. North Am.,* **54** (1974) 915–922.

59. Chamberlain M and Corey-Bloom J. Leptomeningeal metastases: [111]Indium-DTPA CSF flow studies, *Neurology,* **41** (1991) 1765–1769.

60. Berk L. Overview of radiotherapy trials for the treatment of brain metastases, *Oncology,* **9** (1995) 1205–1219.

61. Shapiro W, Young D, and Mehta B. Methotrexate: distribution in cerebrospinal fluid after intravenous ventricular and lumbar injections, *N. Engl. J. Med.,* **293** (1975) 161–166.

62. Nabors M, Grossman S, Burch P, and Eller S. Concentrations of chemotherapeutic agents in brain following lumbar and ventricular administration, *Proc. ASCO,* **8** (1989) 94.

63. Grossman S, Trump D, Chen D, Thompson P, and Camargo E. Cerebrospinal fluid flow abnormalities in patients with neoplastic meningitis, *Am. J. Med.,* **73** (1982) 641–647.

64. Miller K and Wilkinson D. Pharmacokinetics of methotrexate in the cerebrospinal fluid after intracerebroventricular administration in patients with meningeal carcinomatosis and altered cerebrospinal fluid flow dynamics, *Ther. Drug Monitoring,* **11** (1989) 231–237.

65. Burch P, Grossman S, and Reinhard C. Spinal cord penetration of intrathecally administered cytarabine and methotrexate: a quantitative autoradiographic study, *J. Natl. Cancer Inst.,* **80** (1988) 1211–1216.

66. Boogerd W, van der Sande J, and Kröger R. Early diagnosis and treatment of spinal epidural metastasis in breast cancer: a prospective study, *J. Neurol. Neurosurg. Psychiatry,* **55** (1992) 1188–1193.

67. Lishner M, Perrin R, Feld R, et al. Complications associated with ommaya reservoirs in patients with cancer, *Arch. Intern. Med.,* **150** (1990) 173–176.

68. de Waal R, Algra P, Heimans J, Wolbers J, and Scheltens. Methotrexate induced brain necrosis and severe leukoencephalopathy due to disconnection of an ommaya device, *J. Neuro-Oncol.,* **15** (1993) 269–273.

69. Mehta B, Glass J, and Shapiro W. Serum and cerebrospinal fluid distribution of 5-methyltetrahydrofolate after intravenous calcium leucovorin and intra-ommaya methotexate administration in patients with meningeal carcinomatosis, *Cancer Res.,* **43** (1983) 435–438.

70. Siegal T, Lossos A, and Pfeffer M. Leptomeningeal metastases: analysis of 31 patients with sustained off-therapy response following combined-modality therapy, *Neurology,* **44** (1994) 1463–1469.

71. Bleyer W. Clinical pharmacology of intrathecal methotrexate. II. An improved dosage regimen derived from age-related pharmacokinetics, *Cancer Treat. Rep.,* **61** (1977) 1419–1425.

72. Bleyer W, Poplack D, Simon R, et al. "Concentration × Time" methotrexate via a subcutaneous reservoir: a less toxic regimen for intraventricular chemotherapy of central nervous system neoplasms, *Blood,* **51** (1978) 835–842.

73. Fizazi K, Asselain B, Vincent-Salomon A, et al. Meningeal carcinomatosis in patients with breast carcinoma, *Cancer,* **77** (1996) 1315–1323.

74. Sause W, Crowley J, Eyre H, et al. Whole brain irradiation and intrathecal methotrexate in the treatment of solid tumor leptomeningeal metastases: a southwest oncology group study, *J. Neuro-Oncol,* **6** (1988) 107–112.

75. Trump D, Grossman S, Thompson G, Murray K, and Wharam M. Treatment of neoplastic meningitis with intraventricular thiotepa and methotrexate, *Cancer Treat. Rep.,* **66** (1982) 1549–1551.

76. Giannone L, Greco F, and Hainsworth J. Combination intraventricular chemotherapy for meningeal neoplasia, *J. Clin. Oncol.,* **4** (1986) 68–73.

77. Stewart D, Maroun J, Hugenholtz, et al. Combined intraommaya methotrexate, cytosine arabinoside, hydrocortisone and thiotepa form meningeal involvement by malignancies, *J. Neurooncol.,* **5** (1987) 315–322.

78. Gutin P, Weiss H, Wiernik P, and Walker M. Intrathecal N, N′, N″-triethylenethiophosphoramide [Thio-tepa (NSC 6396)] in the treatment of malignant meningeal disease, phase I–II study, *Cancer,* **38** (1976) 1471–1475.

79. Gutin P, Levi J, Wiernik P, and Walker M. Treatment of malignant meningeal disease with intrathecal thiotepa: a phase II study, *Cancer Treat. Rep.,* **61** (1977) 885–887.

80. Chamberlain M, Khatibi S, Kim J, Howell S, Chatelut E, and Kim S. Treatment of leptomeningeal metastasis with intraventricular administration of depot cytarabine (DTC 101), *Arch. Neurol.,* **50** (1993) 261–264.

81. Kim S, Chatelut E, Kim J, et al. Extended CSF cytarabine exposure following intrathecal administration of DTC 101, *J. Clin. Oncol.,* **11** (1993) 2186–2193.

82. Chamberlain M, Kormanik P, Howell S, and Kim S. Pharmacokinetics of intralumbar DTC-101 for the treatment of leptomeningeal metastases, *Arch. Neurol., 52* (1995) 912–917.

83. Berg S, Balis F, Zimm S, et al. Phase I/II trial and pharmacokinetics of intrathecal diaziquone in refractory meningeal malignancies, *J. Clin. Oncol., 10* (1992) 143–148.

84. Levin V, Chamberlain M, Silver P, Rodriguez L, and Prados M. Phase I/II study of intraventricular and intrathecal ACNU for leptomeningeal neoplasia, *Cancer Chemother. Pharmacol., 23* (1989) 301–307.

85. Benjamin J, Moss T, Moseley R, Maxwell R, and Coakham H. Cerebral distribution of immunoconjugate after treatment for neoplastic meningitis using an intrathecal radiolabeled monoclonal antibody, *Neurosurgery, 25* (1989) 253–258.

86. Lashford L, Davies G, Richardson R, et al. Pilot study of ^{131}I monoclonal antibodies in the therapy of leptomeningeal tumors, *Cancer, 61* (1988) 857–868.

87. Moseley R, Benjamin J, Ashpole R, et al. Carcinomatous meningitis: antibody-guided therapy with I-131 HMFG1, *J. Neurol. Neurosurg. Psychiatry, 54* (1991) 260–265.

88. Lien E, Wester K, Lonning P, Solheim E, and Ueland P. Distribution of tamoxifen and metabolites into brain tissue and brain metastases in breast cancer patients, *Br. J. Cancer, 64* (1991) 641–645.

89. Carey R, Davis J, and Zervas T. Tamoxifen-induced regression of cerebral metastases in breast carcinoma, *Cancer Treat. Rep., 65* (1981) 793–795.

90. Salvati M, Cervoni L, Innocenzi G, and Bardella L. Prolonged stabilization of multiple and single brain metastases from breast cancer with tamoxifen. Report of three cases, *Tumori, 79* (1993) 359–362.

91. Hansen S, Galsgard H, von Eyben F, Westergaard-Nielsen V, and Wolf-Jensen J. Tamoxifen for brain metastases from breast cancer, *Ann. Neurol., 20* (1986) 544.

92. Colomer R, Casas D, Del Campo J, Boada M, Rubio D, and Salvador L. Brain metastases from breast cancer may respond to endocrine therapy, *Breast Cancer Res. Treat., 12* (1988) 83–86.

93. van der Gaast A, Alexieva-Figusch J, Vecht C, Verweij J, and Stoter G. Complete remission of a brain metastasis to third-line hormonal treatment with megestrol acetate, *Am. J. Clin. Oncol., 13* (1990) 507–509.

94. Pors H, von Eyben F, Sorenson O, and Larsen M. Long-term remission of multiple brain metastases with tamoxifen. *10* (1991) 173–177.

95. Steward D and Dahrouge S. Response of brain metastases from breast cancer to megestrol acetate: a case report, *J. Neuro-Oncol., 24* (1995) 299–301.

96. Sorensen P, Helweg-Larsen S, Mouridsen H, and Hansen H. Effect of high-dose dexamethasone in carcinomatous metastatic spinal cord compression treated with radiotherapy: a randomised trial, *Eur. J. Cancer, 30A* (1994) 22–27.

97. Vecht C, Hovestadt A, Verbiest H, van Vliet J, and Van Putten W. Dose-effect relationship of dexamethasone on Karnofsky performance in metastatic brain tumors: a randomized study of doses of 4, 8, and 16 mg per day, *Neurology, 44* (1994) 675–680.

98. DeAngelis L. Management of brain metastases, *Cancer Invest., 12* (1994) 156–165.

99. Boogerd W, van der Sande J, and Moffie D. Acute fever and delayed leukoencephalopathy following low dose intraventricular methotrexate, *J. Neurol. Neurosurg. Psychiatry, 51* (1988) 1277–1283.

100. Boogerd W, Moffie D, and Smets L. Early blindness and coma during intrathecal chemotherapy for meningeal carcinomatosis, *Cancer, 65* (1990) 452–457.

21 Regional Chemotherapy for Treatment and Prophylaxis of Meningeal Lymphoma

Brad Pohlman

CONTENTS

SECONDARY CENTRAL NERVOUS SYSTEM LYMPHOMA
PRIMARY CENTRAL NERVOUS SYSTEM LYMPHOMA
REFERENCES

1. SECONDARY CENTRAL NERVOUS SYSTEM LYMPHOMA

Secondary central nervous system lymphoma (SCNSL) refers to lymphoma that initially involves the lymph nodes and, occasionally, extranodal sites, and only subsequently disseminates to the central nervous system (CNS). Many studies have reported the incidence of CNS involvement in patients with non-Hodgkin's lymphoma (1–6). Critical review of these early series is limited by the inclusion of all lymphoma histologies, the discrepancies between old and new lymphoma classifications, the lack of modern imaging modalities, the inclusion of patients with epidural involvement, and the inclusion of patients who received a variety of, and often substandard, chemotherapy regimens. In these large series of unselected patients with non-Hodgkin's lymphoma, approx 5–11% of patients had CNS involvement. Incidence was very low in patients with follicular center, small lymphocytic, and other indolent lymphomas, but incidence was relatively high in patients with diffuse histology, (especially lymphoblastic and Burkitt's lymphoma), young age, poor performance status, more advanced-stage disease, and extranodal involvement (1–7).

SCNSL may occur at any time in the course of the disease (1,2,4,6–9). CNS involvement at the time of diagnosis, and as a first manifestation of relapse, is very uncommon (and often heralds systemic relapse). SCNSL most often occurs in the setting of progressive systemic disease. Patients may be asymptomatic (especially when CNS involvement is present at the time of initial diagnosis). The most common manifestations, however, are headache, altered mental status, and sign/symptoms attributable to cranial nerve and/or spinal nerve root involvement. The diagnosis of SCNSL may be suspected, based on symptoms, neurologic findings, and/or imaging studies, but a definitive diagnosis is made by identifying malignant cells in the cerebral spinal fluid (CSF) and/or brain biopsy. Although neurologic findings and imaging studies may suggest that CNS

From: *Current Clinical Oncology: Regional Chemotherapy: Clinical Research and Practice*
Edited by: M. Markman © Humana Press Inc., Totowa, NJ

involvement is localized, the finding of malignant cells within the CSF, in up to 90% of patients and autopsies that demonstrate multiple sites of leptomeningeal involvement, prove the disseminated nature of this disease (2).

Treatment and prophylaxis of SCNSL has evolved over the past several decades. Most chemotherapy agents that are active in the treatment of lymphoma do not effectively cross the blood–brain barrier. Consequently, therapeutic levels of these drugs cannot be achieved within the CNS by a parenteral route. Intrathecal (IT) administration avoids this obstacle, and theoretically permits higher, potentially therapeutic levels within the CNS. Initially, IT chemotherapy was administered alone; subsequently, systemic chemotherapy (with drugs that cross the blood–brain barrier) has been administered concurrently. In patients with lymphoma, methotrexate (MTX) and cytarabine have been almost the only drugs administered intrathecally.

IT chemotherapy may be administered by lumbar puncture, or directly into the ventricles via an Ommaya reservoir. Intraventricular administration is more convenient and more reliable. Studies have shown that intraventricular administration of MTX provides more consistent distribution within the CSF, and higher concentrations within the ventricles, compared to the lumbar approach (10). However, intraventricular administration has not been proven more effective for either the prophylaxis or treatment of SCNSL than administration by lumbar puncture. The highest and most sustained levels of MTX within the CSF are achieved when the drug is administered intravenously at high doses (with leucovorin rescue), and is then followed by intraventricular administration (11,12). Cytarabine is another drug frequently administered intrathecally for the treatment of SCNSL. Because the CSF has very low levels of the enzyme, cytidine deaminase, cytarabine is not effectively converted to its inactive metabolite; therefore, the CSF level of cytarabine remains above the minimum cytotoxic concentration for 24 h (13).

In various studies, the MTX dose is 6.25–12.5 mg/m^2 (maximum 12–15 mg). MTX is often the only or primary IT drug administered. In more recent studies, cytarabine is also administered either simultaneously or separately. The cytarabine dose is 30–50 mg/m^2. For prophylaxis, these drugs are usually administered 1–3× (maximum of twice weekly) during each cycle or phase of treatment, for a total 5–20 doses. For treatment, these drugs are often administered twice weekly, until malignant cells are no longer present in the CSF. The frequency of administration is decreased to a weekly, and then a monthly, schedule, for a total of 6–12 mo. The optimal schedule for either prophylaxis or treatment is unknown.

Patients treated with IT chemotherapy may develop acute or chronic neurologic complications. MTX may cause an acute chemical arachnoiditis; a subacute neurotoxicity, characterized by motor paralysis, cranial nerve palsies, seizure, and/or coma; and a chronic necrotizing leukoencephalopathy. The risk of these complications may be increased in patients who receive frequent IT injections, concurrent high-dose systemic MTX, and prior or concurrent radiation therapy (RT). Because MTX levels are higher and more sustained in patients with leptomeningeal disease, the risk of complication is higher in patients receiving therapeutic, as opposed to prophylactic, administration (14,15). Cytarabine may also cause arachnoiditis, and, infrequently, myelopathy and necrotizing leukoencephalopathy. These latter complications are more common in patients receiving other intensive CNS therapies (13).

The prognosis for patients with SCNSL is dependent on a number of factors (1,2,4, 6–9): In most studies, the best prognosis is observed in patients with CNS involvement at the time of diagnosis; patients with isolated CNS relapse have an intermediate prognosis; and those patients with progressive systemic disease have the worse prognosis. Some studies suggest that combined modality treatment, which includes high-dose systemic IT chemotherapy, with RT to sites of bulky parenchymal or subarachnoid disease, is superior to IT chemotherapy alone. With treatment, the majority of patients demonstrate clinical improvement or stabilization. Nevertheless, the median survival is only 2–10 mo, with <25% of patients alive at 1 yr. CNS disease is the sole cause of death in only a minority of patients. Most patients succumb to progressive systemic lymphoma.

1.1. Burkitt's Lymphoma

Burkitt's lymphoma is an highly aggressive B-cell malignancy that occurs primarily in children and young adults. The disease is characterized by rapid tumor growth and early dissemination to bone marrow and CNS. All pediatric (and most adult) protocols include CNS prophylaxis. The first successful treatment of Burkitt's lymphoma was in children. In these early studies *(15)*, CNS prophylaxis consisted of IT chemotherapy and cranial irradiation; isolated CNS relapse rates were as high as 15% *(15)*. With the addition of high-dose systemic chemotherapy, several studies *(16–19)* showed that cranial irradiation was not necessary. In most of these studies, patients received several cycles of high-dose MTX and multiple injections of IT MTX and cytarabine. Isolated CNS relapse occurred in 1–3% of patients. At least one study *(20)* has suggested that high-dose MTX alone, without concurrent IT MTX, is inadequate CNS prophylaxis. When these same principles have been applied to the treatment of adults with Burkitt's lymphoma, the incidence of isolated CNS relapse has been similar to pediatric studies *(22,23)*. Patients with CNS involvement at diagnosis have a worse prognosis than those without CNS involvement *(22,24,25)*. These patients usually have other poor prognostic features as well, e.g., elevated lactic dehydrogenase, higher tumor burden, and bone marrow and other extranodal involvement, which may explain their worse prognosis *(24)*. Nevertheless, CNS involvement at diagnosis does not preclude the possibility of long-term, disease-free survival. In fact, 10–67% of these patients may be cured *(16,19,20,22,24)*. The highest success rates appear to be in patients who receive high-dose MTX, high-dose cytarabine, and triple IT chemotherapy (MTX, cytarabine, and hydrocortisone), with or without cranial irradiation *(19,22)*. Similarly, patients with isolated CNS relapse may also be cured *(20,24)*. In contrast, patients with both CNS and systemic relapse have a poor prognosis.

1.2. Lymphoblastic Lymphoma

T-cell lymphoblastic lymphoma (LBL) accounts for approx 30% of childhood lymphoma, and is rare in adults. This disease shares many clinical and biologic features with T-cell acute lymphoblastic leukemia (ALL). The distinction between T-cell LBL and T-cell ALL is arbitrary and many centers now treat these patients identically. SCNSL is uncommon at presentation, but is likely to occur early if CNS prophylaxis is not given. In early studies, CNS prophylaxis consisted of IT MTX and cranial irradiation. More recent studies have included high-dose MTX, with leucovorin rescue, and reserved cranial irradiation for a minority of patients with documented CNS involvement. Because of late relapses, patients generally receive prolonged maintenance systemic and IT therapy. With all these approaches, only 0–3% of patients experience an isolated CNS relapse *(26–31)*. Even with CNS involvement at diagnosis, 30–90% of patients may be long-term survivors *(28,31)*.

1.3. Large-Cell Lymphoma

Large-cell lymphoma is a heterogeneous group of lymphoid neoplasms with a broad range of manifestations. The risk of CNS involvement is very low. Nevertheless, the identification of a subset of patients at increased risk of CNS relapse may allow the administration of CNS prophylaxis. Two recent analyses *(32,33)* determined the risk of leptomeningeal and/or parenchymal CNS relapse in patients with large-cell lymphoma who received modern, doxorubicin-based, combination chemotherapy, and no CNS prophylaxis. In both series, 4% of patients relapsed in the CNS (the majority with leptomeningeal involvement, but some with only parenchymal involvement). Isolated CNS relapse was rare, occurring in <1% of patients. CNS relapse occurred at a median of 6 mo (range 1–44 mo) after diagnosis. Most patients developed either simultaneous CNS and systemic relapse, or developed systemic relapse within 6 mo of CNS relapse. In one study *(30)*, a higher (although not statistically significant) CNS relapse rate was noted in patients with more advanced-stage disease and/or more than one extranodal sites. In the other study *(33)*, multivariate analysis showed that an elevated LDH and involvement of more than one extranodal site at diagnosis were both associated with a statistically significant increased risk of CNS recurrence. Among the 93 patients with both of these risk factors, the risk of CNS recurrence with 1 yr of diagnosis was 17.4%, compared to 2.8% among patients with no risk factors. Based on these studies, patients with newly diagnosed large-cell lymphoma and high-risk features (elevated LDH and more than one extranodal site) may have an especially high risk of CNS relapse, and, therefore, may benefit from CNS prophylaxis. Some authors *(2,34–36)* have noted a significant risk of CNS relapse, and a potential role for CNS prophylaxis in patients with large-cell lymphoma involving specific extranodal sites, e.g., testes, paranasal sinus, and epidural space; others have not *(37–39)*. Consequently, the indications for CNS prophylaxis in patients with large-cell lymphoma must be individualized. Whether CNS prophylaxis in high-risk patients with large-cell lymphoma reduces the incidence of CNS relapse or improves overall survival is unknown.

Data for patients with secondary CNS large-cell lymphoma, either at diagnosis or relapse, who have received modern anthracycline-based induction chemotherapy or salvage chemotherapy, is limited. Treatment of CNS disease in most patients has included IT chemotherapy and/or RT to the brain, and, less often, to sites of gross disease along the vertebral axis. In one recent study *(32)*, three patients presented with CNS involvement at diagnosis: One received IT chemotherapy alone, and two received IT chemotherapy and whole-brain RT. Only one remains disease-free at 26 mo. Nine patients with CNS disease at relapse received RT and IT and/or systemic chemotherapy. The median survival of this group was 7 mo from diagnosis, and 2 mo from the time of CNS relapse. Most patients died from progression of systemic lymphoma.

In another series *(33)*, six patients with leptomeningeal involvement, but no focal neurologic deficits, received IT MTX, cytarabine, and hydrocortisone twice a week–usually via an Ommaya reservoir. Although CSF cytology improved, only one patient experienced symptomatic improvement. Nine patients with focal neurologic deficits, or intraparenchymal lesions in the brain or spinal cord, received only RT to the whole brain and/or involved spinal cord. Six had symptomatic, although transient, responses. The principal cause of treatment failure was progression of CNS disease in five, and systemic disease in four. Five other patients received systemic chemotherapy (DHAP [dexamethasone, cytarabine, and cisplatin]/EHSAP [etoposide, methyl prednisolone, cytarabine and cisplatin] in four, MINE [mitoxantrone, ifosfamide with mesna, and etoposide] in one) combined, in two, with IT treatment. Three patients had CNS responses, and one has a durable remission. Of the 24 patients, only one is currently alive and in remission 1150 d after CNS recurrence. Median survival after CNS recurrence was only 88 d and the probability of survival at 1 yr after diagnosis of CNS recurrence was 25% *(33)*. Again, the treatment of these patients must be individualized, and the optimal therapy is unknown.

1.4. Hodgkin's Disease

CNS involvement by Hodgkin's disease is rare, and usually occurs in patients with progressive systemic disease; however, parenchymal lesions and/or leptomeningeal spread as an isolated site of relapse have been reported *(40,41)*. A few of these patients have been long-term survivors. Treatment has included primarily cranial radiation, chemotherapy directed against systemic disease, and, infrequently, IT chemotherapy. Because of the rarity of this situation, the role of IT chemotherapy cannot be assessed.

2. PRIMARY CENTRAL NERVOUS SYSTEM LYMPHOMA

Primary central nervous system lymphoma (PCNSL) is an uncommon type of extra-nodal lymphoma that involves the brain, eyes, spinal cord, and/or leptomeninges. The pathology is almost always diffuse large B-cell or Burkitt's/Burkitt's-like lymphoma. PCNSL is more common in immunodeficient patients, e.g., congenital immunodeficiency syndromes, HIV+ (AIDS), and organ transplants. By definition, systemic involvement is not part of the initial presentation, and is rare, even with disease progression. The majority of patients present with multifocal parenchymal brain lesions. Malignant cells are identified in the CSF in only 10–25% of patients at diagnosis, yet the leptomeninges are involved at autopsy in nearly all patients. Patients who receive conventional treatment with steroids and RT have a median survival of less than 2 yr and less than 5% are alive at 5 yr. Patients with AIDS have a significantly worse prognosis, and are often not candidates for any therapy but radiation.

Because PCNSL is disseminated throughout the CNS at diagnosis, and relapses occur within the CNS, often at sites remote from the original tumor, a number of investigators have added systemic chemotherapy to RT in an attempt to more effectively treat disseminated disease. At least two studies have also incorporated IT chemotherapy into a multimodality regimen. DeAngelis et al. *(42)* prospectively treated 31 patients with a regimen that included dexamethasone, high-dose MTX, intra-Ommaya MTX, then whole-brain RT, and, finally, high-dose cytarabine. Sixty-four percent of patients responded to MTX prior to initiation of RT. The median survival of these patients was 42.5 mo. Blay et al. *(43)* treated 25 patients with a complex, 3-mo combination chemotherapy regimen, including intravenous cyclophosphamide, vincristine, doxorubicin, cytarabine, high-dose MTX, and IT MTX, and cytarabine, followed by whole-brain RT *(43)*. Seventy percent of patients responded prior to RT. With a median follow-up of 24 mo, the projected 2- and 5-yr overall survivals are 70 and 56%, respectively. No patient in either series experienced acute neurologic toxicity. In one study, delayed dementia and ataxia occurred in 10% of patients *(42)*. Whether the IT administration of chemotherapy used in these two series contributed to the apparent improved survival of these patients is unclear.

REFERENCES

1. Herman TS, Hammond N, Jones S, et al. Involvement of the central nervous system by non-Hodgkin's lymphoma: the Southwest Oncology Group experience, *Cancer,* **43** (1979) 390–397.
2. Young RC, Howser DM, Anderson T, et al. Central nervous system complications of non-Hodgkin's lymphoma: the potential role for prophylactic therapy, *Am. J. Med.,* **66** (1979) 435–443.
3. Litam J, Cabanillas F, Smith TL, et al. Central nervous system relapse in malignant lymphomas: risk factors and implications for prophylaxis, *Blood,* **54** (1979) 1249–1257.
4. Levitt LJ, Dawson DM, Rosenthal DS, and Moloney WC. CNS involvement in the non-Hodgkin's lymphomas, *Cancer,* **45** (1980) 545–552.
5. Johnson GJ, Oken M, Anderson JR, et al. Central nervous system relapse in unfavourable-histology non-Hodgkin's lymphoma: is prophylaxis indicated?, *Lancet,* **2** (1984) 685–687.
6. Mead GM, Kennedy P, Smith JL, et al. Involvement of the central nervous system by non-Hodgkin's lymphoma in adults. A review of 36 cases, *Q. J. Med.,* **60** (1986) 699–714.
7. Mackintosh FR, Colby TV, Podolsky WJ, et al. Central nervous system involvement in non-Hodgkin's lymphoma: an analysis of 105 cases, *Cancer,* **49** (1982) 586–595.
8. Recht L, Straus DJ, Cirrincione C, et al. Central nervous system metastases from non-Hodgkin's lymphoma: treatment and prophylaxis, *Am. J. Med.,* **84** (1988) 425–435.
9. Raz I, Siegal T, Siegal T, and Polliack A. CNS involvement by non-Hodgkin's lymphoma, *Arch. Neurol.,* **41** (1984) 1167–1171.
10. Shapiro WR, Young DF, and Mehta BM. Methotrexate: distribution in cerebrospinal fluid after intravenous, ventricular and lumbar injections, *N. Engl. J. Med.,* **293** (1975) 161–166.
11. Ettinger LJ, Chervinsky DS, Freeman AI, and Creaven PJ. Pharmacokinetics of methotrexate following intravenous and intraventricular administration in acute lymphocytic leukemia and non-Hodgkin's lymphoma, *Cancer,* **50** (1982) 1676–1682.
12. Magrath IT, Janus C, Edwards BK, et al. Effective therapy for both undifferentiated (including Burkitt's) lymphomas and lymphoblastic lymphomas in children and young adults, *Blood,* **63** (1984) 1102–1111.
13. Baker WJ, Royer G, and Weiss R. Cytarabine and neurologic toxicity, *J. Clin. Oncol.,* **9** (1991) 679–693.
14. Nelson RW and Frank T. Intrathecal methotrexate-induced neurotoxicities, *Am. J. Hosp. Pharm.,* **38** (1981) 65–68.
15. Philip T, Lenoir GM, Bryon PA, et al. Burkitt-type lymphoma in France among non-Hodgkin's malignant lymphomas in Caucasian children, *Br. J. Cancer,* **45** (1982) 670–678.
16. Patte C, Philip T, Rodary C, et al. Improved survival rate in children with stage III and IV B cell non-Hodgkin's lymphoma and leukemia using multi-agent chemotherapy: results of a study of 114 children from the French Pediatric Oncology Society, *J. Clin. Oncol.,* **4** (1986) 1219–1226.
17. Patte C, Philip T, Rodary C, et al. High survival rate in advanced-stage B-cell lymphomas and leukemias without CNS involvement with a short intensive polychemotherapy: results from the French Pediatric Oncology Society of a randomized trail of 216 children, *J. Clin. Oncol.,* **9** (1991) 123–132.
18. Mandell LR, Wollner N, and Fuks Z. Is cranial radiation necessary for CNS prophylaxis in pediatric NHL?, *Int. J. Rad. Oncol. Biol. Phys.,* **13** (1987) 359–363.
19. Reiter A, Schrappe M, Parwaresch R, et al. Non-Hodgkin's lymphomas childhood and adolescence: results of a treatment stratified for biologic subtypes and stage. A report of the Berlin-Frankfurt-Munster Group, *J. Clin. Oncol.,* **13** (1995) 359–372.
20. Sariban E, Edwards B, Janus C, and Magrath I. Central nervous system involvement in American Burkitt's lymphoma, *J. Clin. Oncol.,* **1** (1983) 677–681.
21. Lopez TM, Hagemeister FB, McLaughlin P, et al. Small noncleaved cell lymphoma in adults: superior results for stage I–III disease, *J. Clin. Oncol.,* **4** (1990) 615–622.
22. Soussain C, Patte C, Ostronoff M, et al. Small noncleaved cell lymphoma and leukemia in adults. A retrospective study of 65 adults treated with the LMB pediatric protocols, *Blood,* **3** (1995) 664–674.
23. Magrath I, Adde M, Shad A, et al. Adults and children with small non-cleaved-cell lymphoma have a similar excellent outcome when treated with the same chemotherapy regimen, *J. Clin. Oncol.,* **14** (1996) 925–934.
24. Haddy TB, Adde MA, and Magrath IT. CNS involvement in small noncleaved-cell lymphoma: is CNS disease per se a poor prognostic sign?, *J. Clin. Oncol.,* **9** (1991) 1973–1982.
25. Anderson JR, Jenkin DT, Wilson JF, et al. Long-term follow-up of patients treated with COMP or LSA$_2$L$_2$ therapy for childhood non-Hodgkin's lymphoma: a report of CCG-551 from the Childrens Cancer Group, *J. Clin. Oncol.,* **11** (1993) 1024–1032.

26. Slater DE, Mertelsmann R, Koziner B, et al. Lymphoblastic lymphoma in adults, *J. Clin. Oncol.,* **4** (1986) 57–67.
27. Coleman CN, Picozzi VJ, Cox RS, et al. Treatment of lymphoblastic lymphoma in adults, *J. Clin. Oncol.,* **4** (1986) 1628–1637.
28. Hvizdala EV, Berard C, Callihan T, et al. Lymphoblastic lymphoma in children: A randomized trial comparing LSA$_2$-L$_2$ with the A-COP+ therapeutic regimen. A Pediatric Oncology Group study, *J. Clin. Oncol.,* **6** (1988) 26–33.
29. Patte C, Kalifa C, Flamant F, et al. Results of the LMT81 protocol, a modified LSA$_2$I$_2$ protocol with high dose methotrexate, on 84 children with non-B-cell (lymphoblastic) lymphoma, *Med. Pediatr. Oncol.,* **20** (1992) 105–113.
30. Eden OB, Hann I, Imeson J, et al. Treatment of advanced stage T-cell lymphoblastic lymphoma: results of the United Kingdom Childrens Cancer Study Group (UKCCSG) protocol 8503, *Br. J. Haematol.,* **82** (1992) 310–316.
31. Tubergen DG, Krailo MD, Meadow AT, et al. Comparison of treatment regimens for pediatric lymphoblastic non-Hodgkin's lymphoma: a Children's Cancer Group study, *J. Clin. Oncol.,* **13** (1995) 1368–1376.
32. Bashir RM, Bierman P, Vose JM, et al. Central nervous system involvement in patients with diffuse aggressive non-Hodgkin's lymphoma, *Am. J. Clin. Oncol.,* **14** (1991) 478–482.
33. van Besien K, Ha CS, Murphy S, et al. Risk factors, treatment, and outcome of central nervous system recurrence in adults with intermediate-grade and immunoblastic lymphoma, *Blood,* **91** (1998) 1178–1184.
34. Touroutoglou N, Dimopoulos MA, Younes A, et al. Testicular lymphoma: late relapse and poor outcome despite doxorubicin-based therapy, *J. Clin. Oncol.,* **13** (1995) 1361–1367.
35. Jacobs C and Hoppe RT. Non-Hodgkin's lymphomas of the head and neck extranodal sites, *Int. J. Radiat. Oncol. Biol. Phys.,* **11** (1985) 357–364.
36. Epelbaum R, Haim N, Ben-Shahar M, et al. Non-Hodgkin's lymphoma presenting with spinal epidural involvement, *Cancer,* **48** (1986) 2120–2124.
37. Connors JM, Klimo P, Voss N, et al. Testicular lymphoma: improved outcome with early brief chemotherapy, *J. Clin. Oncol.,* **6** (1988) 776–781.
38. Sutcliffe SB and Gospodarowicz MK. Primary extranodal lymphomas, In Canellos GP, Lister TA, Sklar JL (eds), *Lymphomas.* W.B. Saunders, Philadelphia (1998) pp. 449–479.
39. Rathmell AJ, Gospodarowicz MK, Sutcliffe SB, et al. Localized extradural lymphoma: survival, relapse, pattern, and functional outcome. The Princess Margaret Hospital Lymphoma Group, *Radiother. Oncol.,* **24** (1992) 14–20.
40. Sapozink MD, Kaplan HS. Intracranial Hodgkin's disease. A report of 12 cases and review of the literature, *Cancer,* **52** (1983) 1301–1307.
41. Mulligan MJ, Vasu R, Grossi CE, et al. Case report: neoplastic meningitis with eosinophilic pleocytosis in Hodgkin's disease. A case with cerebellar dysfunction and a review of the literature, *Am. J. Med. Sci.,* **296** (1988) 322–326.
42. DeAngelis LM, Yahalam J, Thaler HT, and Zher U. Combined modality therapy for primary CNS lymphoma, *J. Clin. Oncol.,* **10** (1992) 635–643.
43. Blay JY, Bouhour D, Carrie C, et al. C5R protocol: a regimen of high-dose chemotherapy and radiotherapy in primary cerebral non-Hodgkin's lymphoma of patients with no known cause of immunosuppression, *Blood,* **8** (1995) 2922–2929.

22 Regional Chemotherapy for Treatment and Prophylaxis of Meningeal Leukemia

Matt E. Kalaycio

CONTENTS

INTRODUCTION
MENINGEAL LEUKEMIA
OVERT MENINGEAL LEUKEMIA
REGIONAL CHEMOTHERAPY
FUTURE DIRECTIONS
REFERENCES

1. INTRODUCTION

Clinicians recognized the importance of the central nervous system (CNS) as a sanctuary for leukemia cells only when improved treatments began to lengthen the survival of children with acute lymphoblastic leukemia (ALL). Subsequent efforts to treat and prevent meningeal leukemia are partially responsible for the dramatic success in curing childhood ALL. Meningeal leukemia also complicates adult acute leukemia, but higher cure rates have been more elusive in adults. The efforts of early investigators have rendered overt meningeal leukemia uncommon, and recent studies of prophylactic regimens have sought to reduce toxicity, rather than to improve efficacy. However, despite effective prophylaxis, overt meningeal leukemia still occurs, and regional chemotherapy plays an important role in its management.

2. MENINGEAL LEUKEMIA

2.1. Pathogenesis

Price and Johnson *(1)*, who performed autopsy studies, provided valuable insights into the pathogenesis of meningeal leukemia, and suggested appropriate treatment strategies. They found that leukemia originates in the arachnoid blood vessels, rather than deeper CNS capillaries. How the leukemia cells gain access to the arachnoid is uncertain, but the proximity of bone marrow to the cerebrospinal fluid (CSF) suggests direct infiltration as the likely mechanism *(2)*. From their intrusion into the arachnoid, leukemia cells may penetrate the pial-glial membrane over time, and invade the underlying brain parenchyma *(1)*. Intrathecal (IT) chemotherapy does not penetrate brain

From: *Current Clinical Oncology: Regional Chemotherapy: Clinical Research and Practice*
Edited by: M. Markman © Humana Press Inc., Totowa, NJ

parenchyma. Overt meningeal leukemia, then, may not be eradicated with IT administration of chemotherapy alone. The findings of Price and Johnson strongly suggest a role for therapies capable of treating brain parenchyma, such as cranial radiation, in the management of overt meningeal leukemia.

2.2. Diagnosis

The diagnosis of meningeal leukemia may come with the onset of symptoms, or by the detection of leukemic blasts in a routine CSF sample obtained in the absence of symptoms. The most common symptoms reflect the tendency of meningeal leukemia to raise intracranial pressure. Headache and papilledema are frequently noted first, with or without associated cranial nerve palsies (3–5). Other common manifestations include nausea and vomiting, nuchal rigidity, and lethargy, but any neurologic problem in a patient with leukemia may indicate meningeal leukemia, and demands further investigation.

The CSF exam follows a diagnostic lumbar puncture. If ventricular fluid is analyzed instead, one must realize that normal brain may be present and does not necessarily point to a pathologic condition (6). Unlike carcinomatous meningitis, multiple CSF exams do not usually increase diagnostic yield. Nearly all patients will have elevated CSF, when pressure is measured by a manometer, and more than 80% will have CSF leukocytosis (7). Lower CSF glucose and elevated protein levels cannot be relied on for diagnosis. A minority of cases will have normal CSF pressure, leukocyte count, glucose, and protein levels (7). The diagnosis is best made by analyzing a cytospin preparation stained with Wright-Giemsa, which can detect as few as 10^5 leukemic cells, when interpreted by experienced observers (6).

Despite four decades of research, the diagnostic criteria for meningeal leukemia remains controversial (8). A commonly used definition requires a CSF white blood cell (WBC) count >5 mL with "morphologically unequivocal lymphoblasts from a cytocentrifuged sample" (9). There is evidence, however, that the detection of any lymphoblast in the CSF represents meningeal infiltration that requires treatment (10). A CSF sample suspicious for meningeal leukemia can be stained for tDT, or submitted for immunophenotypic analysis (11). Perhaps the easiest method, in the absence of symptoms, however, is simply to repeat the spinal tap in 1 wk, because the number of blasts will not decrease with time. Newer techniques may increase diagnostic sensitivity, but are generally less specific, and are not yet widely available (12–14).

2.3. Incidence

With the advent of effective systemic chemotherapy for childhood ALL, the incidence of overt meningeal leukemia increased to 75% (15). The high incidence suggested that meningeal involvement characterized the disease, and was present at diagnosis. These observations prompted CNS prophylaxis in treatment protocols, and promptly reduced the incidence of overt meningeal leukemia to <15% (16,17). Reflecting the poorer results with systemic chemotherapy in adults, the incidence of meningeal leukemia in adult ALL is only 32%, without, but is reduced to about 10% with, CNS prophylaxis (18,19).

Meningeal leukemia is not a characteristic feature of acute nonlymphoblastic leukemia (ANLL), but may complicate a minority of cases (20,21). ANLL, characterized by inversions or translocations of chromosome 16, and recognized morphologically as acute myelomonocytic leukemia with eosinophilia, is associated with meningeal leukemia when treated with low doses of cytarabine (22). Monocytic leukemia, especially when associated with hyperleukocytosis, may also predispose to meningeal leukemia *(23)*. Relapse rates decrease with CNS prophylaxis, but the impact of prophylaxis on survival is much less certain *(24–26)*.

Other leukemias, such as chronic lymphocytic and hairy cell leukemia, may be complicated by meningeal infiltration, but only rarely *(27–30)*. Neurological signs and symptoms are more often infectious in etiology in these more indolent leukemias.

2.4. Risk Factors

In children, higher WBC counts at diagnosis increase the risk of subsequent meningeal leukemia *(31)*. Low platelet counts and enlarged lymph nodes at diagnosis also predict for subsequent CNS relapse *(32)*. Immunophenotype may also predict for meningeal leukemia. B-cell ALL (Burkitt's lymphoma) and T-cell ALL (lymphoblastic lymphoma) both have a higher incidence of meningeal leukemia than does precursor B-cell ALL *(33–35)*.

Risk factors for meningeal leukemia in adults have not been extensively studied. In a report from M.D. Anderson Cancer Center (MDACC), 153 adult persons with ALL were studied for the development of meningeal leukemia *(36)*. No patient received prophylactic IT CNS chemotherapy, but all received high-dose cytarabine in remission. Thirty-one patients (21%) developed meningeal leukemia. Many characteristics were statistically associated with an increased risk of meningeal leukemia, but not leukocytosis. In a multivariate analysis of significant risk factors, only lactic dehydrogenase levels and the proportion of cells in $S + G_2M$ phase of the cell cycle were shown to independently predict for meningeal leukemia *(36)*.

2.5. Prognosis

Meningeal leukemia responds quickly to appropriate treatment. Relief of symptoms and neurologic deficit usually occurs with one dose of regional chemotherapy *(37)*, with or without radiation therapy (RT). The duration of response, however, depends on presentation, and subsequent CNS directed therapies. Although some reports suggest that patients who relapse with isolated meningeal leukemia have a poor prognosis *(38)*, some patients may achieve long-term disease-free survival, if appropriate treatment is administered *(39,40)*. Even patients who present with neurologic deficits may achieve long-term survival, as long as the leukemia is controlled systemically. Conversely, patients who present with profound neurologic deficits or obtundation have a grim prognosis, even with appropriate treatment *(5)*.

Most patients with ALL are now treated with prophylactic CNS-directed therapies. Meningeal leukemia is uncommon following such treatment, but patients in hematologic remission remain at risk for isolated meningeal relapse. Patients who develop meningeal leukemia while still on therapy, and after receiving CNS prophylaxis, have a poorer prognosis, compared to those relapsing later *(41,42)*. The Netherlands Childhood Leukemia Study Group explored the significance of an isolated CNS relapse in 142 children diagnosed between 1973 and 1985 *(43)*. All had received CNS prophylaxis with IT methotrexate (MTX) and cranial radiation with their induction chemotherapy. The children received a variety of treatments for relapse, and 90% achieved a second complete remission. However, the median duration of second remission was only 14 mo, and no more than 15% of patients were ultimately cured *(43)*. Other reports seem to confirm the morbidity and poor prognosis of patients suffering isolated meningeal relapse *(38,44)*. With aggressive CNS treatment, however, some children may achieve long-term survival, and possibly cure, after an isolated CNS relapse, even when preceded by CNS prophylaxis. The median survival of 35 patients for CNS relapse of ALL, at the Hospital for Sick Children in London between 1970 and 1976, with IT MTX and craniospinal irradiation, was 3 yr *(39)*. The Pediatric Oncology Group (POG) treated 120 children who had isolated meningeal relapse, with IT chemotherapy and cranial radiation. Not only did all patients achieve a second complete remission, but the 4-yr event-free survival was 46% *(45)*. Investigators at the MDACC treated 15 adults for meningeal leukemia with intensive IT or intraventricular chemotherapy and cranial radiation. Although most patients died from systemic relapse, more than 50% achieved CNS remissions lasting longer than 2 yr *(40)*. Clearly, some patients, particularly children, may achieve long-term disease-free survival, and possibly cure, with appropriate therapy *(46)*.

3. OVERT MENINGEAL LEUKEMIA

A diagnosis of meningeal leukemia should prompt an investigation, to rule out hematologic relapse. Systemic relapse frequently occurs simultaneously with, or soon after, meningeal leukemia *(39,47)*. The recognition of hematologic relapse may prompt systemic treatments that will complement regional chemotherapeutic approaches.

The symptomatic patient requires prompt treatment. A diagnostic lumbar puncture is performed, and may by itself relieve symptoms *(37,48,49)*. A dose of chemotherapy may be administered simultaneously, while the cytospin preparation is reviewed to confirm the diagnosis. Dexamethasone administered alone intravenously, or via IT injection, can relieve symptoms, reverse neurologic deficits, and clear the CSF of leukemic blasts, but additional therapy is usually needed to prevent quick relapse *(50)*.

Cranial radiation, usually in conjunction with IT chemotherapy, reverses most cranial nerve palsies *(51)*. Cranial RT alone, however, is inadequate treatment. Neither does adding cranial radiation to IT MTX improve the CNS remission rate *(52)*. Craniospinal radiation effectively induces meningeal leukemia into remission, but is also inadequate alone to prevent relapse *(53)*. CNS radiation is usually applied following remission induction with regional chemotherapy, in order to maintain remission *(49,54,55)*.

4. REGIONAL CHEMOTHERAPY

The treatment of meningeal leukemia represents one of the first attempts to capitalize on the advantages of regional chemotherapy *(56)*. Relatively low doses of active agents are instilled into a defined compartment, achieving high tissue concentrations at the site of disease, with little systemic toxicity. The regional approach to the treatment of meningeal leukemia has been studied mostly in the pediatric population of patients with ALL. However, the results of these studies are probably applicable to adults and patients with ANLL as well.

4.1. Indications

Regional chemotherapy is indicated for the treatment of overt meningeal leukemia, regardless of histologic classification. However, regional chemotherapy is indicated for the prevention of overt leukemia (CNS prophylaxis) only in ALL, including mature B-cell (Burkitt's) leukemia/lymphoma and precursor T-cell ALL/lymphoma (lymphoblastic lymphoma). CNS prophylaxis for monocytic leukemias, particularly when associated with hyperleukocytosis, has been recommended, but no studies document improved survival with this approach *(24–26)*.

Table 1
Chemotherapeutic Agents for Regional Chemotherapy of Meningeal Leukemia

Agent	Clearance	Implication
Methotrexate	From CNS: Bulk flow (delayed) with biphasic $t_{1/2}$ of 4.5 and 14 h Systemically: renal	Prolonged systemic exposure Increased toxicity with renal dysfunction
Cytarabine	Metabolized in systemic circulation	Brief systemic exposure Less systemic toxicity
Diaziquone	Hepatic	Little systemic toxicity with normal hepatic function
6-Mercaptopurine	Metabolized in systemic circulation	Brief systemic exposure Less systemic toxicity
Etoposide	Hepatic and renal	Little systemic toxicity with normal hepatic function

4.2. Route of Administration

Only a few chemotherapeutic agents may be administered by direct instillation into the CSF (Table 1). MTX and cytarabine are the two most commonly used agents. They may be administered by IT injection via lumbar puncture, or by intraventricular injection via a subcutaneously implanted Ommaya reservoir *(57)*. Intraventricular chemotherapy distributes through the CSF in a more uniform fashion than does IT chemotherapy *(58)*. Furthermore, as much as 10% of the administered dose of IT chemotherapy never reaches the CSF *(59)*. Despite the increased incidence of nausea and vomiting *(60)*, risk of leukoencephalopathy *(61,62)*, and risk of infection *(61,63)* with these catheters, potential therapeutic advantages prompted clinical investigations of intraventricular chemotherapy.

Bleyer and Poplack *(64)* treated 10 patients with intraventricular 8–12 mg/m² MTX twice per week, achieving remission in all 10 patients. With maintenance doses of MTX, median survival surpassed 1 yr *(64)*. A prospective trial then randomized 21 patients to either IT or intraventricular MTX *(60)*. The IT dose was 12 mg/m² and the intraventricular dose was 6 mg/m², but both were given twice per week. The remission rate was 88.8% in the intraventricular group, but only an unusually low 33.3% in the IT group. Both arms received cranial radiation in remission, as well as maintenance doses of chemotherapy. The relapse-free survival was 163 wk in the intraventricular chemotherapy group, compared to 75 wk in the IT chemotherapy group ($P = 0.046$).

The relatively brief course of IT chemotherapy for prophylaxis of meningeal leukemia, and the complications of intraventricular shunt placement, typically relegate intraventricular chemotherapy to the treatment of overt meningeal leukemia only *(65)*. A shunt is usually placed after an initial intralumbar treatment, in order to provide long-term access for maintenance regional chemotherapy.

4.3. Technique of Administration

There are no formal studies that investigate the optimal amount of CSF that should be removed prior to injection of IT chemotherapy. Although some authorities suggest allowing one-half of the injection volume to flow out *(66)*, others suggest allowing the entire injection volume to flow out *(54,60)*. The chemotherapy is slowly injected into the CSF, but whether the CSF should be aspirated during injection, to ensure unobstructed flow into the subarachnoid space, is controversial.

Following IT injection of chemotherapy, patients are left supine, or are placed in the Trendelenberg position, to facilitate cephalad flow of drug to the ventricles *(59,66)*. Whether this technique is important clinically has not been tested, but ventricular distribution of MTX is improved 1000× in nonhuman primates kept prone or in Trendelenberg position, compared to those kept upright *(67)*.

4.4. Chemotherapy of Choice

MTX is the prototype for regional chemotherapy of meningeal leukemia. Given alone, IT MTX produces CNS remission rates of 85–100% *(3,48,64,68)*.

Duttera et al. *(52)* randomized 31 patients with meningeal leukemia to either 15 mg/m^2 IT MTX, given every 2–3 d for eight doses, or to MTX in the same dose and schedule plus cranial RT. Six additional doses of MTX were given to the 93% who achieved remission. No advantage could be attributed to the addition of cranial radiation, and patients survived without relapse for a median 125–234 d ($P > 0.1$), depending on initial randomization.

Cytarabine has also proved useful in the treatment of meningeal leukemia. Cytarabine is rapidly cleared from the systemic circulation by the enzyme, cytidine deaminase. This enzyme is nearly absent from the CSF *(69)*, resulting in very slow clearance of cytarabine *(70,71)*. Intraventricular cytarabine, as a result of this favorable distribution of cytidine deaminase, results in little or no systemic toxicity. Wang and Pratt *(72)* treated 13 patients with IT cytarabine for meningeal leukemia. The protocol called for 10 mL/m^2 cytarabine solution (the dose ranged from 5 to 70 mg/m^2) given twice weekly. The remission rate was 63%, but whether this relatively low rate resulted from inadequate dosing or lack of efficacy is uncertain. Band et al. *(73)* treated 10 patients with 4.5–73 mg/m^2 cytarabine given at 3–7-d intervals. Although all patients responded clinically, only two cleared all blasts from the CSF. On the basis of these studies, cytarabine appears to have less efficacy than does MTX in the treatment of meningeal leukemia.

No advantage was demonstrated for the addition of 30 mg/m^2 cytarabine to 15 mg/m^2 MTX and hydrocortisone, given by IT injection every 4–5 d in a prospective randomized trial *(53)*. The combination chemotherapy regimen also failed to significantly improve survival, even when administered at 2, 6, 12, and 20 wk after remission was achieved.

The Southwest Oncology Group (SWOG) compared the combination of MTX and hydrocortisone to MTX, hydrocortisone, and cytarabine, in a prospective, randomized trial of treatment for overt meningeal leukemia. Complete remissions were achieved in 100% of patients with the triple-drug therapy, and 96% of those treated with two drugs. However, the median survival of the patients receiving triple drugs (64.6 wk) was longer than in those receiving just two drugs (47.2 wk). Although the difference was not statistically significant ($P = 0.71$), subsequent SWOG studies have utilized the triple-drug regimen in the design of prophylaxis studies *(74)*. The POG noted a higher-than-expected CNS relapse rate in a clinical trial in low-risk children with ALL receiving IT MTX alone for CNS prophylaxis *(75)*, prompting a change to triple IT chemotherapy in subsequent trials *(76)*. The incidence of CNS relapse was not noticeably different with the three-drug regimen, however *(76)*. Thus, the superiority of triple-drug IT chemotherapy to single-agent MTX has not been established. Nonetheless, as discussed in Subheading 4.8., many modern treatment protocols for childhood ALL use extended triple-IT chemotherapy for CNS prophylaxis *(45,77–83)*.

Table 2
Age-Appropriate Doses of IT Chemotherapy

Age (yr)	Methotrexate (mg)	Hydrocortisone (mg)	Cytarabine (mg)
<1	6	6	12
>1	8	9	16
2	10	10	20
3–8	12	12	24
≥9	12–15	15	30

Adapted with permission from refs. *59* and *66.*

Other agents have also been administered into the CSF. Decadron is effective alone, but is probably better administered with either MTX or cytarabine *(50)*. Thio-TEPA may be administered into the CSF, but is more toxic and less effective than other agents *(84–86)*. Furthermore, thio-TEPA is probably just as effective with less toxicity when administered systemically *(85)*.

Cytarabine has been encapsulated within the aqueous compartments of microscopic (DepoFoam; Depotech, San Diego, CA) particles, to improve its pharmacokinetic profile by increasing its half-life within the CSF *(87,88)*. This formulation appears effective and well-tolerated *(89)*, but whether it offers any real advantage over standard formulations of cytarabine is unknown.

Other agents, such as diaziquone *(90)*, 6-mercaptopurine *(91)*, and etoposide *(92)*, have been tested for use as regional chemotherapy in the CNS, but their use remains investigational.

4.5. Optimal Dose

Some of the early studies *(58,93)* dosed MTX according to body surface area. This approach, however, ignores the fact that the volume of the CSF is uniform in adults, and is not dependent on size. The concentration of MTX in the CSF varies more than 100-fold in patients who receive a dose of 12 mg/m^2.

Age is a more important variable than size in determining the CSF volume. Bleyer et al. *(93)* compared a series of 25 patients treated with 12 mg/m^2 IT MTX to a series of 24 patients treated with a constant dose of 12 mg, and found far less variability in MTX concentrations in patients treated with a constant dose *(93)* (Table 2). An appropriate dose for patients older than age 3 yr is 12 mg MTX in a preservative-free solution. For cytarabine, an appropriate dose is 30 mg *(66)*.

The dose of chemotherapy administered by intraventricular injection is sometimes reduced from that administered by IT injection. Iacoangeli et al. *(60)* showed the superiority of 6 mg intraventricular MTX to 12 mg IT MTX in a randomized study *(60)*. Other studies have not reduced the dose of intraventricular chemotherapy. Green et al. *(61)* gave 12 mg/m^2 MTX, 6 mg/m^2 hydrocortisone, and 25 mg/m^2 cytarabine every 4 d via an Ommaya reservoir, to 11 children, as prophylaxis, and to 16 children, as treatment for overt meningeal leukemia *(61)*. Steinherz et al. treated 39 patients for meningeal leukemia with age-based doses of intraventricular chemotherapy *(54)*. These and other studies suggest that the dose of intraventricular MTX need not be reduced, compared to IT doses, unless neurotoxicity develops *(64,94)*.

Table 3
Studies of Postremission RT Following Isolated CNS Relapse

Ref.	n	Radiation therapy (Gy)	ITC	F/U (mo)	EFS (%)
(68)	15	Craniospinal (25 + 10)	–	NA	47
	14	Cranial (25)			0
(137)	16	None	+	NA	12.5
	16	Intrathecal Radiocolloid	–		0
(55)	14	Craniospinal (30 + 18)	–	36	37
(138)	36	Craniospinal (24 + 14)	–	15	44
	51	Cranial (24)	+		10
(54)	16	Craniospinal (6)	+	24	56
(45)	120	Cranial (24)	+	48	46
(46)	20	Craniospinal (24 + 15)	–	84	70

ITC = maintenance intrathecal chemotherapy; F/U = median follow-up; EFS = event-free survival.

4.6. Optimal Initial Treatment Schedule

A single dose of MTX achieves high response rates, but additional doses are required to prevent quick relapse (48,56). However, the remission rate following doses administered every 2–3 d (3,37,52,95) is not superior to those achieved with doses given once or twice a week (48,53,60,68). Therefore, no more than two doses/wk are generally recommended, to achieve initial remission of meningeal leukemia (49).

Most treatment protocols for overt meningeal leukemia now recommend MTX dosing once or twice weekly, until blasts are cleared from the CSF (3,52,54,60,64,68). However, MTX is cleared slowly from the CSF, and may achieve detectable blood levels for several days following an intraventricular injection (59). This characteristic prompted investigation of a more pharmacokinetically sound dosing schedule. Bleyer et al. (96) compared 1 mg intraventricular MTX administered every 12 h for six doses, to 12 mg/m^2 administered twice weekly, in patients with meningeal leukemia (96). They found equivalent clinical efficacy, with less toxicity, with the 1 mg dose schedule. Whether this "time × concentration" dosing schedule offers an advantage over periodic single-bolus injections of 12 mg is unknown, but there is clearly no reason to exceed a dose of 12 mg, and no need to administer it more often than twice per week in the treatment of meningeal leukemia, with MTX.

4.7. Optimal Maintenance Treatment Schedule

Once CNS remission has been achieved, some form of additional therapy is required to maintain remission (48,56). Early prospective studies of IT MTX alone, given every 4–8 wk for maintenance, showed event-free survival of 7–15 mo for patients in second complete remission (52,53,97). Subsequent studies incorporated RT to improve these results, as indicated in Table 3.

Comparing the studies in Table 3 is difficult. Some studies were performed in the early 1970s and others in the late 1980s. The technique of RT differs from study to study. No allowance is made for simultaneous systemic therapies. These and other problems notwithstanding, the available evidence suggests that RT is an important addition to IT chemotherapy when standard doses of systemic agents are employed, and that long-term survival is possible for selected patients with isolated meningeal relapse.

The largest obstacle to improved survival following a diagnosis of meningeal leukemia is bone marrow relapse. Neither regional chemotherapy nor craniospinal radiation
adequately address this problem. At high-doses, systemic administration of MTX and
cytarabine achieve therapeutic CSF levels, allowing simultaneous treatment of both
the leptomeninges and bone marrow. Balis et al. *(98)* treated 20 children with a loading
dose of 6000 mg/m^2 MTX for a period of 1 hr, followed by an infusion of 1,200 mg/
m^2/h for 23 h. Leucovorin rescue was initiated 12 h after the end of the infusion, with
a loading dose of 200 mg/m^2, followed by 12 mg/m^2 every 3 h for six doses, and then
every 6 h, until the plasma MTX level decreased to less than 1×10^{-7} mol/L. Therapeutic
CSF levels of MTX were achieved, and 80% of patients achieved complete remission.
Lower doses of systemic MTX provide better systemic treatment, but inferior CNS
control, compared to cranial radiation *(99)*. Systemic high-dose cytarabine also achieves
therapeutic CSF levels, and doses of 3 g/m^2, every 12 h for 6–12 doses, are effective
in treating overt meningeal leukemia *(100,101)*. However, the optimal method of combining high-dose systemic therapy with regional chemotherapy, if any, is unknown.

4.8. Optimal Prophylactic Treatment Schedule

The success achieved by oncologists in the cure of childhood ALL can, in large
part, be attributed to the recognition and prevention of overt meningeal leukemia.
Before CNS prophylaxis was routinely administered, standard systemic chemotherapy
delayed, but did not prevent, meningeal leukemia, and resulted in a 5-yr survival of
only 17% *(102)*. Early studies using 24 Gy of cranial RT combined with five weekly
doses of IT MTX, resulted in both a reduction in the incidence of meningeal leukemia
and an increase in 3-yr disease-free survival to 60% *(16)*. CNS prophylaxis is now a
routine component of chemotherapy protocols for childhood ALL *(103)*.

The delivery of prophylaxis has changed, however. The early studies employing 24
Gy of cranial radiation were often complicated by subsequent encephalopathy *(104,105)*
and craniospinal radiation is myelosuppressive, which led to an increased incidence of
infections. Prospective randomized studies then demonstrated that 18 Gy of radiation
was of equivalent efficacy to 24 Gy *(106)*. Cranial radiation plus five doses of IT MTX
became the standard for CNS prophylaxis of childhood ALL.

As factors predictive for meningeal leukemia became better understood, and high-
dose chemotherapy capable of penetrating the CNS became more widely used, the
necessity of cranial radiation was questioned. The POG *(107)* randomized children
with ALL to one of three intensive regimens incorporating prolonged IT chemotherapy,
or to a standard radiation plus five doses of IT MTX strategy. Although the study
indicated that IT MTX can be substituted for RT, many doses of MTX were required.
In a group of children with intermediate-risk ALL, the Children's Cancer Group (CCG)
(108) compared 18 Gy of cranial radiation, combined with early IT MTX to a CNS
prophylaxis regimen of IT MTX alone, administered both early and late, into the
treatment protocol *(108)*. Here, too, RT was found unnecessary. Two European groups
combined their data, to explore the role of cranial radiation in patients undergoing
initial treatment for childhood T-cell ALL *(109)*. Similar systemic chemotherapy was
administered, but the German group used seven doses of IT MTX and 12 Gy of cranial
radiation, while the Italian group substituted extended triple-IT chemotherapy for CNS
prophylaxis. The two regimens were equally effective for patients with WBC <100,000/
µL. However, the event-free survival of patients presenting with a WBC >100,000/µL

was significantly better in the RT regimen, even though no difference in CNS relapse rates could be documented *(109)*.

Other studies took advantage of the benefits of high-dose systemic MTX and cytarabine in treating both systemic and CNS leukemia. These studies eliminated cranial radiation, and achieved low CNS relapse rates *(110,111)*. The Pediatric Branch of the National Cancer Institute randomized patients either to standard doses of systemic chemotherapy with cranial radiation and five doses of IT MTX or to a regimen using high-dose MTX alone. They found that cranial radiation could be replaced by high-dose MTX *(112)*. A study of the CCG, in children with intermediate-risk ALL, found that cranial radiation could be replaced with IT MTX alone, when combined with high-dose systemic chemotherapy *(113)*. Preliminary reports suggest that even high-risk patients can be spared cranial radiation, with high-dose systemic chemotherapy and extended IT chemotherapy *(114)*.

As the systemic chemotherapy for childhood ALL has evolved over the past 30 yr, so has regional chemotherapy. The combination of cranial radiation and five doses of IT MTX has been replaced by high-dose systemic chemotherapy and extended triple-IT chemotherapy for all but the most high-risk children with ALL. Extended triple-IT chemotherapy in this context refers to the combination of MTX, cytarabine, and a glucocorticoid, given in age-adjusted doses (Table 2) every 8 wk through the maintenance phase of treatment, for at least 15 total doses *(82)*. This evolution occurred in response to the recognition of cranial radiation's toxicity, not to its lack of efficacy. As discussed in Subheading 4.9, however, CNS toxicity is not avoided altogether by substituting systemic and regional chemotherapy.

Prophylactic methods in adults have been less well studied. The SWOG randomized 62 evaluable adult patients, who had ALL in first complete remission, to CNS prophylaxis with IT MTX and cranial radiation, or to the identical systemic chemotherapy without CNS prophylaxis. Three of 28 patients receiving CNS prophylaxis (11%) developed meningeal leukemia, compared to 11 of 34 (32%) not receiving prophylaxis ($P = 0.03$) *(19)*. Unfortunately, this benefit of CNS prophylaxis did not translate into either improved relapse-free or overall survival.

Adults appear to be at risk for earlier CNS relapse than are children. The Cancer and Leukemia Group B found that more than half of their patients with CNS relapse were diagnosed before CNS prophylaxis could be given *(115)*. Proponents for early CNS prophylaxis point to a less than 10% relapse rate when CNS prophylaxis is administered during or soon after induction therapy *(17,18,116)*. However, others have noted a similar CNS relapse rate when CNS prophylaxis is given later in the treatment protocol *(19,117)*.

The group at MDACC reviewed their experience with meningeal leukemia in 391 patients treated for ALL on four successive protocols *(18)*. The first protocol (pre-VAD [vincristine, doxorubicin, and dexamethasone]) did not employ CNS prophylaxis. The second protocol (VAD) utilized high-dose systemic chemotherapy. The third protocol (modified-VAD) used the high-dose systemic chemotherapy, but added IT cytarabine for patients at high-risk of CNS relapse. The fourth protocol (hyperCVAD) used high-dose systemic chemotherapy plus alternating IT MTX and cytarabine in all patients (four doses for patients at low-risk, 12 doses for those at high-risk). The results of this review are presented in Table 4. This analysis suffers from its retrospective nature, but strongly suggests that cranial radiation is not necessary to prevent CNS relapse in adult ALL. The study does not, however, answer the question of whether or not CNS prophylaxis improves survival.

Table 4
CNS Prophylaxis for Adult ALL

Protocol	CNS relapse in CR (%)	3-yr event-free survival (%)
Pre-VAD	14	10
VAD	10	26
Modified VAD	5	14
HyperCVAD	0	48

Adapted with permission from ref. *18*.

4.9. Toxicity

Although generally well-tolerated, direct instillation of MTX into the CSF is associated with side effects, the management of which are important for anyone planning to treat meningeal leukemia. The most common side-effect of IT or intraventricular chemotherapy is chemical meningitis *(118)*, which manifests as headache, nausea and vomiting, low-grade fever, nuchal rigidity, and CSF pleiocytosis *(119)*. Bleyer et al. *(120)* demonstrated that high CSF concentrations of MTX contribute to the incidence of acute chemical meningitis *(120)*. Chemical meningitis is more frequent when treating overt meningeal leukemia, compared to prophylactic treatment, because the clearance of MTX is delayed in the presence of active disease *(121)*.

Similarly, adults treated with MTX dosed according to body wt have a higher incidence of chemical meningitis than do those treated with a constant dose, as indicated in Table 2 *(93)*. In one study utilizing 15 mg/m^2 MTX every 2–3 d, the incidence of moderate-to-severe toxicity was 55%. Furthermore, 65% experienced "symptoms severe enough to interfere with their daily life for a period of 48 h or more" *(52)*. In another study *(53)* of IT MTX, given at a dose of 12 mg/m^2, 17 of 26 patients (65%) developed acute toxicity, generally secondary to chemical meningitis. In contrast, studies using no more than 12 mg MTX report acute toxicity in less than 15%. These symptoms can occur within several hours to 2 d after a dose *(59)*.

The symptoms of meningeal irritation may respond to systemic corticosteroids, but chemical meningitis usually resolves over a few days, with analgesics and conservative therapy. However, the possibility of infectious meningitis must be kept in mind, in these immunocompromised hosts.

Serious late toxicity has also been described following regional chemotherapy of the CNS. An encephalopathic reaction occurred in 50% of patients receiving 12 mg/m^2 IT MTX in one study *(96)*. A severe myelopathy, with or without cord necrosis, has also been described *(122–124)*. The spinal cord toxicity of IT chemotherapy may occur after either prophylactic treatment or remission induction of overt meningeal leukemia. The paraplegia or quadriplegia that results may or may not be reversible. In one review of 23 cases *(125)*, only two recovered completely. This devastating complication is, fortunately, rare, with an estimated incidence of less than 3% *(126)*. Seizures may also rarely complicate the syndrome. Strict attention to the dose and agent must be given, to avoid inadvertent overdosage or administration of the wrong agent.

As with any chemotherapy, regional chemotherapy of the CNS can be complicated by accidental overdose. However, the overdosage can be corrected, if recognized in a timely fashion. Not all overdoses require intervention: Doses of MTX up to 25 mg may be well tolerated. Doses higher than 50 mg should probably be treated. If recognized within 1 h of administration, removal of 10–40 cc of CSF will remove significant amounts of MTX, which should limit neurologic toxicity *(127)*. Leucovorin should be given systemically to prevent systemic toxicity. Leucovorin has also been given to ameliorate the occasional systemic side effects of frequently administered IT or intraventricular MTX. However, leucovorin should not be administered intrathecally *(128)*. Large overdoses can be managed by ventriculolumbar perfusion with warmed saline *(129)*.

Although long-term neurologic sequelae resulting from prophylactic IT MTX alone are unusual *(130)*, the addition of cranial radiation appears to increase the incidence of unwanted side effects *(118)*. A severe, acute encephalopathic reaction has been described with the concomitant use of MTX and radiation *(131,132)*. More commonly, the combination of radiation and regional chemotherapy of the CNS results in more subtle CNS effects, such as declines in intellectual function *(133–135)*. However, the encephalopathic process can occasionally be progressive and severe *(105)*. These neurotoxic effects are much less common in adults *(136)* and are not always demonstrable in children *(104)*. The potential for greater neurologic toxicity, coupled with the availability of alternative approaches, argue strongly against the routine application of cranial RT in the prophylaxis of meningeal leukemia, especially in children.

5. FUTURE DIRECTIONS

The historical approach to the treatment of meningeal leukemia provides a database upon which to improve future therapies. The nearly universal success of IT MTX in achieving CNS remission will be difficult to improve on, but new drugs may improve MTX's toxicity profile, or reduce the need for frequent injections. A better understanding of prognostic factors will help select patients with overt meningeal leukemia for potentially curative approaches that combine regional chemotherapy with systemic chemotherapy and RT. Finally, refinements in the delivery of prophylactic CNS therapy promise to reduce toxicity further, while preserving therapeutic efficacy.

REFERENCES

1. Price RA and Johnson WW. Central nervous system in childhood leukemia: I. The arachnoid, *Cancer,* **31** (1973) 520–533.
2. Bleyer WA. Biology and pathogenesis of CNS leukemia, *Am. J. Pediatr. Hematol. Oncol.,* **11** (1989) 57–63.
3. Hardisty RM and Norman PM. Meningeal leukaemia, *Arch. Dis. Child.,* **42** (1967) 441–447.
4. Law IP and Blom J. Adult acute leukemia: frequency of central system involvement in long-term survivors, *Cancer,* **40** (1977) 1304–1306.
5. Stewart DJ, Keating MJ, McCredie KB, et al. Natural history of central nervous system acute leukemia in adults, *Cancer,* **47** (1981) 184–196.
6. Bigner SH. Cerebrospinal fluid (CSF) cytology: current status and diagnostic applications, *J. Neuropathol. Exp. Neurol.,* **51** (1992) 235–45.
7. Hyman CB, Bogle JM, Brubaker CA, Williams K, and Hammond D. Central nervous system involvement by leukemia in children. I. Relationship to systemic leukemia and description of clinical and laboratory manifestations, *Blood,* **25** (1965) 1–12.
8. Lauer SJ, Kirchner PA, and Camitta BM. Identification of leukemic cells in the cerebrospinal fluid from children with acute lymphoblastic leukemia: advances and dilemmas, *Am. J. Pediatr. Hematol. Oncol.,* **11** (1989) 64–73.
9. Mastrangelo R, Poplack D, Bleyer A, Riccardi R, Sather H, and D'Angio G. Report and recommenda-

tions of the Rome workshop concerning poor-prognosis acute lymphoblastic leukemia in children: biologic bases for staging, stratification, and treatment, *Med. Pediatr. Oncol.,* **14** (1986) 191–194.

10. Mahmoud HH, Rivera GK, Hancock ML, et al. Low leukocyte counts with blast cells in cerebrospinal fluid of children with newly diagnosed acute lymphoblastic leukemia, *N. Engl. J. Med.,* **329**(5) (1993) 314–319.

11. Donskoy E, Tausche F, Altman A, Quinn J, and Goldschneider I. Association of immunophenotype with cerebrospinal fluid involvement in childhood B-lineage acute lymphoblastic leukemia, *Am. J. Clin. Pathol.,* **107** (1997) 608–616.

12. Oberg G, Hallgren R, Fenge P. β_2-Microglobulin, lysozyme, and lactoferrin in cerebrospinal fluid in patients with lymphoma or leukaemia: relationship to CNS involvement and the effect of prophylactic intrathecal treatment with methotrexate, *Br. J. Haematol.,* **66** (1987) 315–322.

13. Hansen PB, Kjeldsen L, Dalhoff K, and Olesen B. Cerebrospinal fluid beta-2-microglobulin in adult patients with acute leukemia or lymphoma: a useful marker in early diagnosis and monitoring of CNS involvement, *Acta. Neurol. Scand.,* **85** (1992) 224–227.

14. Kersten MJ, Evers LM, Dellemijn PLI, et al. Elevation of cerebrospinal fluid soluble CD27 levels in patients with meningeal localization of lymphoid malignancies, *Blood,* **87** (1996) 1985–1989.

15. Evans AE, Gilbert ES, and Zandstra R. Increasing incidence of central nervous system leukemia in children, *Cancer,* **26** (1970) 404–409.

16. Aur RJA, Simone J, Hustu O, et al. Central nervous system therapy and combination chemotherapy of childhood lymphocytic leukemia, *Blood,* **37** (1971) 272–281.

17. Gottlieb AJ, Weinberg V, Ellison RR, et al. Efficacy of daunorubicin in the therapy of adult acute lymphocyte leukemia: a prospective randomized trial by the Cancer and Leukemia Group B, *Blood,* **64** (1984) 267–274.

18. Cortes J, O'Brien SM, Pierce S, et al. Value of high-dose systemic chemotherapy and intrathecal therapy for central nervous system prophylaxis in different risk groups of adult acute lymphoblastic leukemia, *Blood,* **86** (1995) 2091–2097.

19. Omura GA, Moffitt S, Vogler WR, and Salter MM. Combination chemotherapy of adult acute lymphoblastic leukemia with randomized central nervous system prophylaxis, *Blood,* **55** (1980) 199–204.

20. Dekker AW, Elderson A, Punt K, and Sixma JJ. Meningeal involvement in patients with acute nonlymphocytic leukemia. Incidence, management, and predictive factors, *Cancer,* **56** (1985) 2078–2082.

21. Brinch L, Evensen SA, Stavem P. Leukemia in the central nervous system, *Acta. Med. Scand.,* **224** (1988) 173–178.

22. Holmes R, Keating M, Cork A, et al. Unique pattern of central nervous system leukemia in acute myelomonocytic leukemia associated with inv(16)(p13q22), *Blood,* **65** (1985) 1071–1078.

23. Tobelem G, Jacquillat C, Chastang C, et al. Acute monoblastic leukemia: a clinical and biologic study of 74 cases, *Blood,* **55** (1980) 71–76.

24. Armitago JO and Burns CP. Maintenance therapy of adult acute nonlymphoblastic leukemia: an argument against the need for central nervous system prophylaxis, *Cancer,* **41** (1978) 697–700.

25. Mandelli F, De Lipsis E, Grignani F, et al. Daunomycin, cytosine arabinoside and 6-thioguanine (DAT) vs vincristine, cytosine arabinoside and 6-thioguanine (VAT) in the induction treatment of acute nonlymphocyte leukemia: a randomized collaborative study, *Med. Pediatr. Oncol.,* **4** (1978) 231–240.

26. Janvier M, Tobelem G, Daniel MT, Bernheim A, Marty M, and Boiron M. Acute monoblastic leukaemia. Clinical, biological data and survival in 45 cases, *Scand. J. Haematol.,* **32** (1984) 385–390.

27. Cash J, Fehir KM, and Pollack MS. Meningeal involvement in early stage chronic lymphocytic leukemia, *Cancer,* **59** (1987) 798–800.

28. Davies GE. Meningeal leukemia complicating chronic lymphocytic leukemia, *Cancer* **50** (1982) 605–606.

29. Liepman MK and Votaw ML. Meningeal leukemia complicating chronic lymphocytic leukemia, *Cancer,* **47** (1981) 2482–2484.

30. Navarrete D and Bodega E. Leukemic meningitis in a patient with hairy cell leukemia. A case report, *Nouv. Rev. Fr. Hematol.,* **29** (1987) 247–249.

31. Melhorn DK, Gross S, Fisher BJ, and Newman AJ. Studies on the use of "prophylactic" intrathecal amethopterin in childhood leukemia, *Blood,* **35** (1970) 55–60.

32. West RJ, Graham-Pole J, Hardisty RM, and Pike MC. Factors in the pathogenesis of central nervous system leukemia, *Br. Med. J.,* **3** (1972) 311–314.

33. Gill PS, Meyer PR, Pavlova Z, and Levine AM. B-cell acute lymphocytic leukemia in adults. Clinical, morphological, and immunologic findings, *J. Clin. Oncol.,* **4** (1986) 737–743.

34. Coleman CN, Cohen JR, Burke JS, and Rosenberg SA. Lymphoblastic lymphoma in adults: results of a pilot protocol, *Blood,* **57** (1981) 679–84.

35. Sweetenham JW, Mead GM, and Whitehouse JM. Adult lymphoblastic lymphoma: high incidence of central nervous system relapse in patients treated with the Stanford University protocol, *Ann. Oncol.,* **3** (1992) 839–841.

36. Kantarjian HM, Walters RS, Smith TL, et al. Identification of risk groups for development of central nervous system leukemia in adults with acute lymphocytic leukemia, *Blood,* **72** (1988) 1784–1789.

37. Hyman CB, Bogle JM, Brubaker CA, Williams K, and Hammond D. Central nervous system involvement by leukemia in children. II. Therapy with intrathecal methotrexate, *Blood,* **25** (1965) 13–22.

38. George SL, Ochs JJ, Mauer AM, and Simone JV. Importance of an isolated central nervous system relapse in children with acute lymphoblastic leukemia, *J. Clin. Oncol.,* **3** (1985) 776–781.

39. Gribbin MA, Hardisty RM, and Chessels JM. Long-term control of central nervous system leukemia, *Arch. Dis. Child.,* **52** (1977) 673–678.

40. Stewart DJ, Smith TL, Keating MJ, et al. Remission from central nervous system involvement in adults with acute leukemia. Effect of intensive therapy and prognostic factors, *Cancer,* **56** (1985) 632–641.

41. Nesbit ME, D'Angio GJ, Sather HN, et al. Effect of isolated central nervous system leukaemia on bone marrow remission and survival in childhood acute lymphoblastic leukaemia, *Lancet,* **1** (1981) 1386–1388.

42. Ortega JA, Nesbit ME, Sather HN, Robison LL, D'Angio GJ, and Hammond GD. Long-term evaluation of a CNS prophylaxis trial—treatment comparisons and outcome after CNS relapse in childhood ALL: a report from the Children's Cancer Study Group, *J. Clin. Oncol.,* **5** (1987) 1646–1654.

43. Behrendt H, van Leeuwen EF, Schuwirth C, et al. Significance of an isolated central nervous system relapse, occurring as first relapse in children with acute lymphoblastic leukemia, *Cancer,* **63** (1989) 2066–2072.

44. Ochs JJ, Rivera G, Aur RJ, Hustu HO, Berg R, and Simone JV. Central nervous system morbidity following an initial isolated central nervous system relapse and its subsequent therapy in childhood acute lymphoblastic leukemia, *J. Clin. Oncol.,* **3** (1985) 622–626.

45. Winick NJ, Smith SD, Shuster J, et al. Treatment of CNS relapse in children with acute lymphoblastic leukemia: a Pediatric Oncology Group study, *J. Clin. Oncol.,* **11** (1993) 271–278.

46. Ribeiro RC, Rivera GK, Hudson M, et al. Intensive re-treatment protocol for children with an isolated CNS relapse of acute lymphoblastic leukemia, *J. Clin. Oncol.,* **13** (1995) 333–338.

47. Nesbit ME Jr., GJ DA, Sather HN, Robison LL, Ortega JA, and Hammond D. Post-induction treatment of childhood acute lymphocytic leukemia, *N. Engl. J. Med.,* **310** (1984) 262–263.

48. Evans AE, D'Angio GJ, and Mitus A. Central nervous system complications of children with acute leukemia, *J. Pediatr.,* **64** (1964) 94–96.

49. Humphrey GB, Krous HF, Filler J, Maxwell JD, and VanHoutte JJ. Treatment of overt CNS leukemia, *Am. J. Pediatr. Hematol.-Oncol.,* **1** (1979) 37–47.

50. Gomez-Almaguer D, Gonzalez-Llano O, Montemayor J, Jaime-Perez JC, and Galindo C. Dexamethasone in the treatment of meningeal leukemia, *Am. J. Hematol.,* **49** (1995) 353–354.

51. Gray JR and Wallner KE. Reversal of cranial nerve dysfunction with radiation therapy in adults with lymphoma and leukemia, *Int. J. Radiat. Oncol. Biol. Phys.,* **19** (1990) 439–444.

52. Duttera MJ, Bleyer WA, Pomeroy TC, Leventhal CM, and Leventhal BG. Irradiation, methotrexate toxicity, and the treatment of meningeal leukemia, *Lancet,* **2** (1973) 703–707.

53. Sullivan MP, Humphrey GB, Vietti TJ, Haggard ME, and Lee E. Superiority of conventional intrathecal methotrexate therapy with maintenance over intensive intrathecal methotrexate therapy, unmaintained, or radiotherapy (2000–2500 rads tumor dose) in treatment for meningeal leukemia, *Cancer,* **35** (1975) 1066–1073.

54. Steinherz P, Jereb B, and Galicich J. Therapy of CNS leukemia with intraventricular chemotherapy and low-dose neuraxis radiotherapy, *J. Clin. Oncol.,* **3** (1985) 1217–26.

55. Kun LE, Camitta BM, Mulhern RK, et al. Treatment of meningeal relapse in childhood acute lymphoblastic leukemia. I. Results of craniospinal irradiation, *J. Clin. Oncol.,* **2** (1984) 359–364.

56. Whiteside JA, Philips FS, Dargeon HW, and Burchenal JH. Intrathecal amethopterin in neurological manifestations of leukemia, *Arch. Intern. Med.,* **101** (1958) 279–285.

57. Ommaya AK. Implantable devices for chronic access and drug delivery to the central nervous system, *Cancer Drug Deliv.,* **1** (1984) 169–179.

58. Shapiro WR, Young DF, and Mehta BM. Methotrexate distribution in cerebrospinal fluid after intravenous, ventricular, and intralumbar injections, *N. Engl. J. Med.,* **293** (1975) 161–166.

59. Balis FM and Poplack DG. Central nervous system pharmacology of antileukemic drugs, *Am. J. Pediatr. Hematol.-Oncol.,* **11** (1989) 74–86.

60. Iacoangeli M, Roselli R, Pagano L, et al. Intrathecal chemotherapy for treatment of overt meningeal leukemia: comparison between intraventricular and traditional intralumbar route, *Ann. Oncol.,* **6** (1995) 377–382.

61. Green DM, West CR, Brecher ML, et al. Use of subcutaneous cerebrospinal fluid reservoirs for the prevention and treatment of meningeal relapse of acute lymphoblastic leukemia, *Am. J. Pediatr. Hematol.-Oncol.,* **4** (1982) 147–154.

62. Colamaria V, Caraballo R, Borgna-Pignatti C, et al. Transient focal leukoencephalopathy following intraventricular methotrexate and cytarabine. A complication of the Ommaya reservoir: case report and review of the literature, *Childs Nerv. Syst.,* **6** (1990) 231–235.

63. Lishner M, Perrin RG, Feld R, et al. Complications associated with Ommaya reservoirs in patients with cancer. The Princess Margaret Hospital experience and a review of the literature, *Arch. Intern. Med.,* **150** (1990) 173–176.

64. Bleyer WA and Poplack DG. Intraventricular versus intralumbar methotrexate for central nervous system leukemia, *Med. Pediatr. Oncol.,* **6** (1979) 207–213.

65. Spiers ASD and Booth AE. Reservoirs for intraventricular chemotherapy, *Lancet* (1973) 1263.

66. Pinkel D and Woo S. Prevention and treatment of meningeal leukemia in children, *Blood,* **84** (1994) 355–366.

67. Echelberger CK, Riccardi R, Bleyer A, Levin AS, and Poplack DG. Influence of body position on ventricular cerebrospinal fluid (CSF) methotrexate (MTX) concentration following intralumbar (IL) administration, *Proc. Am. Soc. Clin. Oncol.,* **22** (1981) 365a.

68. Willoughby MLN. Treatment of overt meningeal leukemia in children: results of second MRC meningeal leukaemia trial, *Br. Med. J.,* **1** (1976) 864–867.

69. Ho DHW. Distribution of kinase and deaminase of 1-βD-arabinofuranosyl-cytosine in tissues of man and mouse, *Cancer Res.,* **33** (1973) 2816–2820.

70. Bekassy AN, Liliemark J, Garwicz S, Wiebe T, Gulliksson H, and Peterson C. Pharmacokinetics of cytosine arabinoside in cerebrospinal fluid and of its metabolite in leukemic cells, *Med. Pediatr. Oncol.,* **18** (1990) 136–142.

71. Zimm S, Collins JM, Miser J, Chatterji D, and Poplack DG. Cytosine arabinoside cerebrospinal fluid kinetics, *Clin. Pharmacol. Ther.,* **35** (1984) 826–30.

72. Wang JJ and Pratt CB. Intrathecal arabinosyl cytosine in meningeal leukemia, *Cancer,* **25** (1970) 531–534.

73. Band PR, Holland JF, Bernard J, Weil M, Walker M, and Rall D. Treatment of central nervous system leukemia with intrathecal cytosine arabinoside, *Cancer,* **32** (1973) 744–748.

74. Komp DM, Fernandez CH, Falleta JM, et al. CNS prophylaxis in acute lymphoblastic leukemia. Comparison of two methods: a Southwest Oncology Group Study, *Cancer,* **50** (1982) 1031–1036.

75. Mahoney DH Jr, Camitta BM, Leventhal BG, et al. Repetitive low dose oral methotrexate and intravenous mercaptopurine treatment for patients with lower risk B-lineage acute lymphoblastic leukemia. A Pediatric Oncology Group pilot study, *Cancer,* **75** (1995) 2623–31.

76. Mahoney DH, Shuster J, Nitschke R, et al. Intermediate-dose intravenous methotrexate with intravenous mercaptopurine is superior to repetitive low-dose oral methotrexate with intravenous mercaptopurine for children with lower risk B-lineage acute lymphoblastic leukemia: a Pediatric Oncology Group Phase III Trial, *J. Clin. Oncol.,* **16** (1998) 246–254.

77. Buhrer C, Hartmann R, Fengler R, et al. Importance of effective central nervous system therapy in isolated bone marrow relapse of childhood acute lymphoblastic leukemia. BFM (Berlin-Frankfurt-Munster) Relapse Study Group, *Blood,* **83** (1994) 3468–72.

78. Giannone L, Greco FA, and Hainsworth JD. Combination intraventricular chemotherapy for meningeal neoplasia, *J. Clin. Oncol.,* **4** (1986) 68–73.

79. Hasle H, Helgestad J, Christensen JK, Jacobsen BB, and Kamper J. Prolonged intrathecal chemotherapy replacing cranial irradiation in high-risk acute lymphatic leukaemia: long-term follow up with cerebral computed tomography scans and endocrinological studies, *Eur. J. Pediatr.,* **154** (1995) 24–29.

80. Hoelzer D, Ludwig WD, Thiel E, et al. Improved outcome in adult B-cell acute lymphoblastic leukemia, *Blood,* **87** (1996) 495–508.

81. Lauer SJ, Camitta BM, Leventhal BG, et al. Intensive alternating drug pairs for treatment of high-risk childhood acute lymphoblastic leukemia. A Pediatric Oncology Group pilot study, *Cancer,* **71** (1993) 2854–2861.

82. Pullen J, Boyett J, Shuster J, et al. Extended triple intrathecal chemotherapy trial for prevention of CNS relapse in good-risk and poor-risk patients with B-progenitor acute lymphoblastic leukemia: a Pediatric Oncology Group study, *J. Clin. Oncol.,* **11** (1993) 839–849.

83. Sullivan MP, Brecher M, Ramirez I, et al. High-dose cyclophosphamide-high-dose methotrexate with coordinated intrathecal therapy for advanced nonlymphoblastic lymphoma of childhood: results of a Pediatric Oncology Group study, *Am. J. Pediatr. Hematol.-Oncol.,* **13** (1991) 288–295.

84. Gutin PH, Levi JA, Wiernik PH, and Walker MD. Treatment of malignant meningeal disease with intrathecal thioTEPA: a phase II study, *Cancer Treat. Rep.,* **61** (1977) 885–887.

85. Strong JM, Collins JM, Lester C, and Poplack DG. Pharmacokinetics of intraventricular and intravenous N,N',N''-triethylenethiophosphoramide (thiotepa) in rhesus monkeys and humans, *Cancer Res.,* **46** (1986) 6101–6104.

86. Trump DL, Grossman SA, Thompson G, Murray K, and Wharam M. Treatment of neoplastic meningitis with intraventricular thiotepa and methotrexate, *Cancer Treat. Rep.,* **66** (1982) 1549–1551.

87. Kim S, Khatibi S, Howell SB, McCully C, Balis FM, and Poplack DG. Prolongation of drug exposure in cerebrospinal fluid by encapsulation into DepoFoam, *Cancer Res.,* **53** (1993) 1596–1598.

88. Kim S, Chatelut E, Kim JC, et al. Extended CSF cytarabine exposure following intrathecal administration of DTC 101, *J. Clin. Oncol.,* **11** (1993) 2186–2193.

89. Chamberlain MC, Khatibi S, Kim JC, Howell SB, Chatelut E, and Kim S. Treatment of leptomeningeal metastasis with intraventricular administration of depot cytarabine (DTC 101). A phase I study, *Arch. Neurol.,* **50** (1993) 261–264.

90. Berg SL, Balis FM, Zimm S, et al. Phase I/II trial and pharmacokinetics of intrathecal diaziquone in refractory meningeal malignancies, *J. Clin. Oncol.,* **10** (1992) 143–148.

91. Adamson PC, Balis FM, Arndt CA, et al. Intrathecal 6-mercaptopurine: preclinical pharmacology, phase I/II trial, and pharmacokinetic study, *Cancer Res.,* **51** (1991) 6079–6083.

92. van der Gaast A, Sonneveld P, Mans DRA, and Splinter TA. Intrathecal administration of etoposide in the treatment of malignant meningitis: feasibility and pharmacokinetic data, *Cancer Chemother. Pharmacol.,* **29** (1992) 335–337.

93. Bleyer WA. Clinical pharmacology of intrathecal methotrexate. II. An improved dosage regimen derived from age-related pharmacokinetics, *Cancer Treat. Rep.,* **61** (1977) 1419–1425.

94. Haghbin M and Galicich JH. Use of the Ommaya reservoir in the prevention and treatment of CNS leukemia, *Am. J. Pediatr. Hematol./Oncol.,* **1** (1979) 111–117.

95. Sullivan MP, Vietti TS, Fernbach DJ, Griffith KM, Haddy TB, and Watkins WL. Clinical investigations in the treatment of meningeal leukemia: radiation therapy regimens vs conventional intrathecal methotrexate, *Blood,* **34** (1969) 301–319.

96. Bleyer WA, Poplack DG, and Simon RM. "Concentration × time" methotrexate via a subcutaneous reservoir: a less toxic regimen for intraventricular chemotherapy of central nervous system neoplasms, *Blood,* **51** (1978) 835–842.

97. Sullivan MP, Vietti TS, Haggard ME, Donaldson MH, Krall JM, and Gehan EA. Remission maintenance therapy for meningeal leukemia: intrathecal methotrexate vs intravenous bis-nitrosurea, *Blood,* **38** (1971) 680–688.

98. Balis FM, Savitch JL, Bleyer WA, Reaman GH, and Poplack DG. Remission induction of meningeal leukemia with high-dose intravenous methotrexate, *J. Clin. Oncol.,* **3** (1985) 485–489.

99. Freeman AI, Boyett JM, Glicksman AS, et al. Intermediate-dose methotrexate versus cranial irradiation in childhood acute lymphoblastic leukemia: a ten-year follow-up, *Med. Pediatr. Oncol.,* **28** (1997) 98–107.

100. Morra E, Lazzarino M, Brusamolino E, et al. Role of systemic high-dose cytarabine in the treatment of central nervous system leukemia. Clinical results in 46 patients, *Cancer,* **72** (1993) 439–445.

101. Frick J, Ritch PS, Hansen RM, and Anderson T. Successful treatment of meningeal leukemia using systemic high-dose cytosine arabinoside, *J. Clin. Oncol.,* **2** (1984) 365–368.

102. Pinkel D, Simone J, Husto O, and Aur RJA. Nine year's experience with "Total Therapy" of childhood acute lymphocytic leukemia, *Pediatrics,* **50** (1972) 246–251.

103. Pinkel D. Ninth annual David Karnofsky Lecture. Treatment of acute lymphocytic leukemia, *Cancer,* **43** (1979) 1128–1137.

104. Soni SS, Marten GW, Pitner SE, Duenas DA, and Powazek M. Effects of central nervous system irradiation on neuropsychologic functioning of children with acute lymphocytic leukemia, *N. Engl. J. Med.,* **293** (1975) 113–118.

105. Price RA and Jamieson PA. Central nervous system in childhood leukemia. II. Subacute leukoencephalopathy, *Cancer,* **35** (1975) 306–318.

106. Nesbit ME Jr, Sather HN, Robison LL, et al. Presymptomatic central nervous system therapy in previously untreated childhood acute lymphoblastic leukaemia: comparison of 1800 rad and 2400 rad. A report for Children's Cancer Study Group, *Lancet,* **1** (1981) 461–466.

107. Sullivan MP, Chen T, Dyment PG, Hvizdala E, and Steuber CP. Equivalence of intrathecal chemotherapy and radiotherapy as central nervous system prophylaxis in children with acute lymphatic leukemia: a Pediatric Oncology Group study, *Blood,* **60** (1982) 948–958.

108. Littman P, Coccia P, Bleyer WA, et al. Central nervous system (CNS) prophylaxis in children with low risk lymphoblastic leukemia (ALL), *Int. J. Radiat. Oncol. Biol. Phys.,* **13** (1987) 1443–1449.

109. Conter V, Schrappe M, Arico M, et al. Role of cranial radiotherapy for childhood T-cell acute lymphoblastic leukemia with high WBC count and good response to prednisone. Associazione Italiana Ematologia Oncologia Pediatrica and the Berlin-Frankfurt-Munster groups, *J. Clin. Oncol.,* **15** (1997) 2786–2791.

110. Krance RA, Newman EM, Ravindranath Y, et al. Pilot study of intermediate-dose methotrexate and cytosine arabinoside, "spread-out" and "up-front," in continuation therapy for childhood non-T, non-B acute lymphoblastic leukemia. A Pediatric Oncology Group study, *Cancer,* **67** (1991) 550–556.

111. Camitta B, Leventhal B, Lauer S, et al. Intermediate-dose intravenous methotrexate and mercaptopurine therapy for non-T, non-B acute lymphocytic leukemia of childhood: a Pediatric Oncology Group study, *J. Clin. Oncol.,* **7** (1989) 1539–1544.

112. Poplack D, Reaman G, Bleyer A, et al. Central nervous system preventive therapy with high-dose methotrexate in acute lymphoblastic leukemia: a preliminary report, *Proc. Am. Soc. Clin. Oncol.,* **3** (1984) 204a.

113. Tubergen DG, Gilchrist GS, O'Brien RT, et al. Prevention of CNS disease in intermediate-risk acute lymphoblastic leukemia: comparison of cranial radiation and intrathecal methotrexate and the importance of systemic therapy: a Childrens Cancer Group report, *J. Clin. Oncol.,* **11** (1993) 520–526.

114. Poplack DG, Reaman GH, Bleyer WA, et al. Successful prevention of central nervous system leukemia without cranial radiation in children with high-risk acute lymphoblastic leukemia, *Proc. Am. Soc. Clin. Oncol.,* **8** (1989) 213a.

115. Ellison RR, Mick R, Cuttner J, et al. Effects of postinduction intensification treatment with cytarabine and daunorubicin in adult acute lymphocytic leukemia: a prospective randomized clinical trial by Cancer and Leukemia Group B, *J. Clin. Oncol.,* **9** (1991) 2002–2015.

116. Lister TA, Whitehouse JMA, Beard MEJ, et al. Combination chemotherapy for acute lymphoblastic leukaemia in adults, *Br. Med. J.,* **1** (1978) 199–203.

117. Henderson ES, Scharlau C, Cooper MR, et al. Combination chemotherapy and radiotherapy for acute lymphocytic leukemia in adults: results of CALGB protocol 7113, *Leukemia Res.,* **3** (1979) 395–407.

118. Ochs JJ. Neurotoxicity due to central nervous system therapy for childhood leukemia, *Am. J. Pediat. Hematol. Oncol.,* **11** (1989) 93–105.

119. Pizzo PA, Poplack DG, and Bleyer WA. Neurotoxicities of current leukemia therapy, *Am. J. Pediatr. Hematol.-Oncol.,* **1** (1979) 127–140.

120. Bleyer WA, Drake JC, and Chabner BA. Neurotoxicity and elevated cerebrospinal-fluid methotrexate concentration in meningeal leukemia, *N. Engl. J. Med.,* **289** (1973) 770–773.

121. Ettinger LJ, Chervinsky DS, Freeman AI, and Creaven PJ. Pharmacokinetics of methotrexate following intravenous and intraventricular administration in acute lymphocytic leukemia and non-Hodgkin's lymphoma, *Cancer,* **50** (1982) 1676–1682.

122. Lopez-Andreu JA, Ferris J, Verdeguer A, Esquembre C, and Castel V. Myelopathy after intrathecal chemotherapy: a case report with unique magnetic resonance imaging changes, *Cancer,* **75** (1995) 1216–1217.

123. McLean DR, Clink HM, Ernst P, et al. Myelopathy after intrathecal chemotherapy. A case report with unique magnetic resonance imaging changes, *Cancer,* **73** (1994) 3037–3040.

124. Watterson J, Toogood I, Nieder M, et al. Excessive spinal cord toxicity from intensive central nervous system-directed therapies, *Cancer,* **74** (1994) 3034–3041.

125. Walker RW. Neurologic complications of leukemia, *Neurol. Clin.,* **9** (1991) 989–999.

126. Werner RA. Paraplegia and quadriplegia after intrathecal chemotherapy, *Arch. Phys. Med. Rehab.,* **69** (1988) 1054–1056.

127. Addiego JE Jr, Ridgway D, and Bleyer WA. Acute management of intrathecal methotrexate overdose: pharmacologic rationale and guidelines, *J. Pediatr.,* **98** (1981) 825–828.
128. Jardine LF, Ingram LC, and Bleyer WA. Intrathecal leucovorin after intrathecal methotrexate overdose, *J. Pediatr. Hematol.-Oncol.,* **18** (1996) 302–304.
129. O'Marcaigh AS, Johnson CM, Smithson WA, et al. Successful treatment of intrathecal methotrexate overdose by using ventriculolumbar perfusion and intrathecal instillation of carboxypeptidase G2, *Mayo Clin. Proc.,* **71** (1996) 161–165.
130. Allen JC. Effects of cancer therapy on the nervous system, *J. Pediatr.,* **93** (1978) 903–909.
131. Casteels-van Daele M and van de Casseye W. Acute encephalopathy after initiation of cranial radiation for meningeal leukemia, *Lancet,* **2** (1978) 834.
132. Oliff A, Bleyer WA, and Poplack DG. Acute encephalopathy after initiation of cranial radiation for meningeal leukemia, *Lancet,* **2** (1978) 13.
133. Jankovic M, Brouwers P, Valsecchi MG, et al. Association of 1800 cGy cranial irradiation with intellectual function in children with acute lymphoblastic leukaemia. International Study Group on Psychosocial Aspects of Childhood Cancer, *Lancet,* **344** (1994) 224–227.
134. Moss HA, Nannis ED, and Poplack DG. Effects of prophylactic treatment of the central nervous system on the intellectual functioning of children with acute lymphocytic leukemia, *Am. J. Med.,* **71** (1981) 47–52.
135. Eiser C. Intellectual abilities among survivors of childhood leukaemia as a function of CNS radiation, *Arch. Dis. Child.,* **53** (1978) 391–395.
136. Tucker J, Prior PF, Green CR, et al. Minimal neuropsychological sequelae following prophylactic treatment of the central nervous system in adult leukemia and lymphoma, *Br. J. Cancer,* **60** (1989) 775–780.
137. Sackmann Muriel F, Schere D, Barengols A, et al. Remission maintenance therapy for meningeal leukemia: intrathecal methotrexate and dexamethasone versus intrathecal craniospinal irradiation with a radiocolloid, *Br. J. Haematol.,* **33** (1976) 119–127.
138. Land VJ, Thomas PRM, Boyett JM, et al. Comparison of maintenance treatment regimens for first central nervous system relapse in children with acute lymphocytic leukemia, *Cancer,* **56** (1985) 81–87.

INDEX